METHODS IN MOLECULAR BIOLOGY

Series Editor
John M. Walker
School of Life and Medical Sciences
University of Hertfordshire
Hatfield, Hertfordshire, UK

For further volumes:
http://www.springer.com/series/7651

For over 35 years, biological scientists have come to rely on the research protocols and methodologies in the critically acclaimed *Methods in Molecular Biology* series. The series was the first to introduce the step-by-step protocols approach that has become the standard in all biomedical protocol publishing. Each protocol is provided in readily-reproducible step-by-step fashion, opening with an introductory overview, a list of the materials and reagents needed to complete the experiment, and followed by a detailed procedure that is supported with a helpful notes section offering tips and tricks of the trade as well as troubleshooting advice. These hallmark features were introduced by series editor Dr. John Walker and constitute the key ingredient in each and every volume of the *Methods in Molecular Biology* series. Tested and trusted, comprehensive and reliable, all protocols from the series are indexed in PubMed.

Retinitis Pigmentosa

Edited by

Stephen H. Tsang

Departments of Ophthalmology, Pathology & Cell Biology Graduate Programs in Nutritional & Metabolic Biology and Neurobiology & Behavior Columbia Stem Cell Initiative, New York, NY, USA

Peter M. J. Quinn

Department of Ophthalmology, Columbia University Medical Center, New York, NY, USA

Humana Press

Editors
Stephen H. Tsang
Departments of Ophthalmology
Pathology & Cell Biology Graduate
Programs in Nutritional & Metabolic
Biology and Neurobiology & Behavior
Columbia Stem Cell Initiative
New York, NY, USA

Peter M. J. Quinn
Department of Ophthalmology
Columbia University Medical Center
New York, NY, USA

ISSN 1064-3745 ISSN 1940-6029 (electronic)
Methods in Molecular Biology
ISBN 978-1-0716-2653-5 ISBN 978-1-0716-2651-1 (eBook)
https://doi.org/10.1007/978-1-0716-2651-1

This Humana imprint is published by the registered company Springer Science+Business Media, LLC, part of Springer Nature.
The registered company address is: 1 New York Plaza, New York, NY 10004, U.S.A.

Foreword

In the past, any disease associated with a diffuse bilateral pigmentary disturbance in the fundus was considered to be retinitis pigmentosa (RP). Today, we no longer entertain this confusing and nonspecific classification. Instead, we know that there are numerous chorioretinal disorders that are associated with chorioretinal pigmentary changes. We also know that RP, itself, is a generic term used to describe a number of inherited retinal dystrophies (IRDs). Furthermore, approximately 25% of these patients will also have non-ocular manifestations complicating their presentation in the clinical setting. Accordingly, pigmentation in the fundus may pose as a diagnostic challenge for an eye physician. Professor Stephen H. Tsang and co-authors have met that challenge in *Retinitis Pigmentosa: Methodologies and Emerging Therapeutics*, a comprehensive text and atlas that has never been previously available. Designed for a broad audience of readers, it begins with the fundamentals and evolves into a digest for the most advanced clinical scientists interested in this group of diseases.

It begins, accordingly, with a description of the retina and the nature of patients with the disease. Beginning in the second or third decade of life, patients with RP experience a decline in peripheral and night vision as a result of photoreceptor degeneration. Typically, this process begins with rod degeneration followed by a wave of cone degradation. Anatomical abnormalities follow the visual dysfunction, which may, in some patients, result in blindness. This group of diseases is considered rare, but it accounts for an estimated 2.5 million cases worldwide with more than 100,000 in the United States alone. The ophthalmic literature in the past was simple in its description of the pigmentary and atrophic findings in the posterior segment of the eye. Thanks to multimodal images of the panoramic fundus and segmental analysis of the stratified retina, retinal physicians now possess a better understanding of the related changes. No longer is each form named in honor of the ophthalmologist or clinician-scientist who first described that dystrophy, as was done for Ushers' syndrome, Leber's congenital amaurosis, or Barde-Beidel syndrome. Instead, we now designate them by their genetic mutations, such as *RHO, RPE-65, RPGR*, or *USH-3*. Accordingly, RP and other IRDs are referred to by their known genetic abnormality. Each of these genetic disturbances—and there are at least 80 known in RP—is responsible for the development of photoreceptor degeneration that is inherited in one of three ways: autosomal recessive, autosomal dominant or sex-linked. In a given patient, these genetic abnormalities may often be traced to one or both parents who may or may not have the features of the disease.

To date, there has not been a definitive text devoted to the methodologies behind identifying and treating this group of diseases. At last, Professor Stephen H. Tsang, Dr. Peter M.J. Quinn and colleagues have assembled a comprehensive review of all of the aspects of this subject. Starting with the fundamentals, the authors present a general overview and then describe the pathophysiological causative factors, clinical manifestations, and functional deficits. The authors have taken advantage of current imaging modalities, advanced biological testing, and existing accumulative knowledge to describe and illustrate the current state for diagnosis and study of this group of diseases. Among the contributors, are a number of indisputable and elite experts in the field, individuals who have earned the respect and admiration of their peers. Their work is an encyclopedic compilation of our current understanding of this heterogenous group of disease. Basic scientists and research personnel will welcome the review of anatomy and pathology as they relate to associated clinical manifestations in the retina. Pathophysiological precursors and techniques which create the basis for emerging and potential therapeutics, as promised by the title of the text. Moreover, readership will be welcomed by all, ranging from interests by casual readers to the most discerning advocates of this subspecialty of retinal diseases.

Nothing fundamental is overlooked. A review of the retina itself begins with a description as a distinct entity. In the visual system, the retina receives light that has passed through the cornea, lens, and vitreous to focus on this thin lining of the ocular fundus. The retina then converts light to neuronal signals which are assembled via the optic nerve to the brain for visual processing. Within the outer retina, there are certain neuroepithelial cells known as rod and cone photoreceptors which are responsible for photoreduction. RP, as a heterogenous group of hereditary diseases, is usually characterized by progressive dysfunction of rods followed by cones with eventual degradation of the retina as a whole. RP patients present in the first or second decade of life with a history of peripheral field loss and night blindness or nyctalopia from rod loss. Ultimately, patients may experience central vision loss or even total blindness. Variable forms of this disease group range from syndromic abnormalities, which may be related to congenital diseases, such as infections with rubella and syphilis, to acquired inflammatory/infectious diseases including toxoplasmosis, tuberculosis, and a nematode infestation. In adults, paraneoplastic disorders with accumulation of melanocytic proliferation, nutritional deficiencies like Vitamin A, idiopathic inflammatory chorioretinal disorders such as multifocal choroiditis, infectious chorioretinal disease, or even trauma may masquerade as an IRD. Other genetic abnormalities have to be ruled out, including mitochondria related syndromes (A3243G) and spinocerebellar ataxia. There is always a challenge for physicians to recognize sex-linked female carriers and modified pigmentary degeneration in the fundus.

When I was in training as an ophthalmologist, there was very little that we could offer a patient with RP. We had some medications for secondary manifestations like macular edema; we had cataract surgery for some predisposed to that development; we even had vitreoretinal surgery for an occasional patient prone to retinal tears and detachment. Most of the time, however, we simply had low vision rehabilitation, primarily magnification, to offer to patients. Not much in the way of benefit, magnification had been around in Europe and the Mediterranean for centuries [1]. As discussed in this text, we now have gene therapy, retinal cell and tissue transplantation, as well as nutritional and drug forms of therapy. In this text, readers will learn that there are innovative forms of therapy currently under investigation, all attractive in concept, yet mostly unproven.

RP, although a devastating disease, is at the forefront of regenerative medicine efforts in ophthalmology. Our understanding of visual processes and retinal degenerations has advanced over the past 50 years, thus elucidating the mechanisms and biochemical causes of retinal degeneration and associated complications. Until recently the exact pathogenesis and etiology of RP has been unknown, but there are currently several hundred clinical studies investigating the use of gene therapy in the treatment of RP. Challenges to gene and cell therapies include the marked genetic heterogeneity of the disease, risks associated with surgical interventions, and immune response following exposure to viral vectors. Despite current barriers to treatment, promising developments in gene editing methodologies and novel gene delivery carriers predict the development of effective therapeutic options in the near future. Given the evolving development in the diagnosis and the array of new therapeutic modalities under investigation for treatment, this is the first text to address them all.

The table of contents clearly indicates, as promised in the title of the volume, emerging forms of therapy for RP addressed generally by the principle figures associated with its biotechnology.

In summary, *Retinitis Pigmentosa: Methodologies and Emerging Therapeutics* is a new and novel addition to our ophthalmic library. It is for novices and experts alike. It includes a detailed history of RP from the discovery of this disease to current treatment options/novel therapies. Research from leaders in the fields of gene editing and stem cell forms of therapy is used to provide context and valuable insights that define the disease and focus on the major recent technological advances including clustered regularly interspaced short palindromic repeats (CRISPR), gene augmentation, genome editing, stem cell therapy, and next-generation sequencing methods. Other topics include the molecular pathways implicated in RP from mutation to rod cell death and may potentially elucidate future targets for new treatment methodologies. Progress within the field is detailed in order for clinicians and researchers alike to find connections and relevant information related to their research and provision of treatment. Overall, the translational applications of gene editing and other therapies for the treatment of RP are all in an effort to direct future care and research relating to RP. The target audience includes researchers, students, clinicians, and biochemists, who will utilize this methods book as a treasured resource due to its applicability to their teaching, research, and patient care. It is an honor to have been invited to write this foreword.

New York, NY, USA *Lawrence A. Yannuzzi*

References

1. Sines G, Sakellarakis YA (1987) Lenses of antiquity. Am J Archaeol 91(2):191–196

Preface

This book provides a history on retinitis pigmentosa and current treatment options. Chapters detail CRISPR, gene therapy, stem cell therapy, next-generation sequencing methods, gene editing, and translational applications of other therapies to the treatment of retinitis pigmentosa.

New York, NY, USA

Stephen H. Tsang
Peter M. J. Quinn

Contents

Contributors

DIVIN O. BADDAM • *Edward S. Harkness Eye Institute, Department of Ophthalmology, Columbia University Irving Medical Center, New York, NY, USA*

SEAN A. BATSON • *Washington Pacific Eye Associates, Seattle, WA, USA*

MARK P. BREAZZANO • *Wilmer Eye Institute—Retina Division, Johns Hopkins Hospital, Baltimore, MD, USA*

SALVATORE MARCO CARUSO • *Edward S. Harkness Eye Institute, Department of Ophthalmology, Columbia University Irving Medical Center, New York, NY, USA*

ALEXANDER H. CHAI • *Yale University, New Haven, CT, USA*

ANGELA Y. CHANG • *Edward S. Harkness Eye Institute, Department of Ophthalmology, Columbia University Irving Medical Center, New York, NY, USA*

YA-JU CHANG • *Edward S. Harkness Eye Institute, Department of Ophthalmology, Columbia University Irving Medical Center, New York, NY, USA*

CHIA-HUA CHENG • *Edward S. Harkness Eye Institute, Department of Ophthalmology, Columbia University Irving Medical Center, New York, NY, USA*

HSU-HSIN CHEN • *Edward S. Harkness Eye Institute, Department of Ophthalmology, Columbia University Irving Medical Center, New York, NY, USA*

NELSON CHEN • *Edward S. Harkness Eye Institute, Department of Ophthalmology, Columbia University Irving Medical Center, New York, NY, USA*

ROYCE W. S. CHEN • *Edward S. Harkness Eye Institute, Department of Ophthalmology, Columbia University Irving Medical Center/New York-Presbyterian Hospital, New York, NY, USA*

AHRA CHO • *Institute of Human Nutrition, Columbia University Irving Medical Center, New York, NY, USA*

RITAH CHUMDERMPADETSUK • *Beth Israel Deaconess Medical Center, Boston, MA, USA*

XUAN CUI • *Edward S. Harkness Eye Institute, Department of Ophthalmology, Columbia University Irving Medical Center, New York, NY, USA*

BRUNA LOPES DA COSTA • *Department of Biomedical Engineering, Columbia University, New York, NY, USA*

AVINASH DHARMADHIKARI • *Clinical Genomics, Department of Clinical Pathology, Children's Hospital Los Angeles, Los Angeles, CA, USA*

VLAD DIACONITA • *Edward S. Harkness Eye Institute, Department of Ophthalmology, Columbia University Irving Medical Center, New York, NY, USA*

JIANHAI DU • *Department of Ophthalmology, Department of Biochemistry, West Virginia University, Morgantown, WV, USA*

ALEXANDRA FEHNEL • *Department of Biomedical Engineering, Columbia University, New York, NY, USA*

MAEHER GREWAL • *Edward S. Harkness Eye Institute, Department of Ophthalmology, Columbia University Irving Medical Center, New York, NY, USA*

SITARA H. HIRJI • *Edward S. Harkness Eye Institute, Department of Ophthalmology, Columbia University Irving Medical Center/New York-Presbyterian Hospital, New York, NY, USA*

WAN-CHUN HUANG • *Edward S. Harkness Eye Institute, Department of Ophthalmology, Columbia University Irving Medical Center, New York, NY, USA*

LAURA A. JENNY • *Edward S. Harkness Eye Institute, Department of Ophthalmology, Columbia University Irving Medical Center, New York, NY, USA*
HA MIN KIM • *Columbia University Vagelos College of Physicians and Surgeons, New York, NY, USA; Department of Ophthalmology, Columbia University Irving Medical Center, New York, NY, USA*
SARAH R. LEVI • *Edward S. Harkness Eye Institute, Department of Ophthalmology, Columbia University Irving Medical Center, New York, NY, USA*
CHAO-YU LIU • *College of Medicine, National Taiwan University, Taipei, Taiwan*
PEI-KANG LIU • *Edward S. Harkness Eye Institute, Department of Ophthalmology, Columbia University Irving Medical Center, New York, NY, USA; Department of Ophthalmology, Kaohsiung Medical University Hospital, Kaohsiung Medical University, Kaohsiung, Taiwan; School of Medicine, College of Medicine, Kaohsiung Medical University, Kaohsiung, Taiwan; Institute of Biomedical Sciences, National Sun Yat-Sen University, Kaohsiung, Taiwan*
YAO LI • *Edward S. Harkness Eye Institute, Department of Ophthalmology, Columbia University Irving Medical Center, New York, NY, USA*
WEI KIONG NGO • *Department of Ophthalmology, New York-Presbyterian Hospital, New York, NY, USA; Jonas Children's Vision Care and Bernard & Shirlee Brown Glaucoma Laboratory, Department of Ophthalmology, Columbia University, New York, NY, USA; National Healthcare Group Eye Institute, Singapore, Singapore*
NICHOLAS D. NOLAN • *Department of Biomedical Engineering, Columbia University, New York, NY, USA*
YAN NUZBROKH • *Steven and Alexandra Cohen Children's Medical Center of New York, Queens, NY, USA*
LAURENCE M. OCCELLI • *Department of Small Animal Clinical Studies, College of Veterinary Medicine, Michigan State University, East Lansing, MI, USA*
JIN KYUN OH • *Edward S. Harkness Eye Institute, Department of Ophthalmology, Columbia University Irving Medical Center/New York-Presbyterian Hospital, New York, NY, USA*
SIMON M. PETERSEN-JONES • *Department of Small Animal Clinical Studies, College of Veterinary Medicine, Michigan State University, East Lansing, MI, USA*
PETER M. J. QUINN • *Department of Ophthalmology Columbia University Medical Center, New York, NY, USA*
SARA D. RAGI • *Department of Ophthalmology, New York-Presbyterian Hospital, New York, NY, USA*
MERRY ZHECHAO RUAN • *Department of Ophthalmology, New York-Presbyterian Hospital, New York, NY, USA*
JOSEPH RYU • *Columbia University Vagelos College of Physicians & Surgeons, New York, NY, USA*
IOANA SCHERBAKOVA • *Edward S. Harkness Eye Institute, Department of Ophthalmology, Columbia University Irving Medical Center, New York, NY, USA*
TARUN SHARMA • *Edward S. Harkness Eye Institute, Department of Ophthalmology, Columbia University Irving Medical Center, New York, NY, USA*
ZACHARY E. SNOW • *Columbia University Vagelos College of Physicians and Surgeons, New York, NY, USA*
MEGAN SOUCY • *Columbia University Irving Medical Center, New York, NY, USA*
AKEMI JOY TANAKA • *Columbia University Irving Medical Center, New York, NY, USA*
ABINAYA THENAPPAN • *Edward S. Harkness Eye Institute, Department of Ophthalmology, Columbia University Irving Medical Center, New York, NY, USA*

MARK D. TRAVOR • *Columbia University Vagelos College of Physicians & Surgeons, New York, NY, USA*
YI-TING TSAI • *Department of Biomedical Engineering, Columbia University, New York, NY, USA*
STEPHEN H. TSANG • *Departments of Ophthalmology, Pathology & Cell Biology Graduate Programs in Nutritional & Metabolic Biology and Neurobiology & Behavior Columbia Stem Cell Initiative, New York, NY, USA*
AMY TSO • *Edward S. Harkness Eye Institute, Department of Ophthalmology, Columbia University Irving Medical Center, New York, NY, USA*
HUNG-HSI WANG • *Edward S. Harkness Eye Institute, Department of Ophthalmology, Columbia University Irving Medical Center, New York, NY, USA*
NAN-KAI WANG • *Edward S. Harkness Eye Institute, Department of Ophthalmology, Columbia University Irving Medical Center, New York, NY, USA*
WEN-HSUAN WU • *Edward S. Harkness Eye Institute, Department of Ophthalmology, Columbia University Irving Medical Center, New York, NY, USA*
CHRISTINE L. XU • *Stanford University School of Medicine, Stanford, CA, USA*
HENRY W. ZHOU • *Columbia University Vagelos College of Physicians & Surgeons, New York, NY, USA*

Chapter 1

Introduction and Discovery of Retinitis Pigmentosa

Hung-Hsi Wang, Nelson Chen, and Nan-Kai Wang

Abstract

Retinitis pigmentosa (RP) is the most common inherited retinal dystrophy. There are three main characteristics of RP: night blindness, retinal pigmentation, and visual field constriction. Among these three features, night blindness was the first to be discovered, which could be dated back to the ancient Egyptians at around 1500 BC. However, the night blindness described at that time was most likely associated with vitamin A deficiency rather than RP. Retinitis pigmentosa was first described in cadaver anatomic dissection before the invention of the ophthalmoscope. However, it was not linked to RP or night blindness. It was not until the invention of the ophthalmoscope that ophthalmologists could truly look into the eye and correlate the retinal pigmentation with clinical symptoms, such as night blindness and visual field constriction. In 1983, at a RP workshop that gathered together many experts, a consensus was reached regarding the terminology and guidelines for the diagnosis of RP. In this chapter, we will introduce the history and discovery of RP along with its characteristics.

Key words Retinitis pigmentosa (RP), Nyctalopia, Night blindness, Retina pigmentation

1 Introduction to Retinitis Pigmentosa

Retinitis pigmentosa (RP) is a set of progressive hereditary disorders that primarily affect photoreceptor and pigment epithelial function [1]. Patients with typical RP usually suffer from the symptoms of night blindness, also known as "nyctalopia," progressive field constriction, and visual loss. Although night blindness is a major symptom of RP, it can also have other causes, such as vitamin A deficiency. Table 1 summarizes the historical landmarks related to RP.

2 Discovery of Night Blindness

Nyctalopia, the term that we use today for night blindness, came from the ancient Greek roots *nykt-* (meaning night) + *alaos-* (meaning blind) + *ops-* (meaning eye) [2]. This term first appeared in the

Stephen H. Tsang and Peter M. J. Quinn (eds.), *Retinitis Pigmentosa*,
Methods in Molecular Biology, vol. 2560, https://doi.org/10.1007/978-1-0716-2651-1_1,

Table 1
Historical landmarks related to retinitis pigmentosa

Year	Author	Description
1500 BC	Egyptians	First discovery of night blindness, used ox liver as treatment
460–379 BC	Hippocrates	First used the word nyctalopia
1836	Bernhard von Langenbeck	First described the pigmentation of the retina of a RP patient
1838	Friedrich August von Ammon	First to draw a colored illustration of the pigmentation of the retina
1853	Adrianus Christophilus van Trigt	First to describe and draw RP by using the ophthalmoscope
1853	Albrecht von Graefe	Also described RP but under the name of morbus Arianus
1857	Franciscus Donders	Named the disease as retinitis pigmentosa
1871	Theodor Leber	First described the disease retinitis pigmentosa sine pigmento
1872	Ludwig Mauthner	Gave the name choroideremia
1877	Theodor Leber	First described congenital stationary night blindness
1882	Mooren	First described retinitis punctate albescens
1888	Jacobsohn	First described gyrate atrophy as atypical retinitis pigmentosa
1895	Cutler	Described gyrate atrophy as retinal chorioideal degeneration
1896	Fuchs	Gave the name gyrate atrophy of the choroid and retina
1973	Simell and Takki	Demonstrated the association of hyperornithinaemia with gyrate atrophy
1858	Albrecht von Graefe	First to discover the association of visual field loss with RP
1901	Gonin	First to describe a typical progression of the visual field loss associated with RP
1945	Karpe	Used ERG on patients with pigmentary retinopathy
1964	Gouras and Carr	Discovered that in early cases of RP, rod damage occurred more than cone damage

works of the well-known Greek physician Hippocrates at around 460–379 BC, and it was often referred to as *nyctalope* and *nyctalopic*. The word "nyctalopia" was discovered in the sixth book of Hippocrates' *Epidemics*, and there has been controversy about whether the term nyctalopia was used to refer to "night blindness" or "day blindness." The reason is that there was evidence that the word "nyctalopia" was used by physicians after Hippocrates to describe both those who cannot see at night and those who cannot see during the day. Galen, an admirer of Hippocrates, in the second century AD wrote, "the word (*nyctalopia*) describes two kinds of diseases: the disease where we do not see at night and the one where we do not see during the day" [3]. Therefore, it is indicated that by the second century, two definitions of the word nyctalopia already existed. In the fourth century, Oribasius wrote: "They call nyctalope, someone who sees well during the day, but when the sun sets sees worse and during the night can see nothing" [4]. During the next century, Palladius commented that those with nyctalopia "see during the day but do not see at night" after studying Hippocrates' works [5]. Later on in the sixth century, Aetius Amidenus, an AD physician, wrote in his *Medical Books*, "they call nyctalopia (the symptom), when someone sees well during the day, worse at sunset and when the night falls can see nothing." He also added that "to some it also happens to see better at night and worse during the day and if the moon is shining to see nothing" [6]. Finally, Ali Abu ibn Sina (1980–1037 AD), also known as Avicenna, wrote that the word nyctalopia was intended to describe the condition of impaired night vision. After much discussion, a conclusion was drawn to this controversy, and the term nyctalopia was used to describe the symptom of impaired dark adaptation [7].

Although the word "nyctalopia" first appeared at around 400 BC, the symptom of night blindness, on the other hand, was first described at around 1500 BC by the Egyptians. However, the cause of this symptom was unlikely to be associated with RP at that time. It is surprising to find that the Papyrus Ebers—that date back to about 1520 BC—recommend using ox liver to treat patients with symptoms of night blindness, even though they likely did not know exactly what the cause of night blindness was. The patients were often instructed to apply roasted ox liver to the eye or eat raw liver. Other treatment options included squeezing out a cooked ox liver and placing the liver juice against the eyes [8]. Later on, the symptom of night blindness and its treatment has been recorded and described throughout different ages in various areas. Hippocrates treated his patients with nyctalopia by instructing them to eat ox or calf liver [9]. Dioscorides instructed his patients to apply the juice of grilled goat liver to the eyes and eat the grilled liver [10]. Galen gave the same instruction as Dioscorides but with the exposure of the night blinded eyes to the steam produced when grilling the liver [11]. Patients with night blindness at ancient times were mostly treated with animal liver; this shows that there must be a relationship between the liver and night blindness. The liver is known to be a rich source of vitamin A, so it is reasonable to assume that the night blindness described by the ancient physicians was due to vitamin A deficiency. Vitamin A deficiency is the lack of vitamin A in the blood and tissue; this can cause impaired rod function that leads to night blindness. It was not until the nineteenth century that scientists recognized that the night blindness described in the ancient times was caused by vitamin A deficiency. Malnutrition, such as vitamin A deficiency, was common during the times of the ancient physicians.

3 Discovery of RP

Before the invention of the ophthalmoscope, eye pathology could only be studied by anatomic dissection and histology from a morbid cadaver. Langenbeck [12] (Fig. 1) first described the pigmentation of the retina in 1836 under the name of "melanosis retinae." Two years later, in 1838, von Ammon [13] (Fig. 2) created the first colored illustration of the pigmented retina (Fig. 3). However, these observations were limited to an anatomico-pathological association, and there was no correlation between the retinal pigmentation and the symptoms of night blindness or what we called RP [8]. Therefore, this accession to our anatomico-pathological knowledge was not applicable to practice and thus provided limited information to a diagnosis without seeing what was going on in the interior of the eye.

After the brilliant discovery of the ophthalmoscope in 1851, ophthalmologists could examine the patient's fundus when they are alive and correlate their symptoms with the changes in the fundus. A.C. van Trigt, a Dutch ophthalmologist, was the first (from accessible material) to describe and draw the fundus of RP of a living patient. He was a student of Dr. Franciscus Cornelius Donders who worked at Donders clinic (in Utrecht) and was assigned to design a table model ophthalmoscope [14]. In 1853, he published his dissertation in Latin entitled "De speculo oculi" [15] with several hand-drawn pictures of the fundi under the ophthalmoscope. In his dissertation, van Trigt described a 42-year-old patient who had been suffering from night blindness with visual field constriction for 20 years. He noted that this patient could only read well with the help of strong light together with facial field restriction. It is amazing how he described and drew the characteristic of the fundus picture in "Fig IV" of his dissertation (Fig. 4). In the legend for "Fig IV," it read: "On the top left is one of the blood vessels covered with pigment. Because of the star-shaped lens opacification, especially the middle part of the retina is seen less sharply."

According to Morren's article [16], Albrecht von Graefe (Fig. 5) had mentioned pigmented retina depositions together with the contraction of the visual file at around the same time as van Trigt. Albrecht von Graefe stated that the deposits of pigment might be regarded as the remains of punctiform hemorrhages. Graefe did not recognize the disease as a type of a particular kind until he saw the occurrence of the pigmentation in the Spanish Marquis Ariani and named the diseased after him as morbus Arianus [16]. In 1857, Donders [17] (Fig. 6) first described "Pigmentbildung in der Netzhaut" (pigmented retina in English translation) as a peculiar disease of the eye-ground, characterized by black points, spots, and lines in the retina, easily detected by ophthalmoscope.

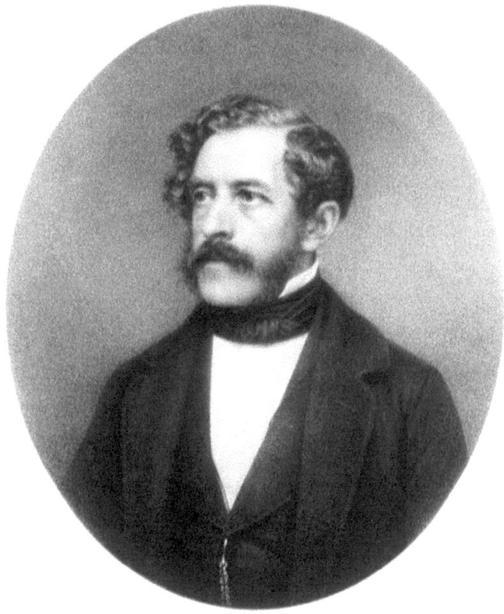

Fig. 1 A portrait of Bernhard von Langenbeck. (Obtained from public domain: https:/en.wikipedia.org/wiki/Bernhard_von_Langenbeck#/media/File:Bernhard_von_Langenbeck.jpg)

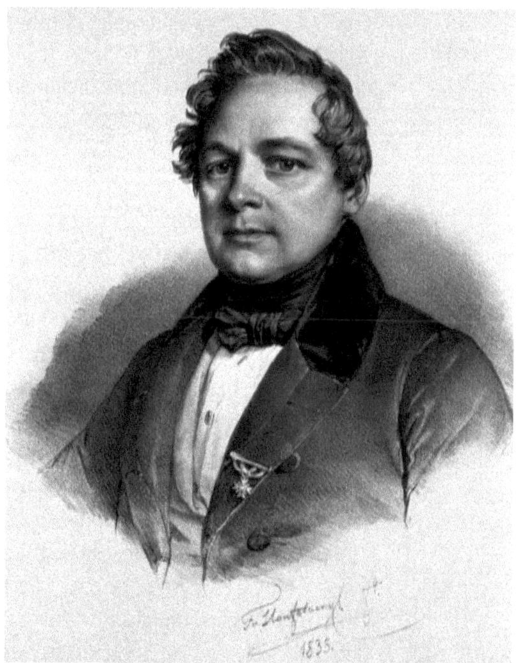

Fig. 2 A portrait of Friedrich August von Ammon. (Obtained from public domain https:/en.wikipedia.org/wiki/Friedrich_August_von_Ammon#/media/File:Friedrich_August_von_Ammon.jpg)

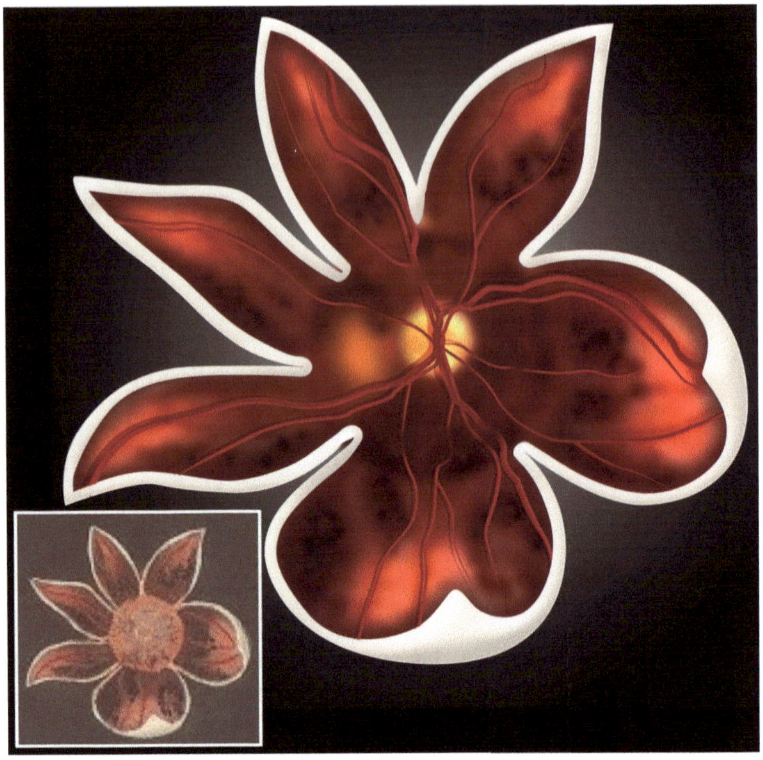

Fig. 3 A pathology illustration of retina pigmentation, recreated from the original work of Friedrich von Ammon in 1838 (lower left image). At the time, the condition was not thought to be linked to the clinical symptom of night blindness. (Obtained from public domain (before 1929))

The case that Donders observed was a 35-year-old man who lost his life in an accident, having been blind from his early youth [18]. Donders found many black points, spots, and lines in the retina of the patient, and he believed that the pigment had developed independently in the retina, raised from an infiltrating exudate, a chronic inflammatory process of the retina [17–19]. Donders put much value on these peculiarities and complications and reasoned that the pigment depended upon an exudation consecutive to retinitis, and this was later coined as "retinitis pigmentosa" [18]. At that period, all observers agreed that the progression of this disease is slow and the limitation of the visual field was always present in the early periods of the disease. However, "retinitis" was later found to be a misnomer because progressive photoreceptor degeneration is no longer thought to have an inflammatory origin.

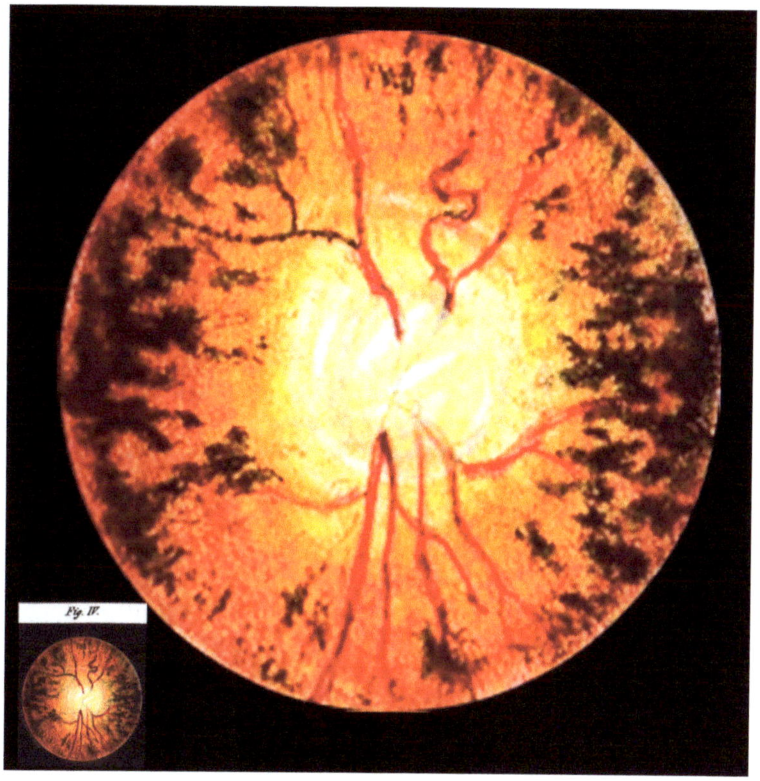

Fig. 4 Recreated image of the first illustration of RP under an ophthalmoscope by van Trigt where he described the pigmentation on the upper left blood vessel in 1853 (lower left image). (Obtained from public domain (before 1929))

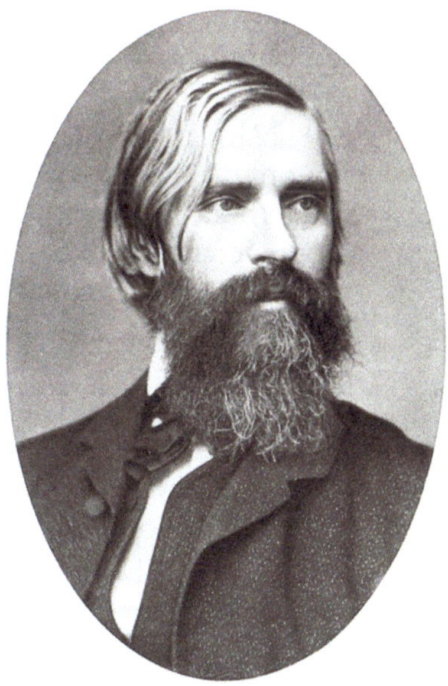

Fig. 5 A portrait of Albrecht von Graefe. (Obtained from public domain https:/en.wikipedia.org/wiki/Albrecht_von_Graefe#/media/File:Albrecht_v_Graefe3.jpg)

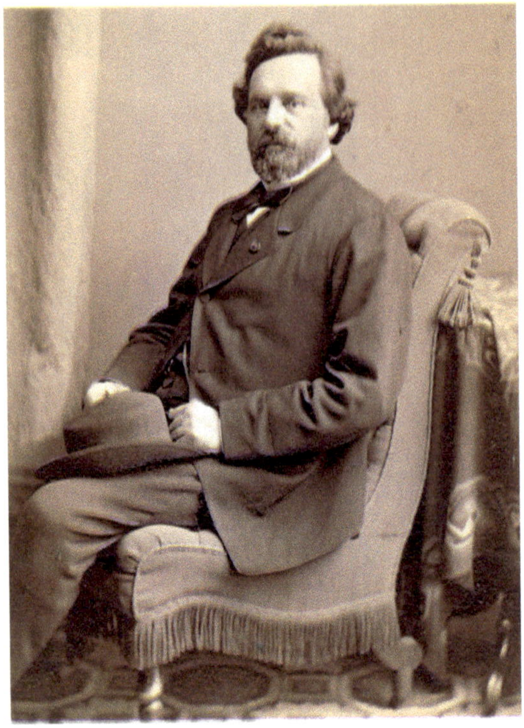

Fig. 6 A portrait of Franciscus Cornelius Donders. (Obtained from public domain https:/en.wikipedia.org/wiki/Franciscus_Donders#/media/File:Donders_Franciscus_Cornelis_(1818_-_1889).jpg)

4 Allied Diseases

Observations of familial night blindness had been described from as early as 1744 by Ovelgun, Riehter in 1828, and Cunier in 1838 [20–22]. However, the causes were unknown during the pre-ophthalmoscope era since the fundus could not be examined while these patients were alive. After the invention of the ophthalmoscope and excluding syphilitic choroiditis as a cause of night blindness, several retinal degenerations also caused night blindness but that presented with different fundus pictures than those seen in RP.

In 1871, Leber (Fig. 7) first described *RP sine pigmento*, where the pigmentation is absent on the retina [23]. However, some doctors believed that the disease described by Leber might have been an early case of RP or mild RP, where the pigmentation had not developed [24–27].

Retinitis punctate albescens was first described by Mooren (Fig. 8) in 1882, which is characterized by numerous discrete white dots which lie underneath the retinal vessels and do not involve the foveal region [28].

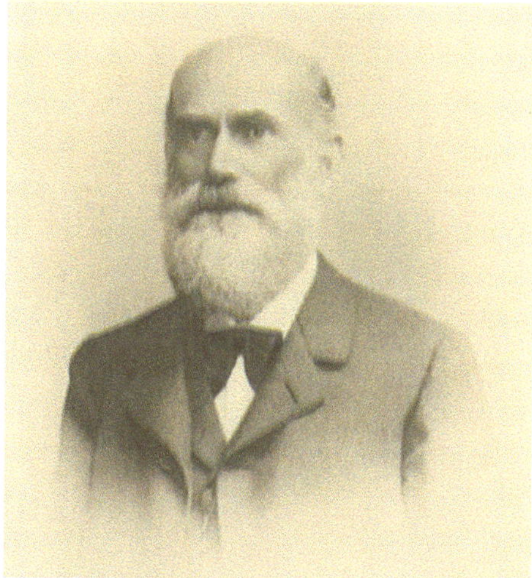

Fig. 7 A portrait of Theodor Leber. (Obtained from public domain https:/en.wikipedia.org/wiki/Theodor_Leber#/media/File:TheodorLeber.JPG)

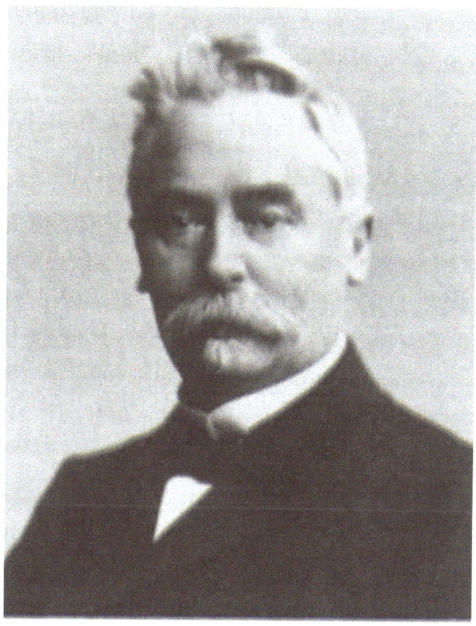

Fig. 8 A portrait of Albert Mooren. (Obtained from public domain https:/de.wikipedia.org/wiki/Albert_Mooren#/media/Datei:Albert_Mooren.jpg)

Gyrate atrophy was initially described as "atypical retinitis pigmentosa" (in German: Retinitis Pigmentosa atypica) by Jacobsohn in 1888 [29] and "retinal chorioideal degeneration" by Cutler in 1895 [30]. Later, it was named as "gyrate atrophy of the choroid and retina" (in German: atrophia gyrata choroideae et retinae) by Fuchs in 1896 [31]. Simell and Takki demonstrated the association of hyperornithinaemia with gyrate atrophy in 1973 [32].

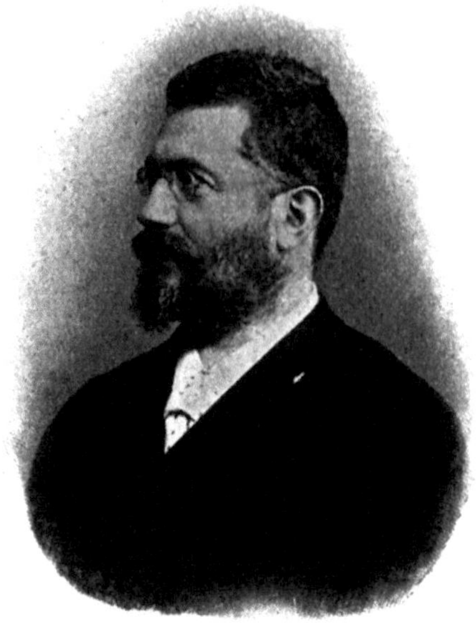

Fig. 9 A portrait of Ludwig Mauthner. (Obtained from public domain https:/en.wikipedia.org/wiki/Ludwig_Mauthner#/media/File:Mauthner.JPG)

Choroideremia was first described by an Austrian ophthalmologist, Ludwig Mauthner (Fig. 9), in 1872 [33]. He interpreted the findings as congenital absence of the choroid and named the disease as "choroideremia," but further observations suggested the progressive choroidal atrophy. In his article in 1872 [33], Mauthner described a 32-year-old German man who had poor vision and night blindness. This patient has eight other siblings. His seven sisters had normal vision, but his 26-year-old brother also had the same disease as him. The visual field in each eye was irregularly contracted to about 10-degree meridian. After looking at the fundus of this patient, Mauthner described the fundus as whitish green along with the normal colored disk and normal distribution of slightly narrow retinal vessels. He also noted that most choroidal vessels were not visible and small masses of pigment were found throughout the fundus. It is interesting to note that when Leber first saw this patient, he classified this case as RP associated with extreme atrophy of the choroid. However, Mauthner argued that the case is choroideremia since the patient had poor vision for as long as he could remember and it was unusual to see so much pigmentation with a nearly normal optic disk. Unfortunately, no drawings were presented [33, 34].

Unlike the other diseases, patients with *congenital stationary night blindness* usually have nearly normal fundus. In 1838, Cunier [20] described a family of seven generations in southern France, where 86 of the family members suffered from night blindness. However, he did not know that the patient he described suffered from what we call congenital stationary night blindness today.

Cunier described a 23-year-old boy who suffered from night blindness which was in the fifth generation of the family [20]. Cunier was able to trace the family tree of the boy and found an ancestor named Jean Nougaret, who also suffered from night blindness. Later on, in the twentieth century, Nettleship continued studying the family that Cunier described. After studying nine generations of the family and 135 who had night blindness, he concluded that the cases Cunier described were truly congenital stationary night blindness and that the disease is not progressive. He also stated that the disease which Cunier described in the family was dominantly inherited [21]. However, Nettleship gave the credit to Leber since Leber was the first to describe no fundus change under the ophthalmoscope in a patient with congenital stationary night blindness [22, 35]. Unlike other diseases mentioned before, patients with congenital stationary night blindness are nonprogressive, and their fundus is nearly normal. The sex-linked, hereditary nature of this disease was reported by Donders in 1855 [36].

5 Visual Field Defect in Retinitis Pigmentosa

A contracted visual field is one of the three major characteristics of RP. However, most patients with this disease rarely noticed any visual field loss in the early stages of RP, but only realized that they had become clumsy [37]. During the nineteenth century, it was hard to determine the visual field of the patient because the results shown could vary upon the different conditions of light and testing, as well as the severity of the diseases [8]. Albrecht von Graefe introduced perimetry and visual field testing to clinical ophthalmology, and he was the first to discover that a contracted visual field was one of the symptoms of RP [38]. At the young age of 30 years, Graefe published an article entitled "Exceptionelles Verhalten des Gesichtsfeldes bei Pigmententartung der Netzhaut" (English translation: Exceptional Behavior of the Visual Field in Pigment Degeneration of the Retina). In this article, Graefe gave a description of the visual disturbances caused by the pigmentary degeneration of the retina. He mentioned night blindness, concentric contraction of the visual fields, and long persisting central vision [38].

In 1901, Gonin published an article in French entitled "Le scotome annulaire dans la dégénérescence pigmentaire de la rétine" (the English translation of this is known as "Ring Scotoma in Pigmentary Degeneration of the Retina"). Gonin was the first to describe a typical progression of the contracted visual field in RP patients [39]. In his article, he stated that the visual field loss began as a partial or complete ring scotoma and, as the disease progressed, the visual field defect increased in size. In the more advanced stages, only a small central visual field remained.

6 Electroretinogram (ERG) in Retinitis Pigmentosa

In 1945, Karpe used the electroretinogram to test photoreceptor function in patients with pigmentary retinopathy and demonstrated that the response could be abnormal to nonrecordable [40, 41]. Karpe stated that this abnormal photoreceptor response could occur before the appearance of clinical symptoms or ophthalmoscopic changes in many patients with pigmentary retinopathy. Later, different ERG protocols were developed to test the rod and cone function separately in patients. Gouras and Carr discovered that in early cases of dominant RP, rod damage occurred more than cone damage [42]. In most of the cases of RP, rod cells are the primary degeneration, and cone cells come after. Therefore, the typical RP is also described as rod-cone dystrophy.

7 Definition of Retinitis Pigmentosa

In 1983, participants and experts in a symposium reached a consensus about the definition of RP and the criteria that should be met before giving the title of RP. The definition of RP is a set of progressive hereditary disorders that diffusely and primarily affect photoreceptor and pigment epithelial function [1]. Four criteria should be reached (Table 2) before concluding the disease as RP: (1) bilateral involvement, (2) loss of peripheral vision, (3) rod dysfunction evidenced by elevated rod final threshold on dark adaption and/or rod responses on ERG that are reduced in amplitude and prolonged in implicit time or are undetectable, (4) and progressive loss in photoreceptor function [37].

Table 2
Criteria of retinitis pigmentosa

1	Bilateral involvement
2	Loss of peripheral vision
3	Rod dysfunction
	(a) Dark adaption: elevated rod final threshold
	(b) Electroretinogram (ERG): rod responses with reduced amplitude and prolonged implicit time or non-detectable
4	Progressive loss in photoreception function

8 The Natural Course of Retinitis Pigmentosa

The sequence of photoreceptor degeneration (rod cells die first and cone cells afterward) explains the initial presentation of night blindness in patients with RP. Since the majority of rod cells are located outside the macular area (peripheral retinal), patients with RP usually present with a contracted visual field in addition to night blindness. When the disease progresses, cone cells die. Because the majority of cone cells are located in the macula area, patients gradually lose central vision in later life.

9 Future Prospective in Retinitis Pigmentosa

Since the discovery of the symptoms and the definition of RP, many physicians and scientists have studied the mechanisms of photoreceptor degenerations. An increasing number of genes related to RP have been identified using modern genetic testing, such as next-generation sequence, whole-exome sequencing, and whole-genome sequence. Several public databases and bioinformatics tools are available for predicting whether the variant is pathogenic or likely benign. There are FDA-approved gene therapy and several ongoing trials targeting disease-causing genes to restore gene function. Recent advances in imaging modalities allow physicians and scientists to characterize RP more specifically and use these image modalities to monitor its progression in nature or after treatment. All of these advances will be discussed later in other chapters of this book.

References

1. Marmor MF, Aguirre G, Arden G, Berson E, Birch DG, Boughman JA, Carr R, Chatrian GE, Del Monte M, Dowling J, Enoch J, Fishman GA, Fulton AB, Garcia CA, Gouras P, Heckenlively J, Hu D-N, Lewis RA, Niemeyer G, Parker JA, Perlman I, Ripps H, Sandberg MA, Siegel I, Weleber RG, Wolf ML, Wu L, Young RSL (1983) Retinitis pigmentosa. A symposium on terminology and methods of examination. Ophthalmology 90(2):126–31
2. Liddell H, Scott R (1940) Greek-English lexicon, 9th edn. Clarendon Press, Oxford
3. Wenkebach E (1956) Hippocratis epidemiarum librum VI commentaria. Corpus Medicorum Graecorum V, 10, 2, 2. Academia litterarum, Berlin, pp 387–390
4. Raeder J (1926) Oribasii synopsis ad eustathium. B. G. Teubner, Leipzig
5. Dietz FR (1834) Scholia in Hippocratis de popularibus morbis librum VI. Königsberg, Borntraeger
6. Olivier A (1950) Aetii Amideni Libri Medicinales V–VIII. Academia litterarum, Berlin
7. Sina AAi (1958) Canon of medicine. Book III, part 3, art.4 §3. Fanlar Nasrioti Academy, Tashkent
8. Bell J (1933) On retinitis pigmentosa and allied diseases. In: K.G.L.f.N.E. Pearson (ed) Treasury of human inheritance. At the University Press, London; Cambridge
9. Joly R (1978) Hippocrate, De la vision. Belles Lettres C.U.F, Paris
10. Goodyer J (1934) Dioscorides De Materia Medica. Oxford University Press, Oxford
11. Kühn KG (1827) Claudii Galeni Opera Omnia. Officina Libraria Car. Cnoblochii, Leipzig, pp 802–803

12. Langenbeck B (1836) De retina observations anatomico-pathologica. Sumtibus Dieterichianis, Göttingen
13. von Ammon FA (1838) Klinische Darstellungen der Krankheiten des menschlichen Auges. G. Reimer, Berlin
14. Den Tonkelaar I, Henkes HE, van Leersum GK (1988) The Utrecht ophthalmic hospital and the development of the ophthalmoscope. Doc Ophthalmol 68(1–2):65–69
15. Trigt ACV (1853) Dissertatio ophthalmologica inauguralis de speculo oculi. Utrecht, Utrecht
16. Mooren A (1863) Ueber retinitis pigmentosa. In: Zehender W (ed) Klinische Monatsblätter für Augenheilkunde. Verlag von Ferdinand Enke, Erlangen, pp 93–106
17. Donders FC (1857) Beiträge zur pathologischen Anatomie des Auges. Arch Ophthalmol 3(1):139–165
18. Homberger J (1861) Retinitis pigmentosa. In: Douglas JH (ed) The Amedican medical monthly, New York, p 180
19. Donders FC (1855) Beiträge zur pathologischen Anatomie des Auges. Arch Ophthalmol 2:106–118
20. Cunier F (1838) Historie d'une hememlopie, hereditaire depuis deux siecles dans un famille de la commune de Vendemian, pres Montpellier. Arm Soc Med de Gand 4:385–395
21. Carr RE (1974) Congenital stationary nightblindness. Trans Am Ophthalmol Soc 72:448–487
22. Nettleship E (1907) A history of congenital stationary nightblindness in nine consecutive generations. Trans Ophthalmol Soc UK 27: 269–293
23. Leber T (1871) Ueber anomale Formen der Retinitis pigmentosa. Albrecht von Graefes Archiv für Ophthalmologie 17:314–341
24. Nettleship E (1908) On retinitis pigmentosa and allied diseases. R Lond Ophthalmol Hosp Rep 17:333–426
25. Nettleship E (1914) A note on the progress of some cases of retinitis pigmentosa sine pigmento and of retinitis punctata albescens. R Lond Ophthalmol Hosp Rep 19:123
26. Usher CH (1914) On the inheritance of retinitis pigmentosa with notes of cases. R Lond Ophthalmol Hosp Rep 19:130–236
27. Bird AC (1988) Clinical investigation of retinitis pigmentosa. Aust N Z J Ophthalmol 16(3): 189–198
28. Mooren A (1882) Fünf Lustren Ophthalmologischer Wirksamkeit. Bergmann, Wiesbaden
29. Jacobsohn E (1888) Ein Fall von Retinitis Pigmentosa atypica. Klin Monatsbl Augenheilkd 26:202–206
30. Cutler C (1895) Drei ungewöhnliche Fälle von Retina-chorioidea Degeneration. Arch Augenheilkd 30:117–122
31. Fuchs E (1896) Ueber zwei der retinitis pigmentosa verwandte krankheiten (retinitis punctata albescens und atrophia gyrata choroideae et retinae). Arch Augenheilkd 32:111–116
32. Simell O, Takki K (1973) Raised plasma-ornithine and gyrate atrophy of the choroid and retina. Lancet 1(7811):1031–1033
33. Mauthner L (1872) Ein Fall von Chorioideremie. Berl Natur-med Ver Innsbruck 2:191
34. Bedell AJ (1937) Choroideremia. JAMA Ophthalmol 17(3):444–467
35. Leber T (1877) Die Krankheiten der Netzhaut und des Sehnerven. In: Handbuch der Gesammten Augenheilkunde, Leipzig, p 649, case 89
36. Donders FC (1855) Torpeur de la retine congenitale heräditaire. Ann Ocul (Paris) 34:270–273
37. Pagon RA (1988) Retinitis pigmentosa. Surv Ophthalmol 33(3):137–177
38. von Graefe A (1858) Vereinzelte Beobachtungen und Bemerkungen. Arch Ophthalmol 4(2):211–276
39. Gonin J (1901) *Le* scotome annulaire dans la dégénérescence pigmentaire de la rétine. Ann Ocul 125:101–130
40. Karpe G, Kornerup T, Wulfing B (1958) The clinical electroretinogram. Acta Ophthalmol 36(2):281–291
41. Heckenlively JR (1987) RP cone-rod degeneration. Trans Am Ophthalmol Soc 85:438–470
42. Gouras P, Carr RE (1964) Electrophysiological studies in early retinitis pigmentosa. Arch Ophthalmol 72:104–110

Chapter 2

Etiology of Retinitis Pigmentosa

Mark P. Breazzano, Maeher R. Grewal, Stephen H. Tsang, and Royce W. S. Chen

Abstract

Retinitis pigmentosa (RP) is a set of symptoms including tunnel vision, night blindness, and progressive vision loss, stemming from a very heterogeneous set of causes—it can result from a several different kinds of mutations (non-syndromic) in conjunction with other symptoms, as part of a larger syndrome (syndromic), or secondary to an organ system disease state (secondary RP). This chapter explores and elucidates these various causes of RP.

Key words Bardet–Biedl syndrome, Leber congenital amaurosis, Non-syndromic retinitis pigmentosa, Rhodopsin, Secondary retinitis pigmentosa, Syndromic retinitis pigmentosa, Usher syndrome

1 Introduction

Retinitis pigmentosa (RP) is not only a disease in and of itself, but it's also a syndrome present in many other diseases. For this reason, RP has many different causes. These causes can largely be broken down into three different categories: non-syndromic (occurring by itself, without any other clinical findings); syndromic (occurring alongside clinical findings such as developmental abnormalities and neurosensory deficits as a part of a larger more complex disorder); and RP secondary to other systemic disease processes such as nephrotic syndrome.

2 Non-syndromic RP

Phototransduction is the process by which light photoreceptors (rod and cone cells) convert light into electrical signals. Inherited genetic abnormalities that interrupt various parts of this phototransduction signaling pathway as well as mutations that disrupt normal metabolism in the supporting retinal pigmentosa epithelial

Stephen H. Tsang and Peter M. J. Quinn (eds.), *Retinitis Pigmentosa*,
Methods in Molecular Biology, vol. 2560, https://doi.org/10.1007/978-1-0716-2651-1_2,

(RPE) layer underlie non-syndromic forms of RP. Mutations in over 50 genes have been identified as causal to non-syndromic RP. In order to grasp why mutations in these genes would result in RP, it is first necessary to understand the basic mechanisms of phototransduction and, more importantly, the cycle of the proteins involved in this pathway and the enzymes responsible for converting them to their active isomers and back.

In rod and cone cells, G-protein-coupled receptors (GPCRs) called opsins contain the chromophore 11-*cis*-retinal. At rest, 11-*cis*-retinal exists as 11-*cis*-retinylidene because it is covalently linked to the opsin receptor forming rhodopsin. When photons hit the eye, 11-*cis*-retinal is converted to its isomer all-trans-retinal and released from the opsin receptor. This change causes a conformational shape change in the opsin GPCR that results in signal transduction. This photon-stimulated pathway closes cGMP-gated ion channels to hyperpolarize the photoreceptors cells. This is the electrical signal in the retina that the optic nerve can interpret, translate, and transmit to the brain [1].

Following this stimulation, all-*trans*-retinal must be converted back to 11-*cis*-retinal and linked back to the opsin receptor to form rhodopsin so further light signals can be transduced (Fig. 1). This conversion first reduces the chromophore from all-trans-retinal to all-trans-retinol via a retinal dehydrogenase (RDH). The trans-retinol then travels to the retinal pigment epithelial (RPE) cells to be recharged to 11-cis-retinal. This recharge occurs in three steps with three different enzymes found in the RPE cells: first, lecithin retinol acyltransferase (LRAT) converts all-trans-retinol into retinyl

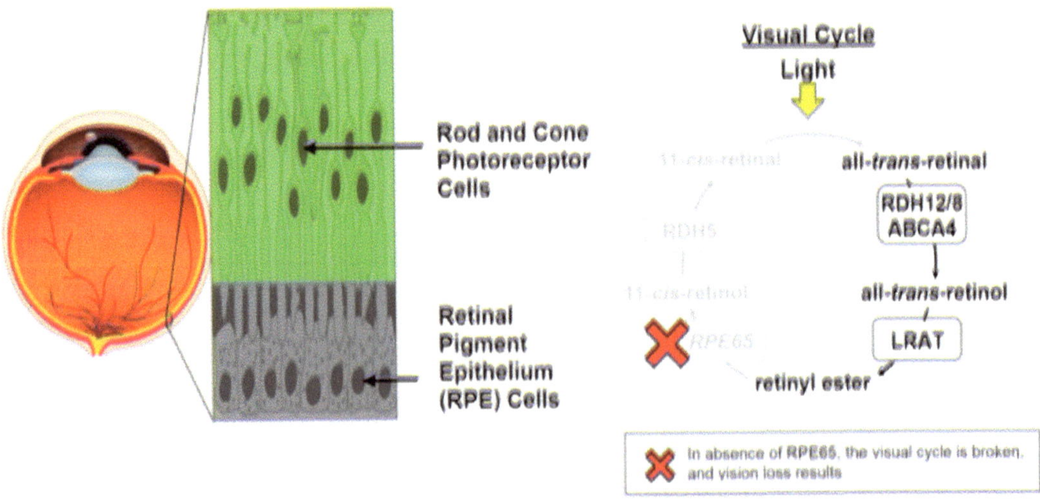

Fig. 1 Recycling of 11-*cis*-retinal is dependent upon *RPE65*. 11-*cis*-retinal is converted to all-*trans*-retinal when hit by photons to transduce signal. The recycling of this molecule back involves a variety of enzymes, importantly including RPE65, that, when mutated, can result in retinitis pigmentosa [3]

ester; then isomerohydrolase retinal pigment epithelium protein kDa 65 (RPE65) converts the retinyl ester into 11-cis-retinol. Finally, a different kind of retinol dehydrogenase (RDH) converts 11-cis-retinol into 11-cis-retinal so that it can travel back to the rod cell and link with opsin to form functional rhodopsin [2]. Mutations in any one of the genes encoding these proteins and enzymes can result in a halt and back-pile of this cycle and consequentially an accumulation of toxic byproducts that damages the photoreceptors and RPE cells. This eventually leads to a progressive loss of rod cells in the back of the eye that results in RP.

The most common mutations resulting in RP involve opsin; since 1990, 150 mutations have been identified. Most of these mutations interrupt proper folding of the protein; the most potent and common in the United States is a missense mutation at codon 23 that exchanges proline for histidine [4]. Mutations that disrupt protein folding do not exclusively involve missense mutations of the rhodopsin itself; however, they involve mutations within the chaperones and spliceosomes responsible for forming rhodopsin properly from its nascent mRNA transcript. Pre-mRNA splicing factor mutations are particularly popular in autosomal dominant forms of RP; even though these proteins are ubiquitously expressed, the retina's eye cell turnover makes it much more vulnerable to aberrant phenotypes from a mutation in one of these factors.

Inheritance patterns of these genetic mutations are broken down as such: 50–60% of RP is inherited in an autosomal recessive pattern; 30–40% of RP is inherited autosomal dominantly; 5–15% of RP shows X-linked inheritance; and a small proportion of cases have been identified with Y-linked or maternal/mitochondrial inheritance patterns [5].

3 Autosomal Recessive Mutations of RP

All of the currently known autosomal recessive mutations (required mutations in both copies of the gene) that can result in RP are listed below [6, 7], both syndromic and non-syndromic varieties; the syndromic forms of RP will be discussed in more detail further in this chapter.

- RP1 results from a mutation in the *ORP1* gene, an oxygen-regulated photoreceptor protein.
- RP4 results from a mutation in the *rhodopsin (RHO)* gene.
- RP12 results from a mutation in *CRB1* involved in cell–cell interaction and maintaining the polarity of the retina.
- RP14 results from a mutation in *TULP1* involved in protein trafficking and rhodopsin transport in the retina.

- RP19 results from a mutation in *ABCA4* involved in removing the toxic byproduct of phototransduction, N-retinylidene-PE, from photoreceptor cells. This form of RP is especially prevalent in Spanish populations.
- RP20 results from a mutation in *RPE65* involved in recycling retinyl ester back into 11-cis-retinol (described above)
- RP25 results from a mutation in *EYS*, a gene expressed in the photoreceptor ciliary pocket and responsible for 5% of AR cases of RP.
- RP26 results from a mutation in *CERKL*, a gene whose protein product is speculated to be a negative regulator of apoptosis in photoreceptor cells.
- RP28 results from a mutation in *FAM161A* involved in the development and progression of retinal progenitor cells during embryogenesis.
- RP35 results from a mutation in *SEMA4A*, a member of the transmembrane semaphorin family, involved in a wide variety of cell functions including migration, axon guidance, and immunomodulation.
- RP36 results from a mutation in *PRCD*, a photoreceptor disc component.
- RP37 results from a mutation in *NR2E3*, part of the nuclear receptor transcription factor family that regulates the expression of many other genes during development and adulthood.
- RP38 results from a mutation in *MERTK*, a proto-oncogene whose protein product is a transmembrane protein; mutations in this gene disrupt normal phagocytosis and turnover of RPE cells.
- RP39 results from a mutation in *USH2A* which encodes usherin, found in the basement membranes of the retina and inner ear; this mutation underlies 10–15% of cases of Usher's syndrome.
- RP40 results from a mutation in *PDE6B*, the phosphodiesterase responsible for activating cGMP in response to photons to close the cGMP-gated ion channels and hyperpolarize the photoreceptor cells to transduce the signal.
- RP41 results from a mutation in *PROM1*, encoding a transmembrane glycoprotein found in adult stem cells to suppress differentiation.
- RP43 results from a mutation in *PDE6A*, a gene of the same phosphodiesterase family as PDE6B responsible for PR40. This protein product modulates rod cell receptor current.
- RP44 results from a mutation in RGR, an opsin subfamily gene; this is a very rare form/cause of RP.

- RP45 results from a mutation in CNGB1 which encodes the beta subunit of the cGMP-gated ion channel in rod photoreceptor cells (*see* RP49 for the alpha subunit mutation).
- RP46 results from a mutation in *IDH3B* involved in the citric acid cycle and thus metabolism in the retina.
- RP47 results from a mutation in *SAG*, an arrest in family gene involved in the desensitization of activated photoreceptor cells.
- RP49 results from a mutation in *CNGA1*, which encodes the alpha subunit of the cGMP-gated ion channel in rod photoreceptor cells (*see* RP45 for the beta subunit mutation).
- RP51 results from a mutation in *TTC8*, a gene implicated in Bardet–Biedl syndrome which is characterized by obesity, learning disabilities, retinal dystrophy, and renal abnormalities. This syndrome is also associated with only retinal dystrophy phenotypes hence its categorization here.
- RP53 results from a mutation in *RHD12*, a retinal dehydrogenase gene associated with Leber congenital amaurosis 13 (LCA13) as well as RP53.
- RP54 results from a mutation in *C2ORF71* whose protein product is associated with the cilia in the outer segment of photoreceptors.
- RP55 results from a mutation in *ARL6* involved in organelle maintenance and cargo trafficking.
- RP56 results from a mutation in *IMPG2* involved in the growth and maintenance of photoreceptor cells.
- RP57 results from a mutation in *PDE6G* which encodes the gamma subunit of the phosphodiesterase responsible for cleaving and activating cGMP in response to photons (*see* RP40 and RP43).
- RP58 results from a mutation in *ZNF513*, a zinc finger protein transcription factor.
- RP59 results from a mutation in *DHDDS* involved in the biosynthesis of glycoproteins.
- RP61 results from a mutation in *CLRN1*, possibly involved in retinal and inner ear homeostasis.
- RP62 results from a mutation in *MAK*, a serine–threonine kinase involved in regulating the cell cycle.
- RP64 results from a mutation in *C8ORF37*, a gene whose function is yet unknown but whose expression is found in the retina, heart, and brain.
- RP65 results from a mutation in *CDHR1*, part of the cadherin adhesive protein family.

- RP66 results from a mutation in RBP3 involved in a retinol binding protein involved in the recycling transport of retinoids between the RPE and photoreceptors.
- RP67 results from a mutation in *NEK2* involved in mitotic regulation.
- RP68 results from a mutation in *SLC7A14* involved in lysosomal regulation.
- RP69 results from a mutation in *KIZ* involved in mitotic spindle formation.
- RP71 results from a mutation in *IFT172* involved in maintaining the cilia.
- RP72 results from a mutation in *ZNF408*, another zinc finger protein.
- RP73 results from a mutation in *HGSNAT* encoding lysosomal acetyltransferase.
- RP74 results from a mutation in *BBS2* involved in Bardet–Biedl syndrome
- RP75 results from a mutation in *AGBL5* whose protein product has deglutamylase activity that may play a role in antiviral immunity.
- RP76 results from a mutation in *POMGNT1*, a Golgi apparatus transmembrane protein.
- RP77 results from a mutation in REEP6 involved in receptor trafficking from the endoplasmic reticulum to the cell surface.
- RP78 results from a mutation in *ARHGEF18*, a Rho GTPase involved in a variety of cell functions including cytoskeletal maneuvering and motility, cell growth, and gene transcription.
- RP79 results from a mutation in *HK1*, the hexokinase enzyme responsible for the first step in glucose metabolism.
- RP80 results from a mutation in *IFT140*, a gene encoding an intraflagellar transport subunit involved in cilia maintenance.
- RP81 results from a mutation in *IFT43*, another intraflagellar transport gene.
- RP82 results from a mutation in *ARL2BP*, an ARF-like protein.
- RP84 results from a mutation in *DHX38*, an RNA helicase active in the splicing process.
- RP85 results from a mutation in *AHR*, a transcription factor that regulates the activity of important metabolic enzymes such as cytochrome P450.

Additionally, although the exact gene has yet to be identified, the loci for RP 22, RP29, and RP32 have been mapped to chromosomes 16, 2, and 1, respectively, in consanguineous families suggesting an autosomal recessive pattern of inheritance in these forms of RP as well [7].

Before moving along to describe autosomal dominant forms of RP, a discussion of juvenile RP is warranted. Childhood onset retinal dystrophy is usually more severe than adult onset forms and involves the loss of both rod and cone photoreceptors together. Juvenile RP is split according to severity—the more severe the cases are known as Leber congenital amaurosis, the less severe the cases are considered RP [8]. The latter can be caused by autosomal recessive mutations *SPATA7* (associated with spermatogenesis), *LRAT* (which esterifies trans-retinol into *trans*-retinyl ester as part of the process to recycle 11-*cis*-retinal), and *TULP1* (*see* RP14 above), as well as an autosomal dominant mutation in *AIPL1* (an aryl-hydrocarbon interacting protein-like).

4 Autosomal Dominant Forms of RP

Autosomal dominant forms of RP only require a mutation in one copy of the gene to result in diseased phenotype. These comprise 30–40% of cases of RP. The known mutations are listed below [6, 7]; those mutations in italics have been shown to be inherited in families in both an autosomal dominant and a recessive manner, depending on the exact mutation in the said gene:

- RP1 results from a mutation in the *ORP1* gene, an oxygen-regulated photoreceptor protein (note that this form of RP can also be inherited autosomal recessively, as listed above).
- RP4 results from a mutation in the *RHO* gene (note that this form of RP can also be inherited autosomal recessively, as listed above).
- RP7 results from a mutation in the peripheral-2 gene involved in stabilizing the myelin sheaths of the peripheral nervous system; other mutations in this same gene are known to cause Charcot–Marie–Tooth disease.
- RP9 results from a mutation in the RP9 gene, which affects alternate splicing.
- RP10 results from a mutation in IMPDH1, which regulates cell growth by catalyzing the conversion of IMP from XMP.
- RP11 results from a mutation in PRPF31, involved in a spliceosome complex.
- RP13 results from a mutation in PRPF8, which is also involved in mRNA splicing.
- RP17 results from a mutation in CA4, a carbonic anhydride.
- RP18 results from a mutation in PRPF3, another mRNA splicing gene.

- RP19 results from a mutation in ABCA4 involved in removing the toxic byproduct of phototransduction, N-retinylidene-PE, from photoreceptor cells. This form of RP is especially prevalent in Spanish populations (note that this form of RP can also be inherited autosomal recessively, as listed above).
- RP27 results from a mutation in *NRL*, encoding neural retina leucine zipper.
- RP30 results from a mutation in *FSCN2*, which encodes a fascin-actin cross linking protein that is critical to photoreceptor disc morphology.
- RP31 results from a mutation in *TOPORS*.
- RP33 results from a mutation in SNRNP200.
- RP35 results from a mutation in SEMA4A, a member of the transmembrane semaphorin family, involved in a wide variety of cell functions including migration, axon guidance, and immunomodulation (note that this form of RP can also be inherited autosomal recessively).
- RP37 results from a mutation in NR2E3, nuclear protein well-documented in RP.
- RP42 results from a mutation in KLHL7 which then disrupts protein degradation.
- RP44 results from a mutation in RGR, an opsin subfamily gene; this is a very rare form/cause of RP (note that this form of RP can also be inherited autosomal recessively, as listed above).
- RP48 results from a mutation in GUCA1B, a guanylate cyclase activator.
- RP50 results from a mutation in BEST1, of the evolutionary genes related to integral membrane proteins such as voltage-gated calcium channels.
- RP53 results from a mutation in RHD12, a retinal dehydrogenase gene associated with Leber congenital amaurosis 13 (LCA13) as well as RP53 (note that this form of RP can also be inherited autosomal recessively).
- RP60 results from a mutation in PRPF6, another pre-mRNA processing factor.
- RP70 results from a mutation in PRPF4, another pre-mRNA processing factor.
- RP83 results from a mutation in ARL3, an ADP-ribosylation factor-like protein associated with GDP and GTP.

As listed above, more than a few of the autosomal dominant mutations associated with RP have to do with pre-mRNA sorting, splicing, and alterations.

5 X-Linked Forms of RP

We now move onto cataloging those mutations on the X chromosome that have been shown to result in RP. These mutations affect males more disproportionally than females and account for 5–15% of all formals of RP [6, 7]:

- RP2 results from a mutation in the *RP2* gene, which interferes with correct folding of photoreceptor beta-tubulin, leading to cell death.
- RP3 and RP15 both are caused by mutations in the *RPGR* gene, which localized to the outer segment of rod cells. It is estimated that 70% of X-linked RP—and 11% of all types of RP—is due to mutations in this gene; RPGR is also implicated in syndromic forms of RP and other eye diseases. Interestingly, while most forms of X-linked RP (XLRP) affects the rod cells predominantly, *RP15* is unique in that carrier females presented with some cone cell involvement.
- RP23 results from a mutation in the *OFD1* gene, a centrosome protein.
- RP6, RP24, and RP34 have all also been mapped to the X chromosome, though their specific gene normative functions are yet unknown.

6 Other Inheritance Patterns of RP

While autosomal recessive, dominant, and X-linked modes of inheritance describe most of the genetic mutations associated with RP, there are a few recorded mutations outside of these descriptors that are rare but interesting anomalies and are worth mentioning.

For example, in 1995, a Chinese family recorded a history with four generations of RP that only presented in males—all sons, no exceptions, were affected, but daughters of affected males were normal. All of the daughters' children (the grandchildren of the affected males), females and males, were healthy as well, negating the hypothesis of X-linked recessive inheritance. Thus geneticists proposed a Y-linked mutation of RP in this family.

RP7 has a double heterozygous mode of inheritance requiring digenic mutations in both the PRPH2 and ROM1 genes, which encode myelin-sheath stabilizing proteins and rod outer segment proteins, respectively [9].

RP8 and RP21 are both syndromic forms of RP inherited through the mitochondria passed down from mother to child. The gene involved in the mutation is MTTS2, a mitochondrial tRNA [10].

Finally, RP5 has been recorded in consanguineous families; it involved a deletion in the long arm of chromosome 6 and is very similar to RP25 (*see* autosomal recessive mutations) [6].

6.1 Syndromic Forms of RP

In addition to mutations that result in only the macular degeneration known as retinitis pigmentosa without the association of any other phenotypes, there are several well-characterized syndromes that include the symptom of retinitis pigmentosa. Eleven of the most common causes of these syndromic types are as follows: Usher syndrome, Bardet–Biedl syndrome, Alport syndrome, Kearns–Sayre syndrome/ragged red fiber myopathy, abetalipoproteinemia, McLeod syndrome, Refsum syndrome, Laurence–Moon syndrome, Cockayne syndrome, Alstrom syndrome, and Leber congenital amaurosis.

6.2 Usher Syndrome

Usher syndrome is a combination of RP-type macular degeneration and hearing loss; this deaf-blindness disorder is currently incurable. It is inherited in an autosomal recessive pattern involving mutations in any 1 of 11 genes, one of which, *USH2A*, was mentioned above. It is usually categorized into three different types according to the genes mutated and the severity of the progress of the disorder, and different types affect different populations disproportionately.

Type I Usher's syndrome patients are born deaf and begin to lose their vision during childhood. As is typical with RP, the vision loss presents as night blindness and tunnel vision first due to loss of rod cells before progressing to eventual total macular degeneration involving cone cells. Mutations comprising type I Usher's syndrome (*CHD23*, *MYO7A*, *PCDH14*, *USH1C*, *USH1G*) involve maintenance of the retinal pigment epithelium and inner ear hair cells; thus, balance is also affected in these individuals. Type I Usher syndrome is more popular in Ashkenazi Jewish populations.

Type II Usher syndrome patients are not born deaf, but only hard of hearing which fortunately is not progressive. In this less severe type of Usher syndrome, vision loss also occurs later, usually in the second or third decades of life. Genes responsible for this type of Usher syndrome include *USH2A*, *GPR98*, and *DFNB31*. *USH2A*, as mentioned above, encodes usherin, which localizes to supportive inner ear and retinal tissue. GPR98 encodes a very large GPCR protein, and DFNB31 encodes whirlin; it is yet unclear how these mutations result in Usher II. Because Usher II is less severe, it is also less diagnosed than Usher I.

Finally, Usher III is the mildest form of Usher syndrome; patients are born with normal hearing and experience progressive hearing loss. Only one gene is currently associated with Usher III, USH3A, encoding a protein involved in synaptic shaping. The vision loss in this form of Usher syndrome is also less severe and has a later onset in life [11].

6.3 Bardet–Biedl Syndrome

Bardet–Biedl syndrome (BBS) affects many more body systems than just Usher syndrome's mere two, although the loss of both vision and hearing for Usher syndrome patients is truly profound and devastating. BBS involves pathogenesis of the cilia that wreaks havoc on metabolism, the renal system, the endocrine system, the sexual system, digit formation, and eyesight. This pleiotropic autosomal recessive condition is characterized by kidney failure, RP, polydactyly, hypogonadism, cardiomyopathy, developmental delay, and diabetes and obesity. Not all patients will experience the same symptoms nor will they experience them to the same degree, because a variety of genes has been shown to cause this syndrome. For those who do experience vision loss as a symptom, it is not present at birth but rather develops in childhood in the expected retinitis pigmentosa pattern—as night blindness and progressive tunnel vision.

So far, 21 genes have been correlated with BBS, and most encode proteins found in the basal bodies of primary cilia; of course, mutations in the proteins comprising cilia would impair their functioning and thus hamper any such organ system relying on cilial motor movement, fluid cycling, and sensation, including the retinal pigment epithelium. These genes include *BBS1*, *BBS2*, *ARL6*, *BBS4*, *BBS5*, *MKKS*, *BBS7*, *TTC8*, *PTHB1*, *BBS10*, *TRIM32*, *BBS12*, *MKS1*, *CEP290*, *WDPCP*, *SD-CCAG8*, *LZTFL1*, *BBIP1*, *IFT27*, *IFT74*, and *C8ORF37*. Note that many of these genes were mentioned in the mutation lists above, including BBS2 responsible for RP74, ARL6 responsible for RP55, TTC8 responsible for RP51, and C8ORF37 responsible for RP64. Additionally, BBS also implicates genes of the IFT family, mentioned above in RP80 and RP81, to be involved with intraflagellar support [12].

6.4 Alport Syndrome

Alport syndrome is another pleiotropic disorder, like Bardet–Biedl syndrome, that is primarily characterized by glomerulonephritis and end-stage kidney disease. Other organ systems that can be involved in Alport syndrome include the eyes and ears, manifesting as vision and hearing loss, though vision loss is the more rare of the two. Alport syndrome is caused by a defect in type IV collagen which is found in the kidneys, ears, and eyes. In the eyes specifically, type IV collagen is an important structural protein found in the basement membranes of the cornea, lens capsule, and retina. Alport syndrome typically manifests in young adulthood, and hearing and vision loss, if present, does not develop until after the kidney symptoms occur. It requires proteinuria and hematuria for diagnosis and is thus primarily a kidney disease; however, increasing severity implicates the sensory systems requiring type IV collagen, and thus it becomes a syndromic cause of RP in very severe patients.

Genes known to cause Alport syndrome if mutated include COL4A3, COL4A4, and COL4A5, three of the six genes encoding type IV collagen basement membrane building blocks. COL4A5 is located on the X chromosome and is responsible for around 85% of cases of Alport syndrome. Males are of course more severely affected; females with one mutated copy may have some hematuria, but this usually does not progress to kidney failure or vision or hearing problems. Mutations in COL4A3 and COL4A4 are located on chromosome 2 and are inherited in an autosomal recessive pattern. As a primarily kidney-centric disease, ACE inhibitors are an effective therapy for the renal symptoms of Alport syndrome; however they are not effective at combatting the vision or hearing loss in more severe patients [13].

6.5 Kearns–Sayre Syndrome/Ragged Red Fiber Myopathy

Kearns–Sayre syndrome, also known as ragged red fiber myopathy, is caused by a deletion in mitochondrial DNA. Because each cell has many mitochondria, this disease is heteroplastic, and its severity can vary across different tissues depending on how many aberrant mitochondria are present in a given cell. The deleted mitochondrial DNA disrupts oxidative phosphorylation and therefore the tissues that require more energy like skeletal muscles are affected more disproportionally. This syndrome is designated ragged red fiber myopathy as this disease affects skeletal muscles the most and gives muscle fibers an abnormal ragged and red appearance in histology. This disease does not only affect muscles however—it can also affect the eyes, heart, cerebellum, ears, and endocrine system resulting in ophthalmoplegia, conduction block, cerebellar ataxia, deafness, diabetes, growth hormone deficiency, and hypoparathyroidism.

In the eyes, specifically, Kearns–Sayre syndrome manifests as pigmentary retinopathy, ptosis, and progressive external ophthalmoplegia due to impaired function of the eyelid and extraocular muscles. In the retina more specifically, bone spicule deposits develop, sometimes in the peripheral pattern characteristic of RP and sometimes in a more macula-centered pattern. Either way, night blindness is common in most KSS patients, and severe vision loss develops in about half of patients. The disease is progressive with onset before age 20; it's inheritance pattern is usually sporadic, but can be autosomal recessive or maternal as well [14].

6.6 Abetalipoproteinemia

Abetalipoproteinemia is a disorder that impairs the normal absorption of fat and fat-soluble vitamins (vitamins A, D, E, and K) from the diet. It results from a mutation in microsomal triglyceride transfer protein (MTTP, autosomal recessive) and thus causes a deficiency in the apolipoproteins B48 and B100, integral in the synthesis and transport of chylomicrons and VLDL (principle cholesterol transporters), respectively. This disease can manifest with a wide variety of symptoms related to the lipoproteins including failure to thrive, steatorrhea, developmental delay, muscle weakness, speech impediment, scoliosis, progressively declining vision, and balance issues. Three signs warn for this condition: acanthocytosis, hypocholesterolemia, and RP. In the eye specifically, it is the deficiency of vitamin A—retinol—which breaks down the retina and can progress to total vision loss [15].

6.7 McLeod Syndrome

McLeod Syndrome is an X-linked recessive neurological disorder of the XK gene. This gene transcribes the Kx protein, which supports the Kell antigen on red blood cells. Mutations in this gene thus impair normal functions of the blood, brain, peripheral nervous system, heart, and muscles. Onset of symptoms usually occurs later in life for men affected who present with peripheral neuropathy, hemolytic anemia, and cardiomyopathy; female carriers remain unaffected. More severe symptoms include seizures, dementia, and behavioral changes. Phenotypically, it is very similar to Huntington's disease, both in behavior and age of onset; some patients even develop the characteristic Huntington's disease chorea and random limb movements. Not all cases of McLeod syndrome include RP as a symptom; in fact, those cases that do often also involve Duchenne muscular dystrophy-type phenotypes. It is thought that a particularly large deletion or mutation in the Kx gene can affect those genes around it on the X chromosome and those neighboring genes then produce the DMD and RP symptoms in severe patients [16].

6.8 Refsum Disease

Refsum disease occurs due to a buildup of phytanic acid in tissues and cells; mutations in PHYH, phytanoyl-CoA hydroxylase, or PEX7, peroxin-7, and peroxisome enzymes responsible for degrading phytanic acid cause this buildup. These mutations are inherited in an autosomal recessive pattern. It is yet unclear the role phytanic acid plays in our functioning, but mice models suggest it may aid in regulating fatty acid metabolism in the liver. Regardless, excess of any substance can be toxin, and excess of this substance is neurologically toxic. Patients experience peripheral neuropathy and cerebellar damage, along with ichthyosis, hearing loss, ataxia, and a variety of vision problems including RP, night blindness, and cataracts. Most patients with Refsum disease will experience vision loss. Both vision and hearing loss problems are due to peripheral nerve damage of the optic and auditory nerves. It is a progressive degenerative disorder with a childhood onset [17].

6.9 Laurence–Moon Syndrome

Laurence–Moon syndrome is very similar to Bardet–Biedl syndrome—it is autosomal recessive and very rare, and patients exhibit symptoms of RP, intellectual disabilities, spastic paraplegia, polydactyly, and diabetes. The vision loss associated with this disorder usually occurs by age 30. There is debate as to whether this disease is the same as Bardet–Biedl syndrome, just of a different order; however, while clinical management for the two is the same, Laurence–Moon syndrome has markedly more random limb movements than BBS. The gene mutated in this syndrome is PNPLA6, which is involved in breaking down cell membranes to drive the growth of further cells [18].

6.10 Cockayne Syndrome

Cockayne syndrome is a fatal, autosomal recessive, neurodegenerative disorder that can affect any and all of the organ systems. Key characteristics include failure to thrive, photosensitivity and other vision issues including RP, and premature aging. Cockayne syndrome is a leukodystrophy, meaning that it involves the degradation of white matter due to a defect in DNA repair; notably, this does not predispose patients to cancer or other infections. Two genes have been linked to this disease: ERCC8, also known as CSA, and ERCC6, also known as CSB. The latter accounts for 70% of cases. Both of the protein products of these genes are involved in transcription-coupled nucleotide excision repair that repairs pyrimidine primers damaged from UV light, radiation, and free radicals. Without this mechanism in place, errors in DNA build up and cause disease [19].

6.11 Alstrom Syndrome

Alstrom syndrome is a very rare, autosomal recessive, childhood disorder characterized by obesity, early-onset type 2 diabetes, dilated cardiomyopathy, developmental delay, sensorineural hearing loss, endocrine dysfunction, and rod-cone dystrophy vision impairment and photosensitivity. It's caused by a mutation in ALMS1, which may play a role in maintaining cilia, which, as has been mentioned before, is important to the upkeep of the retinal pigment epithelium. The vision issues of this disease manifest within 15 months of birth and progressively worsen for the next two decades [20].

6.12 Leber Congenital Amaurosis

Leber congenital amaurosis (LCA) was previously mentioned earlier in this chapter in a discussion of juvenile-onset RP. It is considered the more severe form and usually involves the simultaneous loss of rod and cone cells together, unlike adult forms where rod photoreceptor loss precedes cone loss. LCA is a condition that patients are either born with or develop within the first few months of birth. Besides the RP vision problems, patients also experience nystagmus and sluggish pupillary response. LCA can be caused by up to 18 genes recognized currently, and thus its inheritance can be either autosomal recessive or dominant. The genes, in order, are GUCY2D, RPE65, SPATA7, AIPL1, LCA5, PRGRIP1, CRX, CRB1, NMNAT1, CEP290, IMPDH1, RD3, RDH12, LRAT, TULP1, KCNJ13, GDF6, and PRPH2 [21]. Many of these genes have already been mentioned previously in this chapter.

Additional syndromic causes that are much rarer include Cohen syndrome, Jeanne syndrome, methylmalonic aciduria, Bietti's disease, cystinosis, Zellweger syndrome, Joubert syndrome, and Hallervorden–Spatz syndrome [1]. This wraps up our discussion of common syndromic causes of RP, many of which present with atypical forms of the syndrome; we now move onto a brief look into some of the systemic causes of secondary RP.

7 Secondary RP

Cases of secondary RP arise when diseases affecting other parts of the body progress to encompass ocular deficits similar to those seen in RP, namely, tunnel vision, night blindness, and cone-rod cell atrophy. Diseases that affect the nervous system are the ones that generally fall into this category like Lyme borreliosis which involves cerebral demyelination and syphilis [22]. Additionally, nephrotic syndrome may result in vision impairment and thus RP [23]. These diseases are varied in their biochemical mechanism and the affects they wreak on the body, but no matter the disease, they debilitate the body enough such that photoreceptor cells are unable to maintain themselves.

8 Conclusion

Retinitis pigmentosa describes a set of symptoms that can arise on their own due to aberrant mutations of all forms of inheritance, in conjunction with other symptoms as part of a larger genetic syndrome, or as a result of a systemic disease process that also ends up affecting the eye. All of these causes in some way or another impair the photoreceptors' abilities to maintain themselves by destabilizing the outer segment of the rod cells; by shortening them and exposing them to highly oxygen pressured environments resulting in oxygen toxicity; by interrupting the cell's transcription, translation, or metabolic Kreb's cycle or electron transport chain machinery so that the photoreceptor is no longer able to keep up with the demands of its role and environment; by opening calcium channels and triggering calcium-mediated cell death; or by interfering in the actual turnover of rhodopsin itself. Whether non-syndromic, syndromic, or systemic, RP is ultimately caused by the degeneration of rod and cone photoreceptors.

Conflicts of Interest

Stephen H. Tsang receives financial support from Abeona Therapeutics, Inc and Emendo. He is also the founder of Rejuvitas and is on the scientific and clinical advisory board for Nanoscope Therapeutics.

References

1. (2014) Facts about retinitis pigmentosa. National Eye Institute
2. (2017) Background on Biallelic RPE65 mutation-associated retinal dystrophy. Spark Therapeutics Briefing Document: 35–40
3. (2017) Figure 13: The role of RPE65 in the visual cycle. Spark Therapeutics Briefing Document: 36
4. Hamel C (2006) Retinitis Pigmentosa. Orphanet J Rare Dis
5. Hartong DT et al (2006) Retinitis pigmentosa. Lancet 368:1795–1809
6. Retinitis Pigmentosa; RP #268000. OMIM Database
7. Gene cards: human gene database. Weizmann Institute of Science
8. Gu SM et al (1997) Mutations in RPE65 cause autosomal recessive childhood-onset severe retinal dystrophy. Nat Genet 17:194–197
9. Zhao et al. (1995) Letter. Ophthalmology Genetics: 75–76
10. Mansergh FC et al (1999) Retinitis pigmentosa and progressive sensorineural hearing loss caused by a C12258A mutation in the mitochondrial MTTS2 gene. Am J Hum Genet:971–985
11. (2017) Usher syndrome. Genetics Home Reference, NIH
12. (2013) Bardet-Biedel syndrome. Genetics Home Reference, NIH
13. (2013) Alport syndrome. Genetics Home Reference, NIH
14. (2011) Kearns Sayre syndrome. Genetics Home Reference, NIH
15. (2018) Abetalipoproteinemia. Genetics Home Reference, NIH
16. (2015) McLeod syndrome. Genetics Home Reference, NIH
17. (2016) Refsum disease. Genetics Home Reference, NIH
18. (2018) Laurence-Moon syndrome. National Organization for Rare Disorders
19. (2016) Cockayne syndrome. Genetics Home Reference, NIH
20. (2014) Alstrom syndrome. Genetics Home Reference, NIH
21. (2017). Leber congenital amaurosis. National Organization of Rare Diseases
22. Karma A et al (1993) Secondary retinitis pigmentosa and cerebral demyelination in Lyme borreliosis. Br J Ophthalmol 77:120–122
23. Masugi J et al (1994) Pigmentary retinopathy with nephrotic syndrome, Menetrier's disease, and diabetes mellitus. Intern Med 33:644–648

Chapter 3

Clinical Evaluation of Patients with Retinitis Pigmentosa

Sitara H. Hirji

Abstract

This chapter describes the clinical evaluation process of patients with retinitis pigmentosa (RP). The clinical evaluation consists of a complete history and ophthalmic examination. Here, we outline the aspects of the history and ophthalmic exam that are most important for the evaluation of RP patients. In addition, the expected findings of RP patients and the etiology of these findings are discussed.

Key words Retinitis pigmentosa, Clinical evaluation, Genetic retinopathy, Pigment epithelium, Optic nerve pallor, Vitreous, Cystoid macular edema

1 Introduction

The clinical evaluation of patients with retinitis pigmentosa (RP) includes both a thorough history and a full ophthalmic examination. While the classic clinical presentation is well described, there is a wide range of visual complaints experienced by patients. Additionally, different inheritance patterns of RP such as autosomal dominant and X-linked recessive subtypes may have variations in onset and severity of symptoms [1]. Once a history is provided by the patient, he or she must undergo a full ophthalmic examination. This includes the anterior slit lamp examination, measurement of intraocular pressure, and a dilated fundus examination. Ancillary testing such as dark adaptometry, full-field electroretinography, and multifocal electroretinography is also useful for diagnostic evaluation and will be covered in subsequent chapters. This chapter will describe the methodology for the clinical assessment of RP patients and discuss expected findings for the ophthalmic examination.

1.1 History

A complete history of visual symptoms should start with information about the timing, nature, and severity of the earliest symptoms experienced by the patient. For a majority of patients, the earliest symptom is defective dark adaptation, otherwise known as

Stephen H. Tsang and Peter M. J. Quinn (eds.), *Retinitis Pigmentosa*,
Methods in Molecular Biology, vol. 2560, https://doi.org/10.1007/978-1-0716-2651-1_3,

nyctalopia or night blindness. This symptom is a product of damage to the photoreceptors, specifically the rods, that is characteristic of RP [2]. Age of onset may differ between the genetic subtypes of RP; these differences may aid in early determination of the genetic classification of affected patients. In a retrospective study of patients from 456 families, night blindness occurred at an earlier age in patients with X-linked and autosomal dominant RP as compared to patients with autosomal recessive. By the age of 20, 87% of patients with X-linked RP (XLRP) and 75% of patients with autosomal dominant RP had symptoms, whereas 61% with autosomal recessive inheritance were symptomatic. By the age of 30, 100% of patients with X-linked RP and 89% of patients with autosomal dominant RP were symptomatic, as compared to 74% of autosomal recessive RP patients [3]. If patients do not voluntarily provide night blindness as an experienced symptom, providers may directly ask about speed of dark adaptation which may assist patients in recognizing a deficit. As the disease progresses, patients may also report photophobia with sensitivity to diffuse white light as seen on a bright, cloudy day.

Another classically described symptom of RP is loss of peripheral vision. However, this is not commonly described by the patient with early-stage disease and more often first discovered on visual field testing. If patients are experiencing early loss of peripheral vision, they may describe feeling clumsy as their field of vision narrows. Natural progression of RP is a continuous degradation of the patient's photoreceptors, resulting in the expansion of visual field defects until the patient develops tunnel vision. Ultimately, patients experience loss of central vision, which may cause them difficulty with activities of daily living such as ambulating, reading, and recognizing the faces of people around them [4]. Loss of central vision is also caused by macular complications of RP such as cystoid macular edema (CME) and epiretinal membrane [5, 6].

While most forms of RP are primarily rod degeneration at first followed by reduction in cone sensitivity, there are some patients in which both rods and cones degenerate simultaneously. Rarely, some patients will have cone degeneration primarily prior to decreased rod sensitivity; in these patients, decreased color vision and early loss of visual acuity may be the earliest symptoms [4].

In addition to ascertaining the patient's visual symptoms, family history is crucial to determining the genetic subtype of RP that the patient may have. A multi-generation pedigree should be obtained to help determine the inheritance pattern of the disease. However, as many cases of RP are inherited recessively, patients with a seemingly negative family history may still be at risk for the disease.

Past medical history is important to determine whether the patient has isolated RP or whether it is within the context of a systemic disorder. RP often presents as a syndrome associated with hearing loss, so patients should be asked about subjective hearing loss and may benefit from a quantitative assessment of sensorineural hearing. Syndromes with renal and neurologic involvement are also common, so a careful and comprehensive review of systems is recommended. Additionally, patients should be asked specifically about medical problems that mimic RP such as syphilitic neuroretinitis and Rubella retinopathy and thioridazine-associated retinopathy.

2 Materials

The ocular examination includes the following: visual acuity, refraction, visual fields to confrontation, and intraocular pressure measurement.

1. Refraction.
2. Visual fields to confrontation.
3. Intraocular pressure measurement.
4. Examination of the anterior segment.
5. Dilated fundus exam.

3 Methods

3.1 Visual Acuity

Visual acuity is a product of central visual function, which is usually spared in RP until late in disease. Therefore, patients with RP have generally preserved visual acuity until the disease has progressed to affect the photoreceptors in the central retina. Sandberg et al. demonstrated that retinal thinning due to both loss of photoreceptors and edema are associated with lower visual acuity in patients with RP [7]. Differences in severity of visual acuity loss may be seen between the genetic subtypes of RP. Fishman et al. demonstrated that patients with autosomal dominant disease have the best prognosis in terms of visual acuity, with the majority of patients under 30 years old having a visual acuity of 20/30 or better [8]. In contrast, X-linked recessive RP patients over 50 years all had a visual acuity worse than 20/200 [9]. Additionally, visual prognosis varies between syndromic RP and non-syndromic RP; Usher syndrome type IIa, in which patient have RP alongside sensorineural hearing loss, is associated with earlier and more severe visual acuity impairment than non-syndromic RP [10]. It is important to document severity and progression of visual acuity loss and ensure full use of vision potential with low vision aids and proper refraction. Visual acuity loss is associated with decreased quality of life and emotional states of RP patients [11].

3.2 Refraction

Refractive errors are common in patients with RP (Sieving). Furthermore, they may be a clue to the genetic subtype a patient may have. Patients with autosomal dominant disease are more likely to have hyperopia, whereas patients with X-linked RP are commonly myopic [3, 4]. It is important to ensure proper refraction of patients, especially as they suffer from retinopathy-induced vision loss, to ensure full use of patients' vision potential.

3.3 Visual Fields to Confrontation

As described above, most cases of RP progress from loss of peripheral vision to loss of central vision. Therefore, upon testing of visual fields to confrontation, patients with RP will commonly have deficits found in peripheral fields. These deficits are better characterized using standard automated perimetry.

3.4 Intraocular Pressure Measurement

Intraocular pressure of eyes affected by RP is usually within the normal range, even in late-stage disease [12]. There has been some literature suggesting an association between RP and primary angle closure glaucoma [13, 14]. However, Xu et al. suggest that the relationship is coincidental [15].

3.5 Aqueous Humor

There is evidence that RP is an inflammatory condition; one sign of inflammation seen on slit lamp examination of patients with RP is the presence of aqueous flare. Eyes affected by RP demonstrate increased aqueous flare, indicating impairment of the blood-ocular barrier [16]. Increased flair in patients with RP is associated with CME [16]. Additionally, pro-inflammatory cytokines and chemokines have been shown to be increased in the aqueous humor, providing further evidence of the proposed inflammatory nature of RP [17].

3.6 Lens

On the anterior slit lamp exam, RP patients are commonly found to have posterior subcapsular cataracts (PSC), characterized by yellow, crystalline changes in the peripheral lens cortex; prevalence is reported between 41% and 53% [3, 18, 19]. While the cause of cataract formation is unknown, Fujiwara et al. demonstrated that elevated aqueous flare is a significant risk factor for PSC formation [6]. This supports the literature that has suggested an inflammatory pathogenesis of the cataracts seen in RP patients [20].

3.7 Vitreous

Vitreous abnormalities are seen in a majority of patients with RP. RP patients suffer from a characteristic vitreous degeneration that has been divided into four stages. Stage I is defined as translucent particles throughout the vitreous gel. Stage II is described as translucent particles plus complete vitreous detachment. Stage III is the presence of translucent particles, a vitreous detachment, and the presence of a posterior matrix of dense white opacities and interconnecting fibers. Stage IV is the presence of the particles, vitreous detachment, posterior matrix, and the reduction in the volume of the residual vitreous gel [21]. The degree of vitreous degeneration correlates with the magnitude of retinal destruction. The degeneration of the vitreous is postulated to be the result of progressive loss of hyaluronic acid from the hyaluronic acid collagen complex, as cells responsible for the production of hyaluronic acid are lost from the degeneration of the neurosensory retinal and retinal pigment epithelium [21]. Vitreous detachments are associated with CME caused by vitreomacular adhesion resulting in traction to the macula [22]. In patients with RP, vitreous opacities were first described on slit lamp exam in the early 1900s [21]. More recently, monoclonal antibodies against T cells, B cells, and macrophages were used to characterize the vitreous particles in 14 eyes; all samples contained CD4, T helper, and CD8, suppressor cells, activated T cells, some B cells, and macrophages [23]. Another study demonstrated that of 509 eyes affected by RP, 37.3% eyes exhibited cells in the anterior vitreous cavity and pro-inflammatory cytokines and chemokines were increased in the aqueous humor and the vitreous fluid of RP patients when compared to levels in control patients [17]. Examination of the vitreous for particles, vitreous detachment, and matrix formation may assist in assessing the extent of retinal damage in patients with RP. Vitreous fluorophotometry is also used to quantify the breakdown of the blood-retinal barrier, which provides further information about the extent of disease. Patients with RP show high concentrations of fluorescein within the vitreous due to the compromised blood-retinal barrier, with higher amounts of fluorescein present in later-stage disease [24].

3.8 Fundus Examination

As RP is a disease of the photoreceptors, cells that are located in the retina, the fundus examination is particularly important for clinical evaluation of disease progression. All types of RP classically exhibit a triad of clinical signs on fundus examination: arteriolar attenuation, bone spicule retinal pigmentation, and optic disc pallor. However, these signs represent advanced degeneration of the retina and are usually not present in early stages of disease. Therefore, they are not needed for initial diagnosis of RP. Early retinal changes are more likely to be found using electroretinography to detect defective rod responses.

1. Arteriolar attenuation: The attenuation of retinal arterioles is the earliest clinical sign that is visible on fundus examination in early-stage RP. It is nearly a universal finding in patients with RP, regardless of inheritance pattern [4]. The attenuation is postulated to reflect a decrease in metabolic demand of the degenerating retina in which decreased consumption of oxygen by the retina [12]. The decrease in consumption leads to increased local oxygen levels, resulting in vasoconstriction and reduction in blood flow [25]. Ma et al. demonstrated that the

degree of visual field loss is correlated to the degree of retinal vessel attenuation, as measured by retinal vessel caliber [26]. This finding may be another useful measure for estimating the progression of RP or treatment response. In late-stage RP, pathology demonstrates sclerosis and atrophy of the vasculature [27]. In addition to retinal vasculature being affected, there is loss of all but the largest of choroidal vessels as well [1].

2. Bone spicule retinal pigmentation: Retinal pigmentation is the next clinical sign seen on fundus examination, usually in mid-stage disease. As photoreceptors continue to degenerate, there is increasing loss of pigment from the retinal pigment epithelium. Clumping of melanin in the retina, specifically around the branching retinal blood vessels, causes the characteristic bone spicule appearance. In a histopathologic study of an eye enucleated from a 31-year-old RP patient, two types of pigmented cells were identified: normal retinal pigment epithelial cells that had migrated from the RPE layer and macrophage-like cells that contained melanin [28]. Pigment epithelium was normal in areas where there was no photoreceptor degeneration, suggesting that the pigment epithelium changes were reactive to photoreceptor damage. In response to photoreceptor death, retinal pigment epithelium migrates into the neural retina and forms pigment deposits. Pigment accumulation first appears in the mid-periphery of the retina and eventually appears diffusely, involving the macular in late-stage disease. Macular involvement of pigmentation contributed to the decrease in central visual acuity seen in late-stage disease. Historically, the progression of retinal pigmentation has been described in five stages:
   (a) No changes on fundus examination.
   (b) Pigmentary stippling due to accumulation of pigment granules in the outer layers of the retina.
   (c) Bone spicule formation of pigment.
   (d) Vascular pigmentary sheathing in the mid-periphery of the retina.
   (e) Vascular pigmentary sheathing extending to the disc.
   (f) However, the order of these stages as well as timing of progression may vary depending on the genetic subtype of RP [29].
3. Optic disc pallor: The optic disc of RP patients is commonly described as having a waxy pallor. Most ophthalmic pathologies associated with optic disc pallor are associated with an abnormality in the ganglion cells and retinal nerve fiber layer, such as glaucoma and ischemic optic neuropathies. In the case of RP, the retinal ganglion cells and nerve fiber layer remain intact

until late stages of disease, when extensive loss of photoreceptors causes transneuronal degeneration of ganglion cells [27]. The waxy pallor characteristic of RP has been suggested to be the result of epiretinal membrane formation. Older studies of RP patients describe a preretinal membrane covering the optic nerve that is continuous with Elschnig's membrane [27, 30]. In a series of 108 eyes of different genetic subtypes of RP, 82% had an epiretinal membrane, with an increased percentage seen in eyes of patients aged 60 years or older [31]. More recently, Al Rashaed et al. demonstrated that there is a significant association between optic nerve waxy pallor and the presence of a prelaminar structure such as an preretinal membrane [32]. The membrane originates from fibrous astroglial cells in the optic nerve that migrate through the breaks in the inner limiting lamina of the optic nerve. They may be associated with posterior vitreous detachment frequently observed in RP patients, and contraction of the membranes may cause wrinkling of the inner surface of the retina which is commonly seen in RP patients.

Other findings found on fundus examination include optic nerve atrophy, optic nerve drusen, and CME. Optic nerve atrophy is seen in late-stage disease due to the death of ganglion cells that have undergone transneuronal degeneration. There are two forms of optic nerve head drusen associated with RP: hamartomas and "true drusen" [27]. The hamartomas are found anteriorly in the nerve head and extend into the vitreous. They contain partially calcified astrocytes. The true drusen are laminated, acellular calcifications. The etiology of the drusen is unclear, but it has been suggested that they are derived from material leaked from abnormal blood vessels or from degeneration of retinal ganglion cell axons [33, 34]. These deposits may cause permanent vision loss in RP patients.

One cause of reversible vision loss in RP patients that may be seen on fundus examination is CME. Partial thickness holes or cysts lead to increased capillary permeability. Fluorescein angiography demonstrates that the macula most frequently shows leakage in RP patients and the presence of CME is significantly correlated with a decreased in central visual acuity [35]. The incidence of CME in RP patients is reported as between 10% and 50%. In a systematic review of the treatment of CME secondary to RP, the oral carbonic anhydrase inhibitor acetazolamide was identified as preferred first-line treatment [36]. However, in chronic rebound macular edema characteristic of RP patients, its effectiveness is limited [37]. The identification and treatment of CME in RP patients is especially important as patients are heavily reliant on central vision after the degeneration of their peripheral photoreceptors.

3.9 Summary

RP is an inherited disorder characterized by progressive retinal degeneration. Clinical evaluation of RP patients focuses on symptoms caused by the degeneration of photoreceptors as well as findings seen on slit lamp examination and fundoscopy. Classic symptoms of RP patients are night blindness and loss of peripheral vision due to degeneration of rods. In the late stage of disease, patients note loss of color vision and visual acuity as they experience macular involvement and cone degeneration. Visual acuity and refraction should be determined at each visit. Slit lamp exam is useful for identifying signs of inflammation in the anterior segment, the presence of cataracts, and vitreous abnormalities, among other findings. Fundus examination frequently shows the triad of retinal attenuation, bone spicule pigment accumulation, and waxy optic disc pallor. The fundus should also be evaluated for CME, a secondary diagnosis to RP. Evaluation of patients' signs and symptoms is necessary to assess progression of disease and rate of photoreceptor deterioration. Additionally, providers must ensure full use of vision potential by treating associated pathologies such as subcapsular cataracts and CME.

References

1. Pagon RA (1988) Retinitis pigmentosa. Surv Ophthalmol 33(3):137–177
2. Zeavin BH, Wald G (1956) Rod and cone vision in retinitis pigmentosa. Am J Ophthalmol 42(4):253–269
3. Berson EL, Rosner B, Simonoff E (1980) Risk factors for genetic typing and detection in retinitis pigmentosa. Am J Ophthalmol 89(6): 763–775
4. Hartong DT, Berson EL, Dryja TP (2006) Retinitis pigmentosa. Lancet 368(9549): 1795–1809
5. Hajali M, Fishman GA, Anderson RJ (2008) The prevalence of cystoid macular oedema in retinitis pigmentosa patients determined by optical coherence tomography. Br J Ophthalmol 92(8):1065–1068
6. Fujiwara K, Ikeda Y, Murakami Y, Nakatake S, Tachibana T, Yoshida N et al (2016) Association between aqueous flare and epiretinal membrane in retinitis pigmentosa. Invest Ophthalmol Vis Sci 57(10):4282–4286
7. Sandberg MA, Brockhurst RJ, Gaudio AR, Berson EL (2005) The association between visual acuity and central retinal thickness in retinitis pigmentosa. Invest Ophthalmol Vis Sci 46(9):3349–3354
8. Fishman GA (1978) Retinitis pigmentosa. Visual loss. Arch Ophthalmol 96(7): 1185–1188
9. Fishman GA, Farber MD, Derlacki DJ (1988) X-linked retinitis pigmentosa. Profile of clinical findings. Arch Ophthalmol 106(3):369–375
10. Pierrache LH, Hartel BP, van Wijk E, Meester-Smoor MA, Cremers FP, de Baere E et al (2016) Visual prognosis in USH2A-associated retinitis pigmentosa is worse for patients with usher syndrome type IIa than for those with nonsyndromic retinitis pigmentosa. Ophthalmology 123(5):1151–1160
11. Azoulay L, Chaumet-Riffaud P, Jaron S, Roux C, Sancho S, Berdugo N et al (2015) Threshold levels of visual field and acuity loss related to significant decreases in the quality of life and emotional states of patients with retinitis pigmentosa. Ophthalmic Res 54(2):78–84
12. Grunwald JE, Maguire AM, Dupont J (1996) Retinal hemodynamics in retinitis pigmentosa. Am J Ophthalmol 122(4):502–508
13. Badeeb O, Trope G, Musarella M (1993) Primary angle closure glaucoma and retinitis pigmentosa. Acta Ophthalmol 71(6):727–732
14. Ziaei M, Khalili A, Wormald R (2013) Retinal dystrophy and primary angle-closure glaucoma. Int Ophthalmol 33(6):737–739
15. Xu J, Ouyang Z, Yang Y, Cai X, Wang Z, Lin M et al (2017) Ocular biometry in primary angle-closure glaucoma associated with retinitis pigmentosa. J Ophthalmol 2017:5

16. Küchle M, Nguyen NX, Martus P, Freissler K, Schalnus R (1998) Aqueous flare in retinitis pigmentosa. Graefes Arch Clin Exp Ophthalmol 236(6):426–433
17. Yoshida N, Ikeda Y, Notomi S, Ishikawa K, Murakami Y, Hisatomi T et al (2013) Clinical evidence of sustained chronic inflammatory reaction in retinitis pigmentosa. Ophthalmology 120(1):100–105
18. Heckenlively J (1982) The frequency of posterior subcapsular cataract in the hereditary retinal degenerations. Am J Ophthalmol 93(6):733–738
19. Fishman GA, Anderson RJ, Lourenco P (1985) Prevalence of posterior subcapsular lens opacities in patients with retinitis pigmentosa. Br J Ophthalmol 69(4):263–266
20. Gwon A, Mantras C, Gruber L, Cunanan C (1993) Concanavalin A-induced posterior subcapsular cataract: a new model of cataractogenesis. Invest Ophthalmol Vis Sci 34(13):3483–3488
21. Pruett RC (1975) Retinitis pigmentosa: a biomicroscopical study of vitreous abnormalities. JAMA Ophthalmol 93(8):603–608
22. Schepens CL, Avila MP, Jalkh AE, Trempe CL (1984) Role of the vitreous in cystoid macular edema. Surv Ophthalmol 28(Suppl):499–504
23. Newsome DA, Michels RG (1988) Detection of lymphocytes in the vitreous gel of patients with retinitis pigmentosa. Am J Ophthalmol 105(6):596–602
24. Fishman GA, Cunha-Vaz J, Salzano T (1981) Vitreous fluorophotometry in patients with retinitis pigmentosa. Arch Ophthalmol 99(7):1202–1207
25. Yu DY, Cringle SJ (2005) Retinal degeneration and local oxygen metabolism. Exp Eye Res 80(6):745–751
26. Ma Y, Kawasaki R, Dobson LP, Ruddle JB, Kearns LS, Wong TY, Mackey DA (2012) Quantitative analysis of retinal vessel attenuation in eyes with retinitis pigmentosa. Invest Ophthalmol Vis Sci 53(7):4306–4314
27. Milam AH, Li ZY, Fariss RN (1998) Histopathology of the human retina in retinitis pigmentosa. Prog Retin Eye Res 17(2):175–205
28. Bunt-Milam AH, Kalina RE, Pagon RA (1983) Clinical-ultrastructural study of a retinal dystrophy. Invest Ophthalmol Vis Sci 24(4):458–469
29. Merin S, Auerbach E (1976) Retinitis pigmentosa. Surv Ophthalmol 20(5):303–346
30. Szamier RB (1981) Ultrastructure of the preretinal membrane in retinitis pigmentosa. Invest Ophthalmol Vis Sci 21(2):227–236
31. Sastry SM, Li ZY, Milam AH (1996) Epiretinal membranes in retinitis pigmentosa. Invest Ophthalmol Vis Sci 37(3):4789
32. Al Rashaed S, Khan AO, Nowilaty SR, Edward DP, Kozak I (2016) Spectral-domain optical coherence tomography reveals prelaminar membranes in optic nerve head pallor in eyes with retinitis pigmentosa. Graefes Arch Clin Exp Ophthalmol 254(1):77–81
33. Sacks JG, O'Grady RB, Choromokos E, Leestma J (1977) The pathogenesis of optic nerve drusen. Arch Ophthalmol 95:425–428
34. Puck A, Tso MOM, Fishman GA (1985) Drusenof the optic nerve associated with retinitis pigmentosa. Arch Ophthalmol 103:231–234
35. Newsome DA (1986) Retinal fluorescein leakage in retinitis pigmentosa. Am J Ophthalmol 101(3):354–360
36. Bakthavatchalam M, Lai FHP, Rong SS, Ng DS, Brelen ME (2018) Treatment of cystoid macular edema secondary to retinitis pigmentosa: a systematic review. Surv Ophthalmol 63(3):329–339
37. Cox SN, Hay E, Bird AC (1988) Treatment of chronic macular edema with acetazolamide. JAMA Ophthalmol 106(9):1190–1195

Chapter 4

Molecular Genetic Testing Approaches for Retinitis Pigmentosa

Megan Soucy, Akemi Joy Tanaka, and Avinash Dharmadhikari

Abstract

Retinitis pigmentosa (RP) affects approximately 1 in 4000 individuals. It has many different genetic etiologies and therefore diagnosis can be challenging. Understanding the different testing methodologies is beneficial for clinicians and researchers in order to select the best testing method, whether it be panel testing, whole exome sequencing, or whole genome sequencing for individuals affected with RP. The Methods section also outlines the steps required to complete a WES assay, which has become a popular method for identifying the molecular diagnosis for individuals with RP.

Key words Next-generation sequencing, Retinitis pigmentosa, Whole exome sequencing whole genome sequencing

1 Introduction

Retinitis pigmentosa (RP) is a group of inherited retinal disorders that are characterized by peripheral vision loss and typically a characteristic deposit of intraretinal pigment. These disorders can be classified as nonsyndromic, syndromic, or systemic [1]. RP causes progressive degeneration of the retina that starts in the periphery and moves centrally, where the affected photoreceptor cells undergo apoptosis [2].

The worldwide prevalence of RP is about 1 in 4000 individuals, and it can follow autosomal dominant, autosomal recessive, X-linked, or non-Mendelian inheritance patterns, such as mitochondrial [3]. A clinical diagnosis of RP can be established without identifying the underlying genetic cause. However, knowledge of the molecular etiology may become important for treatment opportunities as the field moves further into precision medicine with the promise of gene therapy.

Stephen H. Tsang and Peter M. J. Quinn (eds.), *Retinitis Pigmentosa*,
Methods in Molecular Biology, vol. 2560, https://doi.org/10.1007/978-1-0716-2651-1_4,

The genetic etiology of RP is complex. Not all pathogenic variations that contribute to RP are currently known. Even within the nonsyndromic subtypes of RP, over 70 genes and loci have been identified to contribute to the phenotype [4]. In addition to the locus heterogeneity, RP has also been shown to have allelic heterogeneity. The *RPGR* gene alone has 195 pathogenic variant entries in ClinVar and over 350 unique variants in LOVD [5, 6]. Additionally, several genes implicated in RP can be causative in other retinal conditions. For example, the *RHO* gene is associated with both autosomal dominant and autosomal recessive RP, autosomal dominant congenital stationary night blindness, and autosomal dominant and autosomal recessive retinitis punctate albescens (OMIM Entry 180380). While genotype–phenotype correlation can be seen with some causative genes, it is not consistent across all genes associated with RP [7]. The genetic complexity of RP contributes to the challenge of selecting the best molecular test for patients in the ever-expanding field of genetics.

Since the completion of the human genome project in 2003, genetic testing has become faster, cheaper, and more accurate. The field evolved from testing a single gene at a time to now sequencing of the entire genome. Providers are now faced with multiple testing options, which is very different from the one or two choices in the past. Understanding the benefits, risks, and limitations of these tests has never been more important in order to select the most appropriate test for each patient and their unique diagnosis. The following addresses the different types of next-generation sequencing testing that aid in the molecular diagnosis for patients with RP and provides protocols for conducting these genetic diagnostic methodologies in a laboratory setting.

1.1 Next-Generation Sequencing

Next-generation sequencing (NGS) refers to a form of sequencing technology that can be utilized in phenotypic driven panels, whole exome sequencing (WES), and whole genome sequencing (WGS). NGS, also known as second-generation sequencing, is characterized by the use of massive parallel sequencing. The exact method of the sequencing depends on the technology platform; however, all NGS sequencing follows the same basic outline of library preparation in which DNA is fragmented, clonal amplification, cyclic array sequencing, alignment to a reference genome, and then variant identification and interpretation [8].

Two of the most important things to clarify as a clinician using NGS are as follows: (1) Was the area of interest sequenced? (2) What is the depth of the coverage? Depth of coverage refers to how many reads of the same region were performed [8]. The typical minimum depth of coverage required for clinical testing is 30×, which means that each nucleotide was sequenced 30 times [9]. When there is insufficient depth of coverage in an area, it may become difficult to determine if a variant is an artifact of the sequencing process or an actual germline mutation. Once a variant is identified, it is then confirmed by Sanger sequencing. While Sanger confirmation used to be standard for all clinical laboratories, the need of this practice is currently being questioned in the field and is no longer practice by some clinical laboratories [10, 11]. The depth of coverage is also important for the analysis of indels and larger deletion/duplication [12]. Not every NGS assay sequences to the depth required to make these calls nor is every NGS assay validated to make those calls. Typically a depth of at least 50× is required in order to call indels [12]. While larger deletions/duplications could be identified by having higher depth, most laboratories are more likely to utilize additional technology to analyze this.

Another crucial part of the sequencing process is how to classify variants that may be disease-causing. While there are guidelines that outline how variants should be classified in a clinical setting, there is still a lot of room for interpretation [13]. There may be different classifications across laboratories for the same variant. As such, finding out how each laboratory classifies their variants and whether a requital process is in place can be important.

NGS as a technology has certain limitations. These limitations may vary depending on the exact type of NGS technique used. One known limitation of the technology is the potential for amplification error or bias [8, 9, 14]. Due to the amplification process, there is a standard minimum amount of DNA that would be required to run each assay. Shorter read lengths can be difficult to map to the reference genome which could cause a misalignment [8, 9, 14]. Areas of the genome with high GC content or very low GC content tend to be more difficult to sequence and have a lower depth of coverage [8, 14, 15]. Similarly areas of the genome that are highly repetitive, like trinucleotide repeat expansions, are difficult to sequence [8, 9, 14]. Some laboratories compensate for these limitations by utilizing other technologies in conjunction with NGS. The best practice is to check with the laboratory for the assay of interest to see what their exact limitations are.

1.2 Panel Testing

NGS panels are curated sets of genes that target a specific phenotype or disease of interest. These panels can vary greatly from laboratory to laboratory. The purpose of a panel is to maximize depth of coverage as well as sensitivity and specificity for the testing of the diagnostic indication [16]. The limited amount of data for mapping and interpretation allows for a greater depth of sequencing to occur in the specific regions and genes of interest. Additionally, laboratories will often utilize additional testing technology to cover areas of interest that would have otherwise been missed by NGS alone, such as intronic variants and repeat expansions. As previously stated in the NGS section, the depth of coverage from the panel will allow the laboratory to call indels [12, 17]. Additional technology can sometimes be added to cover large copy number variants if it is known to be an area of concern.

Diagnostic yields for panels are highly variable due to differences in size, unspecific diagnosis, and additional technology that may or may not be utilize. Currently many labs will also allow for custom panels, in which the provider can add or remove genes from a curated panel or create their own panel. These panels may run on a WES platform, but will often utilize additional technology in order to add the greater depth one would expect from a panel.

1.3 Whole Exome Sequencing

Whole exome sequencing (WES) utilizes NGS to sequence most of the humane exome. The human exome contains all RNA coding regions of the nuclear genome, which is approximately 180,000 exons. While the majority of disease-causing variants are found in the exome, it only comprises 1–2% of the entire genome. The sequencing data is filtered and analyzed based on the phenotypic information provided by the clinician.

WES can be run as either a proband (patient) only or with up to two additional family members for analysis, commonly known as a "trio." Trio testing allows for full sequencing of all three individuals, and the sequence of the family members can be utilized in the interpretation of the proband's results. Detection rate improves when trio analysis is utilized; in some studies detection rate can be improved by as much as 16% [18]. Trio WES can provide information about de novo status and if mutations segregate with disease in the family. This information is vital for mutation classification, especially if the variant is novel.

Since the entire exome is being sequenced, patients also have to make a decision whether they would like to be informed of incidental findings. ACMG has a list of 59 genes that are known to be disease-causing which they recommend all laboratories give patients the option to be informed about [19]. These are all adult-onset conditions for which interventions are currently available. Additionally, a true incidental finding may also arise when data is being analyzed. These refer to known disease-causing mutation in genes completely unrelated to phenotype being tested for and are not on the ACMG list. As such, pre-test and post-test counseling is especially important for patients to make informed decisions about the level of information they would be comfortable receiving.

1.4 Whole Genome Sequencing

Whole genome sequencing (WGS) utilizes NGS technology to sequence the human genome. The human genome encompasses the introns and exons of the over 20,000 nuclear genes and the 37 mitochondrial genes. The technology requires processing of much larger amounts of information than the other testing strategies combined and has been considered the most comprehensive test. Similar to the other testing options, coverage will depend on the technology used, and thus it may be beneficial to contact the laboratories about limitations before selecting the test. One of the benefits of WGS is that many of the technologies do not use PCR for amplification. This allows WGS to typically have more uniform coverage than WES and is able to detect SNVs at lower coverage depths reliably across exons [20, 21]. The same detection benefits of trio testing are available for WGS sequencing as was mentioned for WES.

Secondary findings are also an important consideration for WGS. Sometimes laboratories will also allow for additional interpretation of WGS, such a pharmacogenomics and carrier screening of recessive diseases. Thus, the same importance on pre-test counseling and incidental findings is still very much necessary for this technology.

1.5 Testing Strategies

When choosing a test for RP, there are a few things to consider. Ideally during the appointment when the diagnosis is made, an accurate and detailed family history should be taken. This can provide information about the suspected inerhtiance pattern and identify family members that may be available for either trio analysis or familial segregation/phase testing. An evaluation of the patient's phenotype should also be performed to confirm the confidence in the RP diagnosis is also important. If there is not a high confidence in the RP diagnosis, a broader test may be more appropriate. An idea of how quickly the disease is progressing and if there is any type of clinical intervention is very important. Lastly, the patient's financial situation and availability will inevitably play a significant role in test selection.

Turnaround times (TAT) and prices for panels can vary. Typically, the TAT can be anywhere between 3 and 6 weeks on average. TAT for a particular panel is information that is easily available on almost any brochure or website. What is less transparent is the cost of the testing. NGS panels are generally a cheaper option for patients as they utilize less reagents and generate less data to analyze compared to the other two NGS methodologies. However, the additional technologies that can be utilized to add to the sensitivity can add to costs. For RP there are many sponsored testing panels available, but the quality and size vary greatly between them. However, they remain a very attractive option as it incurs no financial cost for the patients.

Comparatively the TAT for WES is typically 8–16 weeks on average. Cost also varies from laboratory to laboratory and can also very depending if the test is proband only, a duo, or a trio. Insurance may cover some or all of the WES costs, but may be subject to a prior authorization process. It is not uncommon, especially for RP, for insurances to require a tiered approach in which a negative panel testing result may be required before approval for WES.

Clinical WGS on average takes 16 weeks, if not longer for return of results. This test has not yet been approved by insurance in the United States, but some international insurances will reimburse patients for the testing. Few laboratories will offer it as a clinical test due to the lack of reimbursement and the lack of common use in the clinical space. As such, costs typically range from $3,500 to $16,000 depending on the laboratory. Similar to WES, these costs will also depend on the number of individuals being included in the analysis.

One approach for RP is to follow a traditional tiered method, starting with targeted testing through a panel that would then move to WES/WGS. For retinal disorders, including RP, this could be an excellent strategy depending on the panel. For a panel designed to really examine all the required genes and areas of interest for RP, a panel has shown to be more effective than WES with diagnostic yield of 51% [17]. However, a panel is highly variable, and thus clinical judgment is important when considering which panel would be effective to use as a first-tier test.

Many panels commercially available for RP may fall short of the detection rate desired. In this case WES has been examined and proven as an excellent testing option for retinal dystrophies. While diagnostic rates varies for WES, the rates for retinal dystrophy diagnosis have also been shown to be significant with yields between 55% and 71% [22–24]. It is important to note that many studies in this area have a small sample size of patients, individuals undergoing testing, which would influence the diagnostic yield. When more general WES numbers are looked at across indication, the diagnostic rates drop.

WGS testing has been looked at across different subspecialties to evaluate its utility in the clinical space. Overall, diagnostic rates were increased compared to WES and panel testing across subspecialties and in some cases have been shown to be higher [25, 26]. However, when WES reanalysis was introduced, the increased yield of WGS sequencing, while still higher, was shown to be decreased [27]. Value of WGS currently has been in the consistent coverage and in the ability for the raw data to be analyzed in the future. The cost-effectiveness is often cited as an advantage for WGS technology, but as it is not currently covered by insurance in the United States, it may not actually be an advantage for many patients [28].

2 Materials

Laboratory equipment and supplies for WES:

1. Vortex mixer (Baxter Scientific Products).
2. 2100 Bioanalyzer Desktop System (Agilent).

3. PCR Thermal Cycler (Applied Biosystems).
4. LE-220 Sonication System (Covaris).
5. Vacuum DNA concentrator.
6. HiSeq 2500 Sequencer (Illumina).
7. HiSeq Rapid PE Cluster Kit v2 (Illumina).
8. HiSeq Rapid SBS Kit v2 (Illumina).
9. CBot Manifold (Illumina).
10. 7500 Fast Real-Time PCR System (Applied Biosystems).
11. SureSelectXT Library Prep Kit (Agilent).
12. Agencourt AMPure XP Kit (Beckman Coulter).
13. DNA 1000 CHiP Kit (Agilent).
14. Dynabeads MyOne Streptavidin T1 (Thermo Fisher Scientific).
15. Herculase II Fusion DNA Polymerase (Agilent).
16. Library Quantification Kit–Illumina/ABI Prism® (Kapa Biosystems).
17. DNA LoBind tube 1.5 mL (Eppendorf).
18. 1.0 N Sodium hydroxide.
19. 1X Low TE Buffer (10 mM Tris–HCl, pH 8.0, 0.1 mM EDTA).
20. Buffer EB (10 mM Tris–HCl, pH: 8.5).
21. Ethanol 200 proof (absolute) for molecular biology.
22. Sterile, nuclease-free water.

3 Methods

The protocol described here requires high molecular DNA of good quality. Standard commercial DNA extraction kits can be used, for example, AllPrep DNA spin column (Qiagen).

3.1 Library Preparation

This step involves shearing genomic DNA, 3′ end repair by adding an A-base, adapter ligation, and DNA amplification. This is followed by exome capture when performing WES and PCR enrichment to prepare samples for sequencing on an Illumina sequencer (*see* **Note 2**).

3.1.1 DNA Fragmentation

The DNA fragmentation process employs sonication to shear DNA into smaller fragments which will be enriched based on size subsequently.

1. Set up the Covaris instrument.
   (a) Check that the water in the Covaris tank is filled with fresh deionized water to fill line level 15 on the graduated fill line label.

Table 1
Shear settings for Covaris instrument

Setting	Value
Duty cycle	10%
Intensity	5
Cycles per burst	175
Time	360 s
Temperature	4–7 °C

(b) Check that the water covers the visible glass part of the tube.

(c) Set the chiller temperature to between 2 °C and 5 °C to ensure that the temperature reading in the water bath displays 5 °C.

(d) On the instrument control panel, push the Degas button. Degas the instrument for 45 min before use.

2. Dilute 3 μg of high-quality gDNA with 1X Low TE Buffer in a 1.5-mL LoBind tube to a total volume of 130 μL.
3. Use a tapered pipette tip to slowly transfer the 130 μL DNA sample through the pre-split septa of a Covaris MicroTube.
4. Secure the MicroTube and shear the DNA with the settings below (Table 1). The target peak for base pair size is 150–200 bp.
5. While keeping the snap-cap on, insert a pipette tip through the pre-split septa, and then slowly remove the sheared DNA.
6. Transfer the sheared DNA into a new 1.5-mL LoBind tube.
7. To purify the sample, use Agencourt AMPure XP beads. Let the AMPure XP beads come to room temperature for at least 30 min. Mix the reagent well so that the reagent appears homogenous and consistent in color.
8. Add 180 μL of homogenous AMPure XP beads to the 1.5-mL LoBind tube containing the sample. Mix well on a vortex mixer and incubate for 5 min.
9. Put the tube in the magnetic stand. Wait for the solution to clear (approximately 3–5 min).
10. Keep the tube in the magnetic stand. Do not touch the beads while you carefully discard the cleared solution from the tubes.
11. Continue to keep the tube in the magnetic stand while you dispense 500 μL of 70% ethanol in each tube. Use fresh 70% ethanol for optimal result.

12. Let the tube sit for 1 min to allow any disturbed beads to settle and remove the ethanol.
13. Repeat **steps 11** and **12**.
14. Dry the samples at RT for 5 min or until the residual ethanol completely evaporates.
15. Add 50 μL nuclease-free water, mix well on a vortex mixer, and incubate for 2 min at room temperature.
16. Put the tube in the magnetic stand and leave for 3 min, until the solution is clear.
17. Transfer approximately 48 μL of the supernatant to each well of a new LoBind PCR plate, and perform next step end repair. You can discard the beads at this time.
18. Using 1 μL of remaining sheared DNA run a DNA 1000 chip on the Bioanalyzer, verify the size of the fragmented DNA.

3.1.2 End Repair

Subsequent to DNA fragmentation, the ends of DNA have 3′ and 5′ overhangs. For efficient adaptor ligation, these overhangs are repaired by creating blunt-ended fragments.

1. For multiple libraries (prepare on ice): Prepare the reaction mix in Table 2. Mix well on a vortex mixer.
2. Add 52 μL of the reaction mix to each well or tube.
3. Add 48 μL of each DNA sample to each well or tube. Mix by pipetting. Change pipette tips between samples.
4. Incubate in a thermal cycler for 30 min at 20 °C. Do not use a heated lid.

Table 2
End repair mix

Reagent	Volume for 1 library	Volume for 12 libraries (includes excess)
DNA sample	48 μL	
Nuclease-free water	35.2 μL	440 μL
10× End repair buffer (clear cap)	10 μL	125 μL
dNTP Mix (green cap)	1.6 μL	20 μL
T4 DNA Polymerase (purple cap)	1 μL	12.5 μL
Klenow DNA Polymerase (yellow cap)	2 μL	25 μL
T4 Polynucleotide Kinase (orange cap)	2.2 μL	27.5 μL
Total volume	**100 μL**	**650 μL (52 μL/sample)**

3.1.3 AMPure Bead Cleanup

1. Let the AMPure XP beads come to room temperature for at least 30 min.
2. Mix the reagent well so that the reagent appears homogeneous and consistent in color.
3. Add 180 μL of homogenous AMPure XP beads to a 1.5-mL LoBind tube, and add the end-repaired DNA library (~100 μL). Mix well on a vortex mixer and incubate for 5 min.
4. Put the tube in the magnetic stand. Wait for the solution to clear (approximately 3–5 min).
5. Keep the tube in the magnetic stand. Do not touch the beads while you carefully discard the cleared solution from the tubes.
6. Continue to keep the tube in the magnetic stand while you dispense 500 μL of 70% ethanol in each tube. Use fresh 70% ethanol for optimal result.
7. Let the tube sit for 1 min to allow any disturbed beads to settle and remove the ethanol.
8. Repeat **steps 6** and 7 once.
9. Dry the samples at RT for 5 min or until the residual ethanol completely evaporates. Do not dry the bead pellet to the point that the bead pellet appears cracked. Elution efficiency is significantly decreased when the bead pellet is excessively dried.
10. Add 32 μL nuclease-free water, mix well on a vortex mixer, and incubate for 2 min at room temperature.
11. Put the tube in the magnetic stand and leave for 2–3 min, until the solution is clear.
12. Transfer 30 μL of the supernatant to the new row of LoBind PCR plate. You can discard the beads at this time.
13. If you do not continue to next step, seal the plate and store at −20 °C.

3.1.4 Adenylate 3′ Ends

Adapter ligation needs a 3′ A-base. This is achieved using dATPs and Exo (−) Klenow for DNA adenylation.

1. For multiple libraries (prepare on ice):
   (a) Prepare the reaction mix in Table 3. Mix well on a vortex mixer.
   (b) Add 20 μL of the reaction mix to each well or tube.
   (c) Add 30 μL of each DNA sample to each well or tube. Mix by pipetting. Change pipette tips between samples.
2. Incubate in a thermal cycler for 30 min at 37 °C. If you use a heated lid, make sure that the lid temperature does not exceed 50 °C.

Table 3
3′ Adenylation mix

Reagent	Volume for 1 library	Volume for 12 libraries (includes excess)
DNA sample	30 μL	
Nuclease-free water	11 μL	137.5 μL
10× Klenow Polymerase Buffer (blue cap)	5 μL	62.5 μL
dATP (green cap)	1 μL	12.5 μL
Exo (−) Klenow (red cap)	3 μL	37.5 μL
Total volume	**50 μL**	**250 μL (20 μL/sample)**

3. Purify samples using AMPure beads. Let the AMPure XP beads come to room temperature for at least 30 min.
4. Mix the reagent well so that the reagent appears homogeneous and consistent in color.
5. Add 90 μL of homogenous AMPure XP beads to each well containing the A-tailed DNA library (~50 μL). Mix well by pipetting and incubate for 5 min.
6. Put the tube in the magnetic stand. Wait for the solution to clear (approximately 3–5 min).
7. Keep the tube in the magnetic stand. Do not touch the beads while you carefully discard the cleared solution from the tubes.
8. Continue to keep the tube in the magnetic stand while you dispense 200 μL of 70% ethanol in each tube. Use fresh 70% ethanol for optimal result.
9. Let the tube sit for 1 min to allow any disturbed beads to settle and remove the ethanol.
10. Repeat **steps 8** and **9** once.
11. Dry the samples at RT for 5 min or until the residual ethanol completely evaporates. Do not dry the bead pellet to the point that the bead pellet appears cracked. Elution efficiency is significantly decreased when the bead pellet is excessively dried.
12. Add 15 μL of nuclease-free water, mix well on a vortex mixer, and incubate for 2 min at room temperature.
13. Put the tube in the magnetic stand and leave for 2–3 min, until the solution is clear.
14. Transfer 13 μL of the supernatant to a new row of LoBind PCR plate. You can discard the beads at this time.

Table 4
Ligation master mix

Reagent	Volume for 1 library	Volume for 12 libraries (includes excess)
DNA sample	13 μL	
Nuclease-free water	15.5/ 24.5 μL/24.5 μL*	193.75 μL/306.25 μL*
5× T4 DNA ligase buffer	10 μL	125 μL
SureSelect Adaptor Oligo Mix (brown cap)	10 μL/1 μL*	125 μL/12.5 μL*
T4 DNA Ligase (red cap)	1.5 μL	18.75 μL
Total volume	**50 μL**	**462.5 μL (37 μL/sample)**

*low input library

3.1.5 Ligate Adapters

1. For multiple libraries (prepare on ice):
   (a) Prepare the reaction mix in Table 4.
   (b) Add 37 μL of the reaction mix to each well.
   (c) Add 13 μL of each DNA sample to each well. Mix by pipetting. Change pipette tips between samples.
2. Incubate for 15 min at 20 °C on a thermal cycler. Do not use a heated lid.
3. Cleanup the samples using AMPure XP beads. Let the AMPure XP beads come to room temperature for at least 30 min.
4. Mix the reagent well so that the reagent appears homogeneous and consistent in color.
5. Add 90 μL of homogenous AMPure XP beads to each well containing the ligated library (~50 μL). Mix well by pipetting and incubate for 5 min.
6. Put the plate on the magnetic stand. Wait for the solution to clear (approximately 3–5 min).
7. Keep the plate on the magnetic stand. Do not touch the beads while you carefully discard the cleared solution from the tubes.
8. Continue to keep the plate on the magnetic stand while you dispense 200 μL of 70% ethanol in each well. Use fresh 70% ethanol for optimal result.
9. Let the plate sit for 1 min to allow any disturbed beads to settle and remove the ethanol.
10. Repeat **steps 8** and **9** once.
11. Dry the samples at RT for 5 min until the residual ethanol is completely evaporated. Do not dry the bead pellet to the point that the bead pellet appears cracked. Elution efficiency is significantly decreased when the bead pellet is excessively dried.
12. Add 32 μL nuclease-free water, mix well by pipetting, and incubate for 2 min at room temperature.

13. Put the plate on the magnetic stand and leave for 2–3 min, until the solution is clear.
14. For high-input library: Transfer 15 μL of the supernatant to the next row of the LoBind PCR plate for the next step. Transfer the remaining supernatant to a new eight-strip tube, and store them in −20° for future use. For low-input library: Transfer 30 μL of the supernatant to the next row of the LoBind PCR plate. You can discard the beads at this time.

3.1.6 Enrich DNA Fragments

1. For multiple libraries:
   (a) Prepare the reaction mix in Table 5, on ice. Mix well on a vortex mixer.
   (b) Add 35 μL (high input) or 20 μL (low input) of the reaction mix to each well.
   (c) For high-input library prep, add 15 μL of each DNA sample to each well. Mix by pipetting. Change pipette tips between samples.
   (d) For low-input library prep, add 30 μL of each DNA sample to each well, and mix by pipetting.
2. Run the following program in a thermal cycler:
   (a) 98 °C for 2 min.
   (b) Six cycles (high input) or ten cycles (low input) of:
      (i) 98 °C for 30 s
      (ii) 65 °C for 30 s
      (iii) 72 °C for 1 min

Table 5
Components for PCR mix

Reagent	Volume for 1 library	Volume for 12 libraries (includes excess)
Indexing adaptor-ligated library	15 μL (30 μL)	
Nuclease-free water	21 μL (6 μL)	262.5 μL (75 μL)
SureSelect Primer (brown cap)	1.25 μL	15.625 μL
SureSelect ILM Indexing Pre Capture PCR Reverse Primer (clear cap)	1.25 μL	15.625 μL
5× Herculase II Rxn Buffer (clear cap)	10 μL	125 μL
100 mM dNTP Mix (green cap)	0.5 μL	6.25 μL
Herculase II Fusion DNA Polymerase (red cap)	1 μL	12.5 μL
Total volume	**50 μL**	**437.5 μL/250 uL (35 μL/reaction)**

(c) 72 °C for 10 min.

(d) Hold at 4 °C.

3. Purify the sample with Agencourt AMPure XP beads. Let the AMPure XP beads come to room temperature for at least 30 min.

4. Mix the reagent well so that the reagent appears homogeneous and consistent in color.

5. Add 90 μL of homogenous AMPure XP beads to each well of the amplified library (~50 μL). Mix well by pipetting and incubate for 5 min.

   1. Put the plate on the magnetic stand. Wait for the solution to clear (approximately 3–5 min).

6. Keep the plate on the magnetic stand. Do not touch the beads while you carefully discard the cleared solution from the tubes. Continue to keep the plate on the magnetic stand while you dispense 200 μL of 70% ethanol in each well. Use fresh 70% ethanol for optimal result.

   2. Let the plate sit for 1 min to allow any disturbed beads to settle and remove the ethanol.

   3. Repeat **steps** 7 and **8** once.

   4. Dry the samples at RT for 5 min or until the residual ethanol completely evaporates. Do not dry the bead pellet to the point that the bead pellet appears cracked. Elution efficiency is significantly decreased when the bead pellet is excessively dried.

   5. Add 30 μL nuclease-free water, mix well on a vortex mixer, and incubate for 2 min at room temperature.

   6. Put the plate on the magnetic stand and leave for 2–3 min, until the solution is clear.

   7. Transfer 25 μL of the supernatant to a fresh 1.5-mL LoBind tube.

   8. Use the remaining 5 μL to validate the library by Qubit measurement, and run DNA 1000 chip on Bioanalyzer. You can discard the beads at this time.

3.1.7 Validate Library

1. To verify the size of your PCR-enriched fragments, check the template size distribution by running an aliquot of the DNA library on an Agilent Technologies 2100 Bioanalyzer using a DNA 1000 chip (*see* **Note 3**). An example of DNA library size distribution can be seen below (Fig. 1).

2. To verify the DNA library concentration, measure an aliquot of the DNA library using the Qubit fluorometer.

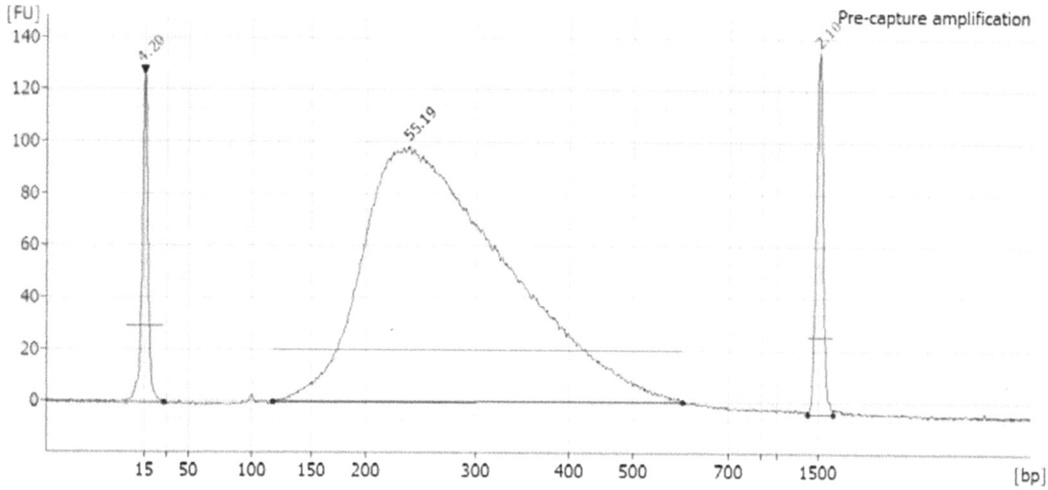

Fig. 1 Example of DNA library size distribution on a DNA 1000 chip

3. If performing whole genome sequencing, proceed to quantifying library by qPCR. If performing exome enrichment, proceed to SureSelect enrichment.

3.1.8 SureSelect Enrichment

1. The hybridization reaction requires 750 ng of DNA with a maximum volume of 3.4 μL. If the prepped library concentration is below 221 ng/μL, use a vacuum concentrator to concentrate the sample at ≤45 °C.
2. Add the entire 2530 μL of prepped library to an Eppendorf tube. Poke one or more holes in the lid with a narrow-gauge needle.
3. Completely lyophilize by using a vacuum concentrator on low heat (less than 45 °C) to dehydrate.
4. Reconstitute with nuclease-free water to bring the final concentration to 221 ng/μL (or greater if sample recovery is of concern). For optimal recovery, pipette up and down along the sides of the tube.
5. Mix well on a vortex mixer and spin in a microfuge for 1 min.
6. Mix the components in Table 6 at room temperature to prepare the hybridization buffer. If precipitate forms, warm the hybridization buffer at 65 °C for 5 min.
7. In a PCR plate, prepare the SureSelect capture library mix for target enrichment. Keep tubes on ice until **step 10**.
8. For each sample, add the amount of SureSelect capture library as listed in Table 7, based on the Mb target size of your design.

Table 6
Hybridization buffer mix

Reagent	Volume for 1 capture (μL), includes excess	Volume for 6 captures (μL), includes excess	Volume for 12 captures (μL), includes excess
SureSelect Hyb #1 (orange cap)	6.6	43.1	86.2
SureSelect Hyb #2 (red cap)	0.2	1.76	0.3
SureSelect Hyb #3 (yellow cap)	2.6	17.23	34.5
SureSelect Hyb #4 (black cap)	3.4	22.42	44.9
Total	**13**	**84.5 (40 μL/sample)**	**169 (13 μL/sample)**

Table 7
SureSelect capture library

Capture size	Volume of SureSelect library	RNase Block dilution (parts RNase Block: parts water)	Volume of RNase Block dilution to add
<3.0 Mb	2 μL	1:9 (10%)	5 μL
≥3.0 Mb	5 μL	1:3 (25%)	2 μL

Table 8
SureSelect block mix

Reagent	Volume for 1 reaction	Volume for 12 reactions (includes excess)
SureSelect Indexing Block #1 (green cap)	2.5 μL	31.25 μL
SureSelect Block #2 (blue cap)	2.5 μL	31.25 μL
SureSelect Indexing Block #3 (brown cap)	0.6 μL	7.5 μL
Total	**5.6 μL**	**70 μL**

(a) Use nuclease-free water to prepare a dilution of the SureSelect RNase Block (purple cap) as listed in Table 7. Prepare enough RNase Block dilution for all samples, plus excess.

(b) Add the amount of diluted SureSelect RNase Block (purple cap) listed in Table 7 to each capture library, and mix by pipetting.

9. Mix the contents in Table 8 to make the correct amount of SureSelect Block mix for the number of samples used.

10. In a separate PCR plate, prepare the prepped library for target enrichment.
    (a) Add 3.4 μL of 221 ng/μL prepped library to the "B" row in the PCR plate. Put each sample into a separate well.
    (b) Add 5.6 μL of the SureSelect Block Mix to each well in row B.
    (c) Mix by pipetting up and down.
    (a) Seal the wells of row "B" with caps and put the PCR plate in the thermal cycler.
11. During this step you will only heat the preppared library with blockers; you will not heat the hybridization buffer or capture library yet.
    (a) Start the following thermal cycler program:
        (i) 95 °C for 5 min.
        (ii) Hold at 65 °C.
    (b) Use a heated lid on the thermal cycler at 105 °C to hold the temperature of the plate on the thermal cycler at 65 °C.
12. Maintain the plate at 65 °C while you prepare the mix of 13 μL of hybridization buffer with 2-μL diluted RNAse Block and 5-μL SureSelect library probe so each sample will have 20 μL of the capture library hybridization mix. Make sure that the plate is at 65 °C for a minimum of 5 min before you go to the next step.
13. While maintaining the plate at 65 °C, use a multichannel pipette to add the 20-μL capture library mix from **step 6** to each sample well of the PCR plate:
    (a) Mix well by slowly pipetting up and down eight to ten times. The hybridization mixture is now 27–29 μL, depending on the degree of evaporation during the pre-incubations.
    (b) Seal the wells with strip caps or double adhesive film. Use new adhesive seals or strip caps. The structural integrity of the seals and caps can be compromised during the previous incubation steps.
14. Make sure all wells are completely sealed.
15. Incubate the hybridization mixture for 16–24 h at 65 °C with a heated lid at 105 °C.

3.1.9 Magnetic Bead Preparation

1. Pre-warm SureSelect Wash 2 at 65 °C in a circulating water bath or heat block for use in "Subheading 3.1.10."
2. Vigorously resuspend the Dynabeads MyOne Streptavidin T1 on a vortex mixer.

   (a) Magnetic beads settle during storage.
3. For each hybridization, add 50 μL of Dynabeads MyOne Streptavidin T1 to a 1.5-mL microfuge tube.
4. Wash the beads:
   (a) Add 200 μL of SureSelect Binding Buffer.
   (b) Mix the beads on a vortex mixer for 5 s.
   (c) Put the tubes into the Dynal magnetic separator.
   (d) Remove and discard the supernatant.
   (e) Repeat step "a" through step "d" for a total of three washes.
5. Resuspend the beads in 200 μL of SureSelect Binding Buffer.

3.1.10 Select Hybrid Capture with SureSelect

1. Keep the PCR plate or tubes at 65 °C in the PCR machine while you add the hybridization mixture directly from the thermal cycler to the bead solution. Invert the tube to mix three to five times.
2. Incubate the hybrid capture/bead solution on a Nutator or equivalent for 30 min at room temperature. Make sure the sample is properly mixing in the tube.
3. Briefly spin in a centrifuge.
4. Separate the beads and buffer on a magnetic separator and remove the supernatant.
5. Resuspend the beads in 500 μL of SureSelect Wash 1 by mixing on a vortex mixer for 5 s.
6. Incubate the samples for 15 min at room temperature. Occasionally mix on a vortex mixer.
7. Briefly spin in a centrifuge.
8. Separate the beads and buffer on a magnetic separator and remove the supernatant.
9. Wash the beads.
   (a) Resuspend the beads in 500 μL of 65 °C pre-warmed SureSelect Wash 2, and mix on a vortex mixer for 5 s to resuspend the beads.
   (b) Incubate the samples for 10 min at 65 °C in a recirculating water bath, heat block, or equivalent.
   (c) Occasionally mix on a vortex mixer.
   (d) Invert the tube to mix. The beads may have settled.
   (e) Briefly spin in a centrifuge.
   (f) Separate the beads and buffer on a magnetic separator and remove the supernatant.

Table 9
Herculase II master mix

Reagent	Volume for 1 reaction	Volume for 12 reactions (includes excess)
Captured on-bead DNA	14 μL	
Nuclease-free water	18.5 μL	231.25 μL
5× Herculase II Rxn Buffer (clear cap)	10 μL	125 μL
100-mM dNTP Mix (green cap)	0.5 μL	6.25 μL
Herculase II Fusion DNA Polymerase (red cap)	1 μL	12.5 μL
SureSelect ILM Indexing Post Capture Forward PCR Primer (orange cap)	1 μL	12.5 μL
PCR Primer Index 1 through Index 16 (clear caps)	1 μL	
Total	**50 μL**	**387.5 μL (35 μL/reaction)**

(g) Repeat step "a" through step "e" for a total of three washes. Make sure all of the wash buffer has been removed.

(h) Mix the beads with 30 μL of nuclease-free water on a vortex mixer for 5 s to resuspend the beads.

3.1.11 Amplify the Captured Library to Add Index Tags

1. For multiple libraries:
   (a) Prepare the reaction mix in Table 9, on ice. Mix well on a vortex mixer.
   (b) Add 31 μL of the reaction mix to each well or tube.
   (c) Add 5 μL of the appropriate index PCR Primer Index 1 through Index 16 (clear caps) from the SureSelect Library Prep Kit ILM to each well, and mix by pipetting.
   (d) Pipette each DNA sample up and down to make sure that the bead solution is homogenous.
   (e) Use a pipette to add 14 μL of each DNA sample to each well or tube. Mix by pipetting. Change pipette tips between samples to avoid cross-contamination.
2. Put the tubes in a thermal cycler and run the program below:
   (a) 98 °C for 2 min.
   (b) 10–16 cycles* of the following:
      (i) 98 °C for 30 s
      (ii) 57 °C for 30 s
      (iii) 72 °C for 1 min

Table 10
Cycle times

Capture size	Cycles
1 kb up to 0.5 Mb	16 cycles
0.5 Mb up to 1.49 Mb	14 cycles
>1.5 Mb	12 cycles
All exon	10–12 cycles

[a]Use the optimal cycle number to repeat PCR at the 50-μL reaction scale. *See* Table 10 for approximate number of cycles for a given library size

(c) 72 °C for 10 min.

(d) Hold at 4 °C (Table 10).

3.1.12 Sample Purification Using Agencourt AMPure XP Beads (see Note 1)

1. Let the AMPure XP beads come to room temperature for at least 30 min.
2. Mix the reagent well so that the reagent appears homogeneous and consistent in color.
3. Add 90 μL of homogenous AMPure beads to each well of amplified library (~50 μL). Mix well by pipetting and incubate for 5 min.
4. Put the plate on the magnetic stand. Wait for the solution to clear (approximately 3–5 min).
5. Keep the plate on the magnetic stand. Do not touch the beads while you carefully discard the cleared solution from the wells.
6. Continue to keep the tube in the magnetic stand while you dispense 200 μL of 70% ethanol in each well. Use fresh 70% ethanol for optimal result.
7. Let the plate sit for 1 min to allow any disturbed beads to settle and remove the ethanol.
8. Repeat **step 6** and **step 7** once.
9. Dry the samples at room temperature for 5 min or until the residual ethanol is completely evaporated. Do not dry the bead pellet to the point that the bead pellet appears cracked. Elution efficiency is significantly decreased when the bead pellet is excessively dried.
10. Add 30 μL nuclease-free water, mix well by pipetting, and incubate for 2 min at room temperature.
11. Put the plate on the magnetic stand and leave for 2–3 min, until the solution is clear.
12. Transfer the supernatant (~30 μL) to a fresh 1.5-mL LoBind tube. You can discard the beads at this time.

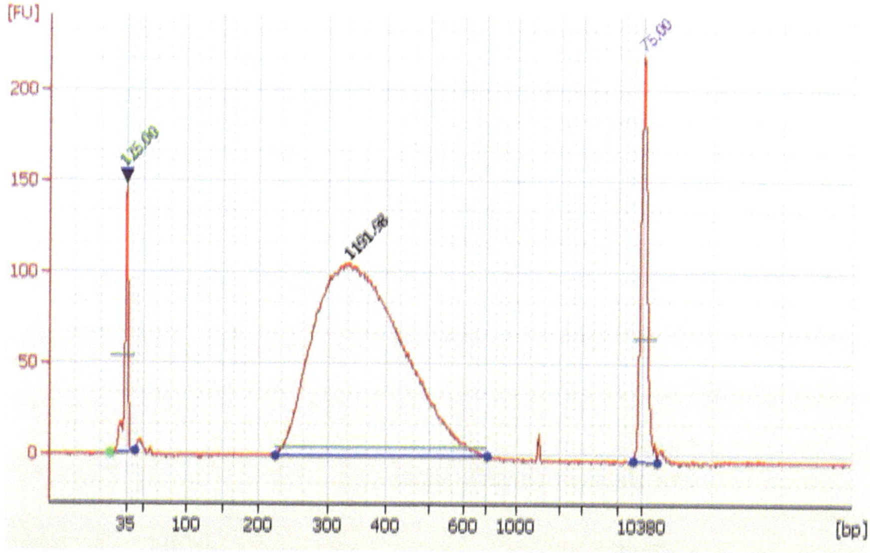

Fig. 2 Example of DNA library size distribution on a high-sensitivity chip

3.1.13 Validation of Enriched Library

1. To verify the size of your PCR-enriched fragments, check the template size distribution by running an aliquot of the DNA library on an Agilent Technologies 2100 Bioanalyzer using a high-sensitivity chip. An example of DNA library size distribution can be seen below (Fig. 2).
2. Proceed to *Library Quantification by qPCR.*

3.1.14 Library Quantification by qPCR

1. Before qPCR reaction setup, add 1-mL Primer Premix (10X) to the 5-mL bottle of KAPA SYBR® FAST qPCR Master Mix (2X), and mix by vortexing for 10 s. Record the date of Primer Premix addition on the KAPA SYBR® FAST qPCR Master Mix bottle.
2. Ensure that all components are completely thawed and thoroughly mixed prior to use.
3. Perform a 1:10,000 dilution of each library in Elution Buffer. Mix thoroughly by vortexing for 10 s.
4. qPCR reactions for the six standards and each library dilution must be set up in triplicate.
5. Load each well of the qPCR plate as indicated below (Table 11), for a total reaction volume of 20 μL. Ensure that the qPCR plate is sealed.
6. Collect all components in the bottom of the wells by brief centrifugation.
7. Place the reactions in the real-time thermocycler, programmed with the following qPCR protocol:

Table 11
qPCR Master Mix

Reagent	Volume (μL)
KAPA SYBR® FAST qPCR Master (mix containing primer premix)	12
PCR-grade water	4
Diluted library DNA or DNA standard (1–6)	4
Total volume per sample	**20**

Table 12
DNA standard concentrations

Sample name	dsDNA concentrations (pM)
Standard 1	20
Standard 2	2
Standard 3	0.2
Standard 4	0.02
Standard 5	0.002
Standard 6	0.0002

(a) 95 °C for 5 min

(b) 35 cycles of:

(i) 95 °C for 30 s

(ii) 60 °C for 45 s

8. Annotate the DNA standards as follows (Table 12) before analyzing the data according to the qPCR instrument guidelines.
9. Confirm that the reaction efficiency calculated for the DNA Standard dilution series falls within the range of 90–110%.

3.2 DNA Sequencing

This step involves performing an initial cluster generation run followed by the sequencing run as per standard Illumina protocols for HiSeq sequencing.

3.2.1 Denature Template DNA

1. Using the adjusted library concentration as calculated from the qPCR results, dilute the library to a concentration of 2 nM.
2. If clustering SureSelect enrichment samples, libraries can be pooled before denaturing. Combine 10 μL of each 2-nM library in a separate PCR well.

3. Combine the following volumes of pooled template DNA and 0.1-N NaOH in a microcentrifuge tube:
   (a) 2-nM template DNA (10 μL)
   (b) 0.1-N NaOH (10 μL)
4. Vortex briefly to mix the template solution.
5. Centrifuge the template solution to 280 × *g* for 1 min.
6. Incubate for 5 min at room temperature to denature the template into single strands.
7. Transfer 20 μL of denatured template to a tube containing 980 μL of pre-chilled HT1 (hybridization buffer).
8. Place the denatured template DNA on ice until you are ready to proceed to final dilution.

3.2.2 Dilute Denatured DNA

1. Dilute the denatured DNA to 15 pM by combining the following volumes in a microcentrifuge tube:
   (a) 20-pM denatured DNA (750 μL)
   (b) Pre-chilled HT1 (250 μL)
2. Invert several times to mix, and then pulse centrifuge the template solution.
3. Place the denatured and diluted template DNA on ice until you are ready to prepare the eight-tube strip.

3.2.3 Denature and Dilute PhiX Control

1. Combine the following volumes to dilute the PhiX library to 2 nM:
   (a) 10-nM PhiX library (2 μL)
   (b) Elution Buffer (8 μL)
2. Combine the following volumes of 2-nM PhiX library and 0.1-N NaOH in a microcentrifuge tube to result in a 1-nM PhiX library:
   (a) 2-nM PhiX library (10 μL)
   (b) 0.1-N NaOH (10 μL)
3. Vortex briefly to mix the 1-nM PhiX library solution.
4. Centrifuge the template solution to 280 × *g* for 1 min.
5. Incubate for 5 min at room temperature to denature the PhiX library into single strands.
6. Transfer 980 μL of pre-chilled HT1 (hybridization buffer) to the tube containing 20 μL of denatured PhiX library to result in a 20-pM PhiX library.
7. Dilute the denatured 20-pM PhiX library to 18 pM as follows:
   (a) 20-pM denatured PhiX library (900 μL).
   (b) Pre-chilled HT1 (100 μL).

(c) Place the denatured PhiX library on ice until you are ready to mix it with the sample library.

3.2.4 Mixing of Sample Library and PhiX Control

1. Combine the following volumes of denatured PhiX control library and your denatured sample library to result in a 1% volume ratio:
   (a) Denatured sample library (990 μL)
   (b) Denatured PhiX control (10 μL)
2. Set the combined sample library and PhiX control aside on ice until you are ready to prepare the eight-tube strip.
3. Perform a cBot cluster generation loading the samples into the flow cell as per the manufacturer's protocol. The libraries are loaded at a coverage of 100X. Once the cluster generation run is performed, the flow cell is now ready to be loaded on the Illumina HiSeq2500 as per standard Illumina HiSeq sequencing protocols.
4. The following QC metrics should be met for a run to be deemed successful:
   (a) Estimated yield per sample >10 GB for whole exome
   (b) Q30 score > or equal to 70%

3.3 Data Analysis

This consists of four steps:

1. Primary analysis: This first step involves demultiplexing of raw sequencing data in the binary base call (BCL) format to FASTQ format using the Illumina Casava software.
2. Secondary analysis: This step includes mapping of paired end 2 × 150 bp reads to the reference genome which converts FASTQ to BAM files, calculation of coverage, tagging duplicate reads, variant calling, and joint analysis to generate variant call format (vcf) files using the Burrows-Wheeler aligner (BWA) [29], Picard tools [http://broadinstitute.github.io/picard], and Genome Analysis Toolkit (GATK) [30], respectively.
3. Tertiary analysis: The third analysis step is variant annotation consisting of adding variant-level and gene-level annotations using the Ensemble Variant Effect Predictor (VEP) [31]. This includes variant effect categories, gnomAD allele frequencies, in silico damaging predictions, and OMIM and ClinVar associations.
4. Interpretation: Finally, variants are prioritized and filtered based on a combination of allele frequency, familial segregation if samples are available, mode of inheritance, and associated phenotypes. Candidate variants are subsequently classified as per the ACMG guidelines for sequence interpretation [13].

4 Conclusion

The NGS testing approach should be a partnered decision between the physician and patient to determine which testing strategy satisfies their individual goals. RP has many additional challenges to consider such as genetic heterogeneity. This adds additional complexity in selecting an effective panel for many providers. Meanwhile, WES and WGS strategies have been proven to be effective for diagnosis but may be cost prohibitive with insurance constraints.

Currently, there is a transition within medicine to move WES to a first-tier test, with the thought that WGS will follow. During this transition period, a more individual approach may be necessary than a blanket statement that WES/WGS would be best for each patient first. Having a thorough knowledge of the genetics behind RP will be beneficial in evaluating panel options when WES is not an option.

5 Notes

1. For low-input DNA library preps, skip Agencourt AMPure purification step.
2. Illumina sequencing guide (https://www.illumina.com/science/technology/next-generation-sequencing/beginners.html).
3. Agilent library guide for sequencing (https://www.agilent.com/cs/library/applications/ NGS_Sequencer_Guide.pdf).

References

1. Fahim AT, Daiger SP, Weleber RG (1993) In: Adam MP et al (eds) Nonsyndromic retinitis pigmentosa overview, GeneReviews® [Internet]. Seattle (WA): University of Washington, Seattle; 1993–2022. Available from: https://www.ncbi.nlm.nih.gov/books/NBK1417/
2. Ferrari S et al (2011) Retinitis pigmentosa: genes and disease mechanisms. Curr Genomics 12(4):238–249
3. Hartong DT, Berson EL, Dryja TP (2006) Retinitis pigmentosa. Lancet 368(9549): 1795–1809
4. Daiger SP (2020) RetNet retinal information network. The University of Texas Health Science Center, Houston
5. ClinVar. National Center of Biotechnology Information (NCBI). [cited 2019
6. Fokkema I, Den-Dunnen JT, Taschner P (2009) RPGR. Available from: rpgr.hgu.mrc.ac.uk/index.php?select_db=RPGR
7. Chang S et al (2011) Diagnostic challenges in retinitis pigmentosa: genotypic multiplicity and phenotypic variability. Curr Genomics 12(4): 267–275
8. Hui P (2014) Next generation sequencing: chemistry, technology and applications. Top Curr Chem 336:1–18
9. Priest JR (2017) A primer to clinical genome sequencing. Curr Opin Pediatr 29(5):513–519
10. Mu W et al (2016) Sanger confirmation is required to achieve optimal sensitivity and specificity in next-generation sequencing panel testing. J Mol Diagn 18(6):923–932
11. Sikkema-Raddatz B et al (2013) Targeted next-generation sequencing can replace Sanger

sequencing in clinical diagnostics. Hum Mutat 34(7):1035–1042

12. Muzzey D, Evans EA, Lieber C (2015) Understanding the basics of NGS: from mechanism to variant calling. Curr Genet Med Rep 3(4): 158–165
13. Richards S et al (2015) Standards and guidelines for the interpretation of sequence variants: a joint consensus recommendation of the American College of Medical Genetics and Genomics and the Association for Molecular Pathology. Genet Med 17(5):405–424
14. Caspar SM et al (2018) Clinical sequencing: from raw data to diagnosis with lifetime value. Clin Genet 93(3):508–519
15. Rieber N et al (2013) Coverage bias and sensitivity of variant calling for four whole-genome sequencing technologies. PLoS One 8(6): e66621
16. Adams DR, Eng CM (2018) Next-generation sequencing to diagnose suspected genetic disorders. N Engl J Med 379(14):1353–1362
17. Consugar MB et al (2015) Panel-based genetic diagnostic testing for inherited eye diseases is highly accurate and reproducible, and more sensitive for variant detection, than exome sequencing. Genet Med 17(4):253–261
18. Farwell KD et al (2015) Enhanced utility of family-centered diagnostic exome sequencing with inheritance model-based analysis: results from 500 unselected families with undiagnosed genetic conditions. Genet Med 17(7):578–586
19. Kalia SS et al (2017) Recommendations for reporting of secondary findings in clinical exome and genome sequencing, 2016 update (ACMG SF v2.0): a policy statement of the American College of Medical Genetics and Genomics. Genet Med 19(2):249–255
20. Meienberg J et al (2016) Clinical sequencing: is WGS the better WES? Hum Genet 135(3): 359–362
21. Meynert AM et al (2014) Variant detection sensitivity and biases in whole genome and exome sequencing. BMC Bioinformatics 15: 247
22. Riera M et al (2017) Whole exome sequencing using Ion Proton system enables reliable genetic diagnosis of inherited retinal dystrophies. Sci Rep 7:42078
23. de Castro-Miro M et al (2016) Novel candidate genes and a wide spectrum of structural and point mutations responsible for inherited retinal dystrophies revealed by exome sequencing. PLoS One 11(12):e0168966
24. Lee K et al (2015) High diagnostic yield of whole exome sequencing in participants with retinal dystrophies in a clinical ophthalmology setting. Am J Ophthalmol 160(2):354–363 e9
25. Lionel AC et al (2018) Improved diagnostic yield compared with targeted gene sequencing panels suggests a role for whole-genome sequencing as a first-tier genetic test. Genet Med 20(4):435–443
26. Carss KJ et al (2017) Comprehensive rare variant analysis via whole-genome sequencing to determine the molecular pathology of inherited retinal disease. Am J Hum Genet 100(1): 75–90
27. Alfares A et al (2018) Whole-genome sequencing offers additional but limited clinical utility compared with reanalysis of whole-exome sequencing. Genet Med 20(11):1328–1333
28. Schwarze K et al (2018) Are whole-exome and whole-genome sequencing approaches cost-effective? A systematic review of the literature. Genet Med 20(10):1122–1130
29. Li H, Durbin R (2009) Fast and accurate short read alignment with Burrows-Wheeler transform. Bioinformatics 25(14):1754–1760
30. McKenna A et al (2010) The Genome Analysis Toolkit: a MapReduce framework for analyzing next-generation DNA sequencing data. Genome Res 20(9):1297–1303
31. McLaren W et al (2016) The Ensembl variant effect predictor. Genome Biol 17(1):122

Chapter 5

Pedigree Analysis of Families and Patients Affected by Retinitis Pigmentosa

Ioana Scherbakova and Sara D. Ragi

Abstract

Family pedigrees allow for a more thorough understanding of human genetic disorders. They are used to help establish patterns of inheritance and to identify individuals at risk of disease. Pedigree analysis can be helpful in identifying genetic disorders that demonstrate mechanisms such autosomal dominant or recessive inheritance, X-linked inheritance, and anticipation.

Key words Pedigrees, Patterns of inheritance, Retinitis pigmentosa, Inherited retinal disorders, Autosomal dominant RP, Autosomal recessive RP, X-Linked RP

1 Introduction

Retinitis pigmentosa (RP) refers to a large group of retinal degenerative disorders that can be inherited or can occur de novo. These disorders are caused by progressive dysfunction and loss of rod and cone photoreceptors. Clinically, RP is characterized by progressive night blindness (nyctalopia), peripherally constricted visual fields, electroretinograms with reduced or absent retinal function, and a characteristic fundus appearance with pale optic discs, attenuated arterioles, mottled RPE, and peripheral retinal pigment clumping. More than 70 genes have been known to cause RP, which can occur sporadically or be inherited in an autosomal dominant, autosomal recessive, X-linked, or simplex form (inheritance not known). The simplex form accounts for almost half of cases [1]. Many cases are due to mutations in the gene for rhodopsin (the rod photopigment), the gene for peripherin (a glycoprotein located in the photoreceptor outer segment), or genes associated with the structure and function of cilia [2]. There are also rare, syndromic forms of RP that occur in association with systemic diseases (e.g., Usher syndrome, abetalipoproteinemia, Kearns-Sayre syndrome, and Refsum syndrome).

Stephen H. Tsang and Peter M. J. Quinn (eds.), *Retinitis Pigmentosa*,
Methods in Molecular Biology, vol. 2560, https://doi.org/10.1007/978-1-0716-2651-1_5,

Family pedigrees can be highly informative in cases of RP and can facilitate genetic counseling. Although RP is often inherited in a Mendelian fashion, atypical pedigrees are common and can reflect sporadic disease resulting from a de novo mutation or the involvement of multiple genes with different modes of inheritance.

2 Materials

1. Paper and writing utensil (or computer software equivalent).
2. Tools to make proper symbols associated with genders.
3. List of questions to interview the proband/their family (*see* Subheading 3).

3 Methods

3.1 Protocol

1. Obtain the patient's family medical history. Important questions to ask are as follows: Has anyone in your family had a condition similar to yours? Do any medical problems seem to run in your family? Are any of your family members related by blood? Parental consanguinity can suggest autosomal recessive inheritance.
2. After obtaining a general family history, systematically ask the patient about all immediate relatives (parents, siblings, and offspring). Ask if they are living or dead and whether they have or had any health concerns. Ask about each pregnancy a woman may have had so as not to overlook miscarriages or stillbirths. If the patient has offspring, ask about the health of the person with whom they had children.
3. In a pedigree, females are represented by circles and males by squares. Unions are indicated by a horizontal line joining two symbols, and children of a union are indicated with a vertical line descending from the horizontal line. Siblings are connected by horizontal lines above their corresponding symbols. Siblings are drawn in birth order from left (first born) to right (youngest).
4. Consanguineous unions are indicated by a double horizontal line. The degree of consanguinity can be written above the relationship line (e.g., "first cousins").
5. Each generation is numbered with Roman numerals, and each individual within a generation is numbered consecutively with Arabic numerals. Thus, III-4 indicates the fourth person in the third generation of a family.
6. Deceased individuals are marked with a horizontal line through their corresponding symbol.
7. Individuals affected with a given disorder are represented by shaded-in symbols. Unaffected carriers of a genetic variant are

marked by a black dot in the center of the corresponding symbol.

8. The first person with disease who presented to medical attention is referred to as the proband. The proband is indicated by an arrow near the individual's symbol.
9. Label the proband with all relevant information (e.g., name/initials, current age, disease and age of onset, genetic variant, etc.).
10. If other indicators are necessary, such as whether an individual has undergone genetic testing, this can be represented with a chosen marker (e.g., an asterisk can be used to indicate that the individual has undergone genetic evaluation). Create a key to label all of the markers used in the pedigree.

3.2 Examples of Pedigrees Containing IRDs Can Be Seen in Figs. 1, 2, and 3

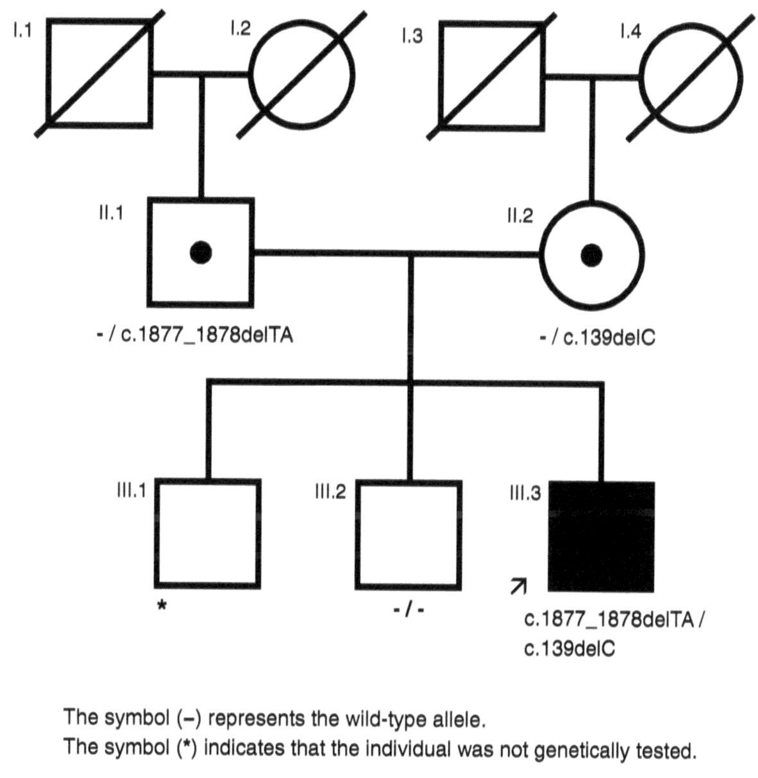

Fig. 1 The family pedigree of a 15-year-old boy with Leber congenital amaurosis due to compound heterozygous mutation in the *PROM1* gene. The proband inherited two heterozygous frameshift variants in the *PROM1* gene

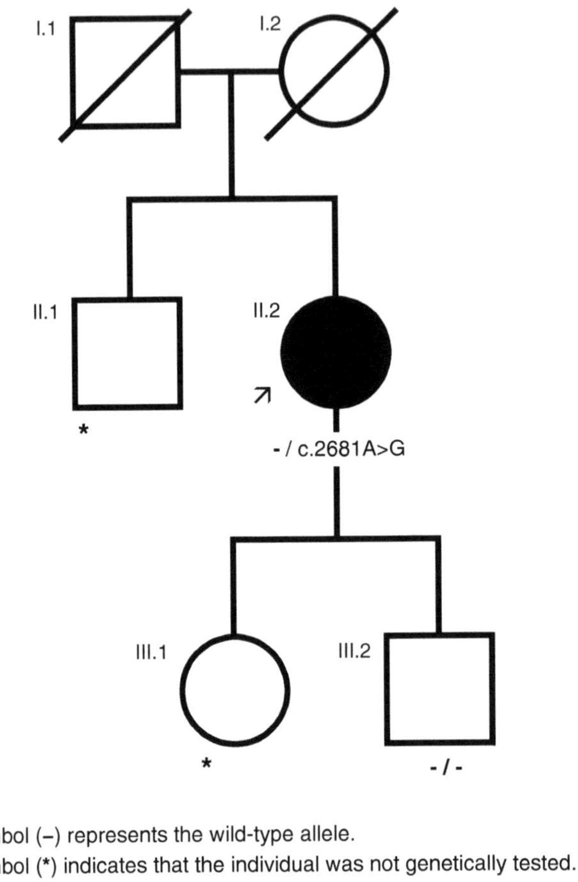

Fig. 2 The family pedigree of a 57-year-old woman with pattern macular dystrophy due to a heterozygous missense point mutation in the *CRB1* gene. Her daughter does not yet have genetic testing, and her son has two normal *CRB1* alleles

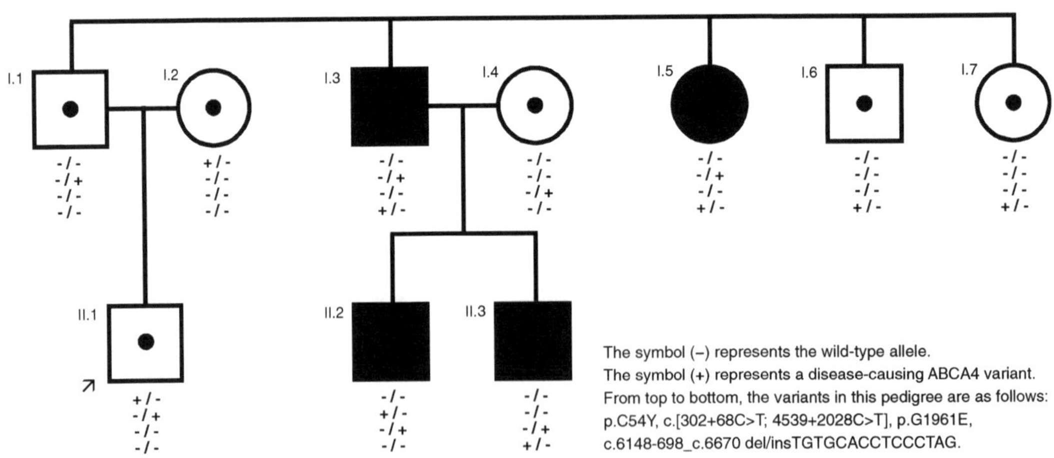

Fig. 3 The family pedigree of a 43-year-old man with Stargardt disease due to two different disease-causing alleles of the *ABCA4* gene. The pedigree illustrates the segregation of four different pathogenic alleles within the family. The mother of the proband had pattern macular dystrophy [3]

3.3 Conclusion

Identifying patients at risk of a heritable disease can lead to closer monitoring, earlier diagnosis, and earlier introduction to clinical services and assistance. Creating and analyzing family pedigrees for individuals with RP can help uncover disease-related mutations and allow for better understanding of the causes of RP. This may allow for enrollment in clinical trials and the development of new strategies for the diagnosis, treatment, and prevention of inherited retinopathies.

References

1. Tsang S, Sharma T (2018) Autosomal dominant retinitis pigmentosa. In: Tsang S, Sharma T (eds) Atlas of inherited retinal diseases, Advances in experimental medicine and biology, vol 1085. Springer, Cham
2. Alkuraya FS (2014) Retinitis pigmentosa. In: Murray MF, Babyatsky MW, Giovanni MA et al (eds) Clinical genomics: practical applications in adult patient care, 1st edn. McGraw-Hill, New York
3. Lee W, Xie Y, Zernant J et al (2016) Complex inheritance of ABCA4 disease: four mutations in a family with multiple macular phenotypes. Hum Genet 135(1):9–19

Chapter 6

Whole Genome Sequencing for Detection of Structural Variants in Patients with Retinitis Pigmentosa

Alexander H. Chai

Abstract

Retinitis pigmentosa (RP) is a group of inherited retinal diseases characterized by the progressive degeneration of rod then cone photoreceptors. Most of the known mutations that cause RP reside in the protein-coding portions of DNA; however, a growing number of pathogenic mutations have been identified within the non-coding portions. This chapter details a brief method for the detection of structural variants throughout the genome for the identification of novel mutations and to ultimately provide patients with a precise molecular diagnosis.

Key words Retinitis pigmentosa, Structural variants, Whole genome sequencing, PacBio Sequel, pbsv (Pacific Biosciences structural variant calling and analysis tools), ngmlr (coNvex Gap-cost alignMents for Long Reads)

1 Introduction

Retinitis pigmentosa (RP) is a group of inherited retinal diseases characterized by the progressive degeneration of rod then cone photoreceptors. It is caused by any one mutation in over 80 different genes [1]. Given the diversity of each gene's underlying pathophysiology, current treatment options remain highly personalized to each gene [2].

The precise identification of a molecular diagnosis is imperative for the individualized treatment of patients with inherited retinal dystrophies (IRDs). The advent of next-generation sequencing (NGS) technologies has significantly lowered the cost and time of genetic screenings for these patients, and subsequently, over 3000 pathogenic mutations have been identified [1]. These findings have led to significant advances in the field of gene therapy for the treatment of otherwise incurable patients. However, many patients

Stephen H. Tsang and Peter M. J. Quinn (eds.), *Retinitis Pigmentosa*,
Methods in Molecular Biology, vol. 2560, https://doi.org/10.1007/978-1-0716-2651-1_6,

are still left without a molecular diagnosis, and therefore no treatment can be developed for them. This can, in part, be attributed to the fact that most IRD studies have focused on the coding regions of DNA [3]. Recent studies suggest that mutations in the intronic regions of DNA may play a larger role in disease than was previously thought, suggesting that the use of whole genome sequencing for research and diagnosis in the clinic may reveal the molecular pathogeneses of previously unsolved IRD [3].

PacBio's Sequel systems use a long-read technology that is more expensive and has a lower throughput than that of other competing technologies. However, long-read technologies have several advantages over short-read technologies, especially in the detection of structural variants. Short-read technologies have been reported to only detect 10% [4] to 70% [5, 6] of variants and report a false positive read up to 89% of the time [5, 7–9]. There is evidence that suggests that long-read technologies can identify some diseases that short-read sequencing technologies may not have detected, can directly sequence repeat expansions and regions with high GC content, can resolve variant phasing, and can distinguish a gene of interest from its pseudogenes [10–12].

One persistent issue with long-read sequencing technologies has been its high sequencing error, which is about 10–15% for PacBio machines [13]. These errors typically show up as short insertion/deletion (indel) mutations; however, biological indels are typically much larger than this. To overcome this sequencing error, the alignment software used in this protocol (ngmlr) uses a scoring algorithm called a convex gap-cost model, which seeks to compute a proper alignment by penalizing indel mutations on a logarithmic scale rather than a linear scale, as seen in Fig. 1 [11]. This encourages long series of gaps or insertions to be recognized as one large mutation rather than a number of small ones. These variants are then identified by PacBio's pbsv software to be displayed.

This chapter details a brief methodology for the detection of structural variants located through the genome using Pacific Biosciences® Whole Genome Sequencing technologies, with its workflow shown in Fig. 2. Using the PacBio Sequel sequencing system and the SMRTLink analysis software, one can easily identify insertions, deletions, inversions, and translocations. It is recommended to use PacBio's library preparation kit for the Sequel to simplify the process.

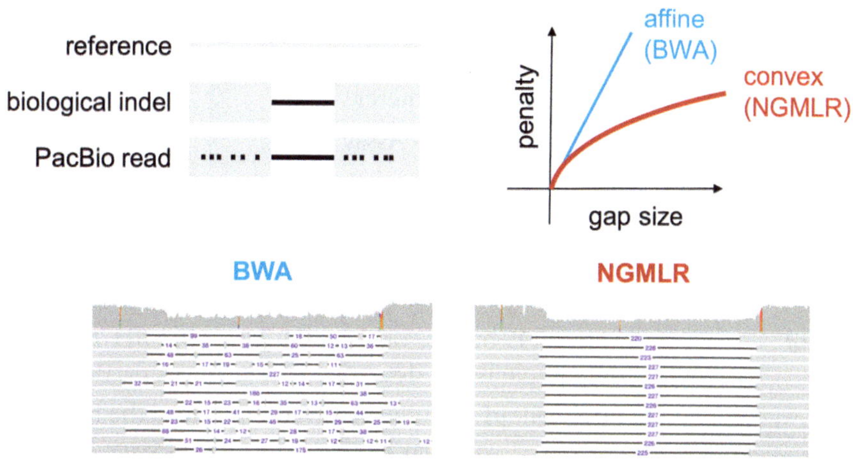

Fig. 1 Ngmlr alignment software uses a scoring algorithm called a convex gap-cost model, which seeks to compute a proper alignment by penalizing indel mutations on a logarithmic scale rather than a linear scale [11]

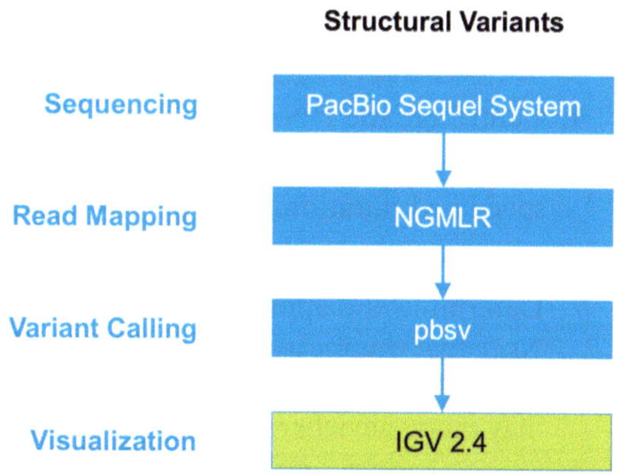

Fig. 2 Schematic outlining the methodology used for the detection of structural variants located through the genome using Pacific Biosciences® Whole Genome Sequencing technologies

2 Materials

1. PacBio Sequel System.
2. PacBio SMRT Link Software (open-source).
3. PacBio SMRTbell® Express Template Preparation Kit.
4. PacBio AMPure® PB Beads.
5. Covaris® g-TUBE® DNA Shearing Device.
6. Eppendorf® DNA LoBind tubes (1.5 mL).
7. Eppendorf® Minispin plus Centrifuge.
8. BluePippin Size-Selection System.

9. BluePippin Gel Cassette and DNA Marker S1 Kit.
10. VWR Tube Rotator.
11. Qubit 3.0 Fluorometer.
12. Qubit dsDNA HS Assay Kit.

3 Methods

3.1 Library Preparation and Sequencing

3.1.1 Fragment DNA

1. Dissolve at least 5 μg of non-degraded DNA sample in DI water, TE buffer, or 10 mM Tris–HCl pH 8.5. Ensure that the sample is not degraded and is free of particulate matter.
2. Place 150 μL of fully dissolved DNA into the top of a Covaris® g-TUBE®; you may load multiple if necessary. Screw the cap on very firmly (*see* **Note 1**).
3. Load the g-TUBEs into an Eppendorf® MiniSpin plus centrifuge with the screw cap facing up.
   (a) If a different centrifuge is used, RPM values may require alteration to obtain a ~20-kbp shear. Follow manufacturer instructions.
4. Centrifuge the DNA sample at a rate of 5700 RPM for 60 s.
5. Invert the g-TUBEs and repeat centrifugation at the same speed and duration.
6. Unscrew the tube body and recover the samples.
7. Determine the approximate size range of the DNA samples. Note that the sheared fragment size is largely dependent on the quality of the original gDNA and that the sheared fragments may range anywhere between 6 kbp and 20 kbp.
8. Concentrate the DNA sample using 0.45X volume of AMPure PB magnetic beads at room temperature in a LoBind microcentrifuge tube. Refer to the manufacturer guide for details.

3.1.2 Repair DNA Damage and Ends

1. Thaw the repair reagent components on ice.
2. Dilute stock DNA Prep Additive in a 1:5 ratio by adding 1 μL of additive with 4 μL of the Enzyme Dilution Buffer in the kit [14].
3. To remove single-strand overhangs, add the following reagents to a LoBind microcentrifuge tube:
   (a) 7.0 μL of DNA Prep Buffer
   (b) 45.0 μL of sheared DNA
   (c) 1.0 μL of NAD
   (d) 1.0 μL of diluted DNA Prep Additive
   (e) 1.0 μL of DNA Prep Enzyme
4. Mix reagents well, and then spin down the tube contents in a microfuge.

5. For 15 min, incubate at 37 °C, and then return the reaction to 4 °C.
6. Add 2.0 μL of DNA Damage Repair Mix v2 to the 55.0 μL of DNA.
7. Mix the reaction well ten times using wide-bore pipette tips, and then spin down the tube contents in a microfuge.
8. For 30 min, incubate at 37 °C, and then return the reaction to 4 °C.
9. To the previous mixture, add 3.0 μL of the End Prep Mix to repair ends. Pipette mix ten times for thorough mixing. Spin down the contents quickly with a microfuge.
10. Incubate at 20 °C for 10 min, then incubate at 65 °C for 30 min, and then return to 4 °C.

3.1.3 Ligate SMRTbell™ Adapters and Purify Templates

1. In a LoBind microcentrifuge tube on ice, add the following reagents in the order shown:
   (a) 60.0 μL of end-repaired DNA mixture
   (b) 5.0 μL of Overhang Adapter v3
   (c) 30.0 μL of Ligation Mix
   (d) 1.0 μL of Ligation Additive
   (e) 1.0 μL of Ligation Enhancer
2. Mix with wide-bore pipette tips 10×.
3. Quickly spin down contents in a microfuge.
4. Incubate at 20 °C for 60 min, and then return the reaction to 4 °C.
5. Add 44 μL (0.45X concentration) volume of AMPure PB beads.
6. Mix solution thoroughly 15 times with wide-bore pipette.
7. Quickly spin down contents in a microfuge.
8. Incubate at room temperature for 5 min.
9. Spin down the solution once again to collect the beads.
10. Place tube in magnetic bead rack to collect the AMPure beads. Pipette the supernatant into another tube without disturbing the beads.
11. Wash the beads with freshly prepared 80% ethanol for 30 s, then pipette out, and discard the ethanol. Repeat once (*see* **Note 2**).
12. Remove the residual ethanol by removing the tube from the magnetic bead rack and spinning it down. Place the tube back into the magnetic rack, and pipette out the remaining ethanol, which should be at the bottom of the tube. If any remains, repeat this step.

13. A 11 μL of Elution Buffer to the DNA sample. Pipette mix 15 times, and then incubate at 37 °C for 15 min.
14. Briefly spin down the tube.
15. Fully separate the beads on the magnetic bead rack, and then transfer the supernatant to a clean 1.5-mL LoBind tube. You may discard the beads.
16. Verify DNA sample quality and concentration to ensure all steps thus far have succeeded and for use in calculating sequencing primer volumes.

3.1.4 Anneal Sequencing Primer and Bind Polymerase

1. This step can be done easily using SMRT Link's Sample Setup software. Access SMRT Link using the Chrome web browser, then navigate to the Sample Setup, and begin a new calculation.
2. Enter all requested information, making sure to select CLR (continuous long reads) as the sequencing mode. Use the Ctrl-P command to print the customized calculations and instructions for annealing sequencing primers and binding polymerases, and then follow the directions. Use Sequencing Primer v4 and the diffusion loading method.

3.2 Read Mapping/ Calling Structural Variants

1. Navigate to the analysis section of the SMRTLink software.
2. Create a new analysis. Make sure that the selected analysis application is the Structural Variant Calling protocol and that a minimum of two reads and 20% of reads support the confirmation of a variant.
3. Run the analysis using input data from the Sequel system. The reads will be aligned to the selected reference genome, and then structural variants will be specifically called using PacBio's pbsv software.
4. Export the .vcf file containing the indexed structural variants, and then export the aligned reads of the whole genome in .bam format.

3.3 Visualization of Results

1. Import the .vcf file of the structural variants and the .bam file of the aligned read from SMRTLink software into the Broad Institute's Integrative Genomics Viewer [15].
2. From this interface, one can view the structural variations that were output by ngmlr/pbsv in SMRTLink.

4 Notes

1. Because this method directly sequences the starting DNA without any type of amplification, the sequencing quality is highly dependent on the original DNA sample's quality and

purity. Ensure that the DNA is double-stranded, has not been exposed to extreme conditions (pH, temperature, or UV radiation), and is free of contaminants.

2. The ethanol must be prepared freshly due to its hygroscopic properties. The ethanol should not be stored for any more than 3 days in a tightly sealed polypropylene tube.

References

1. Duncan JL et al (2018) Inherited retinal degenerations: current landscape and knowledge gaps. Transl Vis Sci Technol 7(4):6. https://doi.org/10.1167/tvst.7.4.6
2. Koch SF et al (2015) Halting progressive neurodegeneration in advanced retinitis pigmentosa. J Clin Invest 125(9):3704–3713. https://doi.org/10.1172/JCI82462
3. Sudmant PH et al (2015) An integrated map of structural variation in 2,504 human genomes. Nature 526(7571):75–81. https://doi.org/10.1038/nature15394
4. Teo SM et al (2012) Statistical challenges associated with detecting copy number variations with next-generation sequencing. Bioinformatics 28(21):2711–2718. https://doi.org/10.1093/bioinformatics/bts535
5. Robinson JT et al (2011) Integrative genomics viewer. Nat Biotechnol 29(1):24–26. https://doi.org/10.1038/nbt.1754
6. Travers KJ et al (2010) A flexible and efficient template format for circular consensus sequencing and SNP detection. Nucleic Acids Res 38(15):e159. https://doi.org/10.1093/nar/gkq543
7. Goodwin S, McPherson JD, McCombie WR (2016) Coming of age: ten years of next-generation sequencing technologies. Nat Rev Genet 17(6):333–351. https://doi.org/10.1038/nrg.2016.49
8. Biosciences P (2021) pbsv - PacBio structural variant (SV) calling and analysis tools. Available from: https://github.com/PacificBiosciences/pbsv
9. Tattini L, D'Aurizio R, Magi A (2015) Detection of genomic structural variants from next-generation sequencing data. Front Bioeng Biotechnol 3:92. https://doi.org/10.3389/fbioe.2015.00092
10. Huddleston J et al (2017) Discovery and genotyping of structural variation from long-read haploid genome sequence data. Genome Res 27(5):677–685. https://doi.org/10.1101/gr.214007.116
11. Spielmann M, Mundlos S (2016) Looking beyond the genes: the role of non-coding variants in human disease. Hum Mol Genet 25 (R2):R157–R165. https://doi.org/10.1093/hmg/ddw205
12. Procedure & checklist – Preparing gDNA libraries using the SMRTbell® express template preparation kit 2.0. 2019
13. Mills RE et al (2011) Mapping copy number variation by population-scale genome sequencing. Nature 470(7332):59–65. https://doi.org/10.1038/nature09708
14. Roberts RJ, Carneiro MO, Schatz MC (2013) The advantages of SMRT sequencing. Genome Biol 14(7):405. https://doi.org/10.1186/gb-2013-14-6-405
15. User Manual: g-TUBE. 2016

Chapter 7

Fundus Photography Methodologies to Assess RP Patients

Jin Kyun Oh, Joseph Ryu, and Stephen H. Tsang

Abstract

The development of fundus photography and imaging has improved our ability to diagnose and monitor inherited retinal degenerations. Nowadays, color fundus photography has become a staple in evaluating patients with retinitis pigmentosa (RP). Other important multimodal forms of fundus photography used today include red-free fundus photography, short-wavelength autofluorescence, and near-infrared autofluorescence. These photography methodologies provide valuable information on the natural history of disease progression, which in turn can lead to the identification of viable outcome measurements for current and future therapeutic trials. Further advances and developments in the field of fundus imaging will help in our understanding of RP and allied disorders.

Key words Fundus photography, Red-free photography, Short-wavelength autofluorescence, Near-infrared autofluorescence, Quantitative autofluorescence

1 Introduction

The ability to visualize and evaluate the human retina was first made possible by the development of the ophthalmoscope in 1851 by Hermann von Helmholtz, allowing for the study and management of previously blinding eye diseases, such as retinal detachments, tears, and tumors [1, 2]. Four decades after the development of the ophthalmoscope, A.C. van Trigt first described the phenotypic features of a rare, inherited retinal disease, which was later named retinitis pigmentosa (RP) [3, 4]. Despite its genetic and phenotypic heterogeneity, RP is characterized by a distinct pathophysiology involving rod photoreceptor death followed by cone photoreceptor death. Clinically, RP patients present with a waxy optic disc pallor, arteriolar attenuation, and intraretinal pigment migration in a bone spicule pattern within the fundus. Some features such as the bone spicules are now known to become more prominent with disease progression [5, 6].

Stephen H. Tsang and Peter M. J. Quinn (eds.), *Retinitis Pigmentosa*,
Methods in Molecular Biology, vol. 2560, https://doi.org/10.1007/978-1-0716-2651-1_7,

In 1886, Jackman and Webster obtained the first successful photograph of a human fundus, thereby allowing for the documentation and recording of retinal examination [7]. Although the quality of these initial images was limited by long exposure times and prominent corneal reflexes, they set the stage for the future commercialization and widespread use of fundus photography in the study of retinal diseases. The field of fundus photography has since rapidly developed with the advent of digital photography, the expansion of field of view capabilities to 200°, rapid acquisition times, the ability to capture high-quality images without dilation, and the introduction of modalities that help capture different physiological and pathological characteristics of retinal disorders [8].

Fundus photographs have played a crucial role in the diagnosis and monitoring of inherited retinal dystrophies such as RP. While color fundus photographs are vital for capturing the characteristic features of the disorder, RP is a retinal disease with a wide range of complex phenotypes that can vary depending on the underlying pathogenic mutation. Other modalities of fundus imaging, including red-free fundus photography, short-wavelength autofluorescence, and near-infrared autofluorescence, have been essential in the study and understanding of initially unrecognized manifestations of RP and similar allied diseases.

2 Materials

Various multimodal imaging techniques are to be used including:

1. Color fundus photography.
   - Capable of characterizing degeneration of photoreceptors and retinal pigment epithelium (RPE).
   - Displays presence of bone spicules, vascular attenuation, and optic nerve pallor.
2. Red-free fundus photography.
   - Filter that blocks 500 nm red light.
3. Fundus autofluorescence.
   - Short-wavelength autofluorescence (SW-AF): Blue light autofluorescence obtained with excitation at wavelengths between 400 nm and 590 nm.
   - Near-infrared autofluorescence (NIR-AF): Obtained with excitation at a wavelength of 788 nm.
   - Quantitative autofluorescence (qAF): Imaging analysis that corrects for laser power and the sensitivity of the internal detector by using an internal reference capable of compensating for such variations.

3 Methods

3.1 Color Fundus Photography

RP is an inherited retinal disease characterized by the progressive degeneration of rod and cone photoreceptors as well as the RPE [9]. Clinically, the disease is characterized by three hallmark features—bone spicules, vascular attenuation, and optic nerve pallor—all of which can be visualized on color fundus photography (Fig. 1a). However, in early stages of disease, the fundus may appear normal as the RPE can take an average of 5 years to appear following symptomatic onset, and the optic disc and ophthalmic vasculature may not be visibly affected (Fig. 1b) [6]. Color fundus photography can therefore be used to document subtle changes in the fundus appearance over time that may be missed on other forms of multimodal imaging such as fundus autofluorescence [10]. In an estimated 20% of cases, the characteristic bone spicule pigmentation may not develop at all, and the disease is then referred to as retinitis pigmentosa sine pigmento [5].

Other abnormalities of the fundus associated with RP can also be detected by color fundus photography. Due to the genetic heterogeneity of RP, different etiologies of the disease can present with noticeably different phenotypes. For example, RP caused by mutations in ceramide kinase-like (*CERKL*) may be characterized by the presence of degenerative lacunae in the peripheral retina (Fig. 2a), while RP caused by mutations in RPE-retinal G protein-coupled receptor (*RGR*) may present with areas of nummular subretinal pigment as opposed to the classic RPE (Fig. 2b) [11]. Some forms of RP may only demonstrate subtle changes on color fundus photographs, such as the salt-and-pepper mottling of

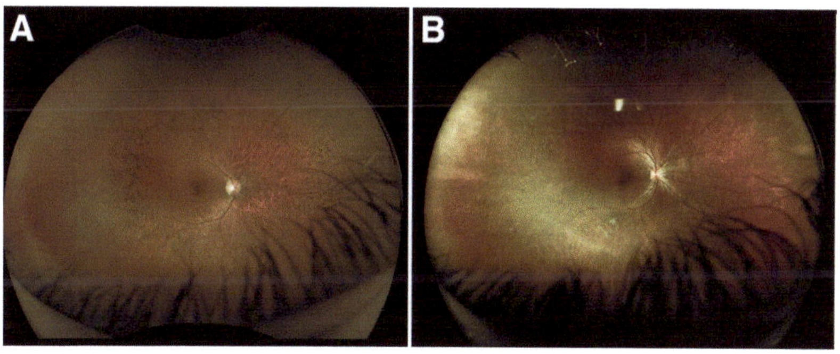

Fig. 1 Color fundus photographs of patients with retinitis pigmentosa and retinitis pigmentosa sine pigmento. (**a**) A color fundus photograph of the right eye of a woman with autosomal dominant retinitis pigmentosa caused by a mutation in the rhodopsin (*RHO*) gene. Imaging revealed the classic features of intraretinal pigment migration, vascular attenuation, and waxy pallor of the optic disc. (**b**) A color fundus photograph of the right eye of a woman with autosomal recessive retinitis pigmentosa caused by mutations in the protocadherin-15 (*PCDH15*) gene. Imaging revealed mottling of the retinal pigment epithelium without the presence of intraretinal pigment migration

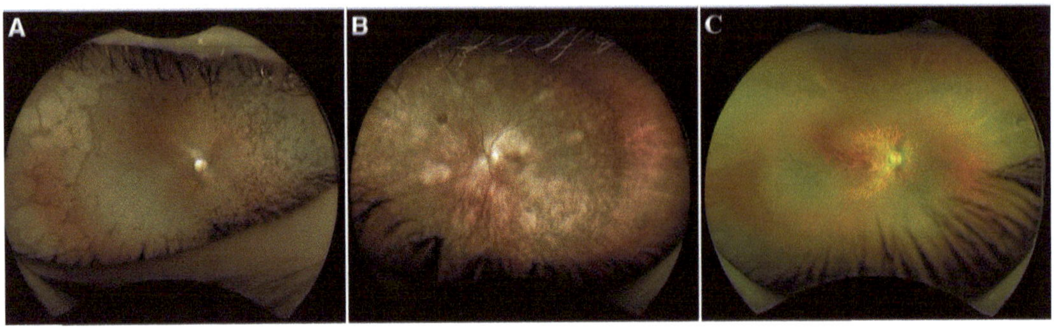

Fig. 2 Color fundus photographs of the phenotypic heterogeneity seen in retinitis pigmentosa. (**a**) The color fundus photograph of the right eye of a woman with autosomal recessive retinitis pigmentosa caused by mutations in ceramide kinase-like (*CERKL*). This image showed the presence of dense intraretinal pigment migration as well as patches of lacunar atrophy in the temporal retina. (**b**) A color fundus photograph of the left eye of a woman with autosomal dominant retinitis pigmentosa caused by a mutation in retinal G protein-coupled receptor (*RGR*). This image demonstrated the presence of subretinal pigment migration and retinal pigment epithelium atrophy. (**c**) Color fundus photography of the right eye of a woman with mutations in retinoid isomerohydrolase (*RPE65*) demonstrates significant mottling of the retinal pigment epithelium and vascular attenuation without the presence of intraretinal pigment migration

the RPE seen in patients with biallelic mutations in retinoid isomerohydrolase (*RPE65*) (Fig. 2c) [12, 13]. This mottling is understood to be caused by localized processes occurring at the level of the retinal pigment epithelium.

In addition to the clinical features associated with RP, color fundus photographs can be used to evaluate conditions that are associated with the disorder such as cystoid macular edema and epiretinal membrane formation. Cystoid macular edema is estimated to occur in half of all RP patients and can be visualized on color fundus images as petaloid lesions within the central macula [14, 15]. Epiretinal membranes are estimated to occur in roughly a quarter of RP patients and can be visualized as subtle reflective irregularities of the normal macular reflex [14, 16].

Despite its many utilities in the diagnosis and monitoring of RP, color fundus photography also has a number of limitations. One such constraint is the color of the fundus—its natural red hue makes it difficult to detect subtle changes [17, 18]. This is compounded by the fact that color fundus photographs require illumination and the visualization of specific parts of retinal anatomy are affected by the wavelength of light used [18, 19, 20]. When it comes to evaluating age-related macular degeneration, Hubbard et al. have suggested that digital fundus images can be too dim or too bright and have poorer color contrast and balance [21]. Consequently, color fundus photographs may not accurately reflect the true color of the retina, and subtle changes may be missed.

Another limitation of color fundus photographs is that they are a two-dimensional representation of three-dimensional anatomy [22]. In the case of RP, this is especially problematic in the evaluation and monitoring of conditions such as cystoid macular edema, which creates a three-dimensional swelling of the macula that may be missed on color fundus photographs [23]. Attempts to address this constraint have included the use of photographs from multiple angles to construct an approximate three-dimensional view of the retina [24]. Recently, the development of confocal scanning laser ophthalmoscopes which utilize several horizontal and vertical scanning mirrors across different depths of the retina has further improved three-dimensional estimation [22]. However, resolution of three-dimensional anatomy using confocal scanning ophthalmoscopes is limited to depths of 100 μm and is affected by patient position, eye movements, and variable focus [22, 25].

Finally, the lack of standardization and the qualitative interpretation of color fundus photography limit its use in the monitoring of RP in the setting of clinical trials and natural history studies [12]. Typically, such studies look for outcome measurements that are quantifiable using imaging modalities such as optical coherence tomography or autofluorescence imaging. To date, there are no common and reliable outcome measurements that are detectable through color fundus images.

3.2 Red-Free Fundus Photography

While color photographs are the most commonly utilized form of fundus photography, other modes of examination have also been adapted to better elucidate retinal pathology, including red-free fundus photography. Red-free fundus photography was first described in 1968 by Mizuno et al. to describe fundus photos obtained using a filter that blocked 500-nm red light [26]. This form of photography has since become widely utilized to monitor neovascularization and abnormalities of the nerve fibers within the retina [26, 27]. Specifically in the case of RP, red-free fundus photographs fill a specific niche as a diagnostic indicator of the tapetal-like reflex seen in female carriers of X-linked RP.

First described by W.A. Frost in 1902, the tapetal-like reflex is a shining, reflective phenomenon similar to the reflex of the tapetum lucidum seen in the eyes of animals [28]. This feature was first associated with X-linked RP by Falls et al. in female carriers of the disease and was hypothesized to be caused by skewed X-inactivation within the retina [29, 30]. Although the tapetal-like reflex has classically been associated with carriers of X-linked RP caused by mutations in retinitis pigmentosa GTPase regulator (*RPGR*), cases of the tapetal reflex have also been documented in carriers of mutations in the RP2 gene (*RP2*) [9, 31]. Acton et al. evaluated multimodal imaging in these carriers and suggested that while this tapetal reflex may be seen on color fundus photographs or on autofluorescence imaging, the greatest visualization was achieved using red-free color fundus photography using a green light filter at 488 nm to block out red light [32]. The capture of this tapetal reflex serves an important role in the diagnosis of male family members with RP as well as carriers themselves, as studies suggest even heterozygous carriers of X-linked RP may experience retinal degeneration in later life [32].

3.3 Fundus Autofluorescence

Fundus autofluorescence is a noninvasive form of fundus imaging that captures endogenous fluorescence that is emitted when the retina is excited by specific wavelengths [33–35]. In patients with RP, fundus autofluorescence images reveal morphological characteristics that may help in the diagnosis and monitoring of the many heterogeneous forms of RP. The two most commonly used subtypes of fundus autofluorescence include SW-AF and NIR-AF.

SW-AF, or blue light autofluorescence, is obtained with excitation at wavelengths between 400 nm and 590 nm [33, 34]. Peak fluorescence is noted to occur between 490 and 510 nm, and most confocal scanning laser ophthalmoscopes acquire images using an excitation of 488 nm [33–35]. The biochemical source of this innate autofluorescence is an amalgam of bisretinoid compounds found within the RPE as the result of nonenzymatic reactions of aldehyde adducts that occur in photoreceptor outer segments [36, 37]. In contrast, NIR-AF signal is obtained with excitation at a wavelength of 788 nm, and the source of this autofluorescence is believed to originate from melanin within the RPE and melanocytes within the choroid [38, 39].

The first study of short-wavelength autofluorescence phenotypes in RP patients was performed in 2003 by Holder et al. who described the presence of an abnormal, perifoveal hyperautofluorescent ring on imaging that demarcates the boundary between healthy and degenerated photoreceptors [40]. The boundary of the inner border of the ring has been shown to delineate the area of preserved retinal function [41]. Many studies have examined the utility of SW-AF images in monitoring the progression of RP and have suggested strong correlations between the diameter of the hyperautofluorescent ring on SW-AF and the width of the ellipsoid zone on spectral domain optical coherence tomography, as well as correlations between the area of the hyperautofluorescent ring on SW-AF and retinal function on microperimetry and multifocal electroretinogram [42–45].

Clinically, the progressive shrinking of the hyperautofluorescent ring on SW-AF has been shown to be most rapid in patients with X-linked RP followed by autosomal recessive RP and then autosomal dominant RP [46]. The slower deterioration seen in autosomal dominant RP is consistent with studies that suggest autosomal dominant RP is the mildest form of disease, while the quick deterioration seen in X-linked RP is consistent with observations that X-linked RP is the most severe [47, 48]. Because of the strong association between the hyperautofluorescent phenotype on SW-AF imaging and other measurements of retinal health, changes to the hyperautofluorescent ring have been suggested and used as primary and secondary outcome measurements in therapeutic trials for RP [42, 46].

However, while SW-AF images of RP patients provide valuable clinical data, these images are confounded by factors such as laser power and the sensitivity of the internal detector. In 2011, Delori et al. developed a formula that took into consideration these factors and equipped confocal scanning laser ophthalmoscopes with an internal reference that can compensate for such variations in order to produce quantitative measures of autofluorescence [49]. Images are acquired in high-speed video mode following a specific protocol as summarized by Sparrow et al., and images are analyzed in a custom software written in IGOR (Wavemetrics, Lake Oswego, OR) or HEYEX software (Heidelberg Engineering) [49–53]. Image gray levels are then standardized to the internal reference, and a quantitative autofluorescence (qAF) value can be computed from the mean qAF measured across three concentric rings divided into eight segments around the central fovea [49, 50].

Studies of qAF have demonstrated that the hyperautofluorescent ring seen in RP patients represents a true increase in autofluorescence intensity as opposed to the appearance of an increase in autofluorescence caused by a relative decrease in SW-AF intensity in the surrounding retina [53]. Additionally, qAF may be particularly valuable for monitoring disease progression and therapeutic outcomes in trials for RP caused by mutations in genes involved in the canonical visual cycle, such as retinoid isomerohydrolase (*RPE65*) or lecithin retinol acyltransferase (*LRAT*) [50]. Qualitative studies have noted that SW-AF images are dark or difficult to obtain in such patients [54]. The ability to indirectly quantify changes in bisretinoid levels over time may be useful in characterizing disease progression or therapeutic improvement following treatment.

Finally, NIR-AF is a less frequently used modality of autofluorescence imaging which has been valuable in the evaluation and diagnosis of RP patients. Duncker et al. demonstrated that the prominent hyperautofluorescent ring found in the NIR-AF images of RP patients correlates spatially with the ring seen on SW-AF images [55]. A study by Jauregui et al. revealed that the progressive constriction of the hyperautofluorescent ring is also consistent between these two imaging modalities [56]. The similar findings seen between these imaging modalities remain puzzling as the source of autofluorescence emission is currently known to be different between the two [50, 55, 56]. Clinically, NIR-AF images appear to be just as valuable as SW-AF images in the diagnosis and monitoring of disease in RP patients with the added benefit of being more tolerable for the patient and thus increasing patient cooperativity.

Conflicts of Interest

Stephen H. Tsang receives financial support from Abeona Therapeutics, Inc and Emendo. He is also the founder of Rejuvitas and is on the scientific and clinical advisory board for Nanoscope Therapeutics.

References

1. Letocha C (1994) Hermann von Helmholtz: a century later. Arch Ophthalmol 112(12): 1524–1525
2. Tasman W (1996) History of retina 1896-1996. Ophthalmology 103(8 Suppl):S143–S152
3. Van Trigt AC. De oogspiegel *Nederlandisch Lancet*, third series, Utrecht, 1852–1853;2d:417–509
4. Donders FC (1855) Beitrage zur pathologischen Anatomic des Auges. Graefes Arch Klin Exp Ophthalmol 2:106–118; 1857;1: 139–165
5. Pearlman JT, Flood SR, Seiff SR (1976) Retinitis pigmentosa without pigment. Am J Ophthalmol 81(4):417–419
6. Takahashi VKL, Takiuti JT, Jauregui R, Mahajan VB, Tsang SH (2018) Rates of bone spicule pigment appearance in patients with retinitis pigmentosa sine pigmento. Am J Ophthalmol 195:176–180
7. Jackman WT, Webster JD (1886) On photographing the retina of the living human eye. Philadel Photogr 23:340–341
8. Panwar N, Huang P, Lee J et al (2016) Fundus photography in the 21st century – a review of recent technological advances and their implications for worldwide healthcare. Telemed J E Health 22(3):198–208. https://doi.org/10.1089/tmj.2015.0068
9. Verbakel SK, van Huet RAC, Boon CJF et al (2018) Non-syndromic retinitis pigmentosa. Prog Retin Eye Res 66:157–186
10. Schuerch K, Marsiglia M, Lee W, Tsang SH, Sparrow JR (2016) Multimodal imaging of disease-associated pigmentary changes in retinitis pigmentosa. Retina 36 Suppl 1(Suppl 1): S147–S158
11. Sengillo JD, Cho GY, Paavo M et al (2019) Hyperautofluorescent dots are characteristic in ceramide kinase like-associated retinal degeneration. Sci Rep 9(1):876. Published 2019 Jan 29
12. Chung DC, Bertelsen M, Lorenz B et al (2019) The natural history of inherited retinal dystrophy due to biallelic mutations in the RPE65 gene. Am J Ophthalmol 199:58–70
13. Chao DL, Burr A, Pennesi M (2019) RPE65-Related Leber Congenital Amaurosis / Early-Onset Severe Retinal Dystrophy. In: Adam MP, Mirzaa GM, Pagon RA, et al., eds. GeneReviews®. Seattle (WA): University of Washington, Seattle; November 14
14. Liew G, Strong S, Bradley P et al (2019) Prevalence of cystoid macular oedema, epiretinal membrane and cataract in retinitis pigmentosa. Br J Ophthalmol 103(8):1163–1166
15. Rotsos TG, Moschos MM (2008) Cystoid macular edema. Clin Ophthalmol 2(4): 919–930. https://doi.org/10.2147/opth.s4033
16. Stevenson W, Prospero Ponce CM, Agarwal DR, Gelman R, Christoforidis JB (2016) Epiretinal membrane: optical coherence tomography-based diagnosis and classification. Clin Ophthalmol 10:527–534. Published 2016 Mar 29. https://doi.org/10.2147/OPTH.S97722
17. Uji A, Muraoka Y, Yoshimura N (2019) Hidden information in color fundus photographs is revealed by the decorrelation stretching method. Retin Cases Brief Rep 13(2): 176–180
18. Bernardes R, Serranho P, Lobo C (2011) Digital ocular fundus imaging: a review. Ophthalmologica 226(4):161–181
19. Elsner A, Burns S, Weiter J, Delori F (1996) Infrared imaging of sub-retinal structures in the human ocular fundus. Vis Res 36:191–205
20. Fernández E, Unterhuber A, Považay B, Hermann B, Artal P, Drexler W (2006) Chromatic aberration correction of the human eye for retinal imaging in the near infrared. Opt Express 14:6213–6225
21. Hubbard L, Danis R, Neider M, Thayer D, Wabers H, White J, Pugliese A, Pugliese M (2008) Group ARED2R: brightness, contrast, and color balance of digital versus film retinal images in the Age-Related Eye Disease Study 2. Invest Ophthalmol Vis Sci 49:3269–3282
22. Abràmoff MD, Garvin MK, Sonka M (2010) Retinal imaging and image analysis. IEEE Rev Biomed Eng 3:169–208. https://doi.org/10.1109/RBME.2010.2084567

23. Hirakawa H, Iijima H, Gohdo T, Tsukahara S (1999) Optical coherence tomography of cystoid macular edema associated with retinitis pigmentosa. Am J Ophthalmol 128(2): 185–191
24. Allen L (1964) Ocular fundus photography: suggestions for achieving consistently good pictures and instructions for stereoscopic photography. Am J Ophthalmol 57:13–28
25. Webb RH, Hughes GW (1981) Scanning laser ophthalmoscope. IEEE Trans Biomed Eng 28(4):488–492
26. Mizuno K, Majima A, Ozawa K, Ito H (1968) Red-free light fundus photography. Photographic optogram. Invest Ophthalmol 7(3): 241–249
27. Venkatesh P, Sharma R, Vashist N, Vohra R, Garg S (2015) Detection of retinal lesions in diabetic retinopathy: comparative evaluation of 7-field digital color photography versus red-free photography. Int Ophthalmol 35(5): 635–640
28. Frost WA (1902) Unusually well-marked retinal reflex. Trans Ophthalmol Soc UK 22: 208–209
29. Falls HF, Cotterman CW (1948) Choroidal degeneration: a sex-linked form in which heterozygous women exhibit a tapetal-like retinal reflex. Arch Ophthalmol 40:685–703
30. Cideciyan AV, Jacobson SG (1994) Image analysis of the tapetal-like reflex in carriers of X-linked retinitis pigmentosa. Invest Ophthalmol Vis Sci 35(11):3812–3824
31. Flaxel CJ, Jay M, Thiselton DL et al (1999) Difference between RP2 and RP3 phenotypes in X linked retinitis pigmentosa. Br J Ophthalmol 83(10):1144–1148
32. Acton JH, Greenberg JP, Greenstein VC et al (2013) Evaluation of multimodal imaging in carriers of X-linked retinitis pigmentosa. Exp Eye Res 113:41–48
33. Delori FC, Dorey CK, Staurenghi G, Arend O, Goger DG, Weiter JJ (1995) In vivo fluorescence of the ocular fundus exhibits retinal pigment epithelium lipofuscin characteristics. Invest Ophthalmol Vis Sci 36(3):718–729
34. Von Ruckmann A, Fitzke FW, Bird AC (1996) Distribution of fundus autofluorescence with a scanning laser ophthalmoscope. Ophthalmic Lit 1(49):33
35. Von Ruckmann A, Fitzke FW, Bird AC (1997) Fundus autofluorescence in age-related macular disease imaged with a laser scanning ophthalmoscope. Invest Ophthalmol Vis Sci 38(2): 478–486
36. Sparrow JR, Wu Y, Kim CY, Zhou J (2010) Phospholipid meets all-trans-retinal: the making of RPE bisretinoids. J Lipid Res 51(2):247–261
37. Sparrow JR, Yoon KD, Wu Y, Yamamoto K (2010) Interpretations of fundus autofluorescence from studies of the bisretinoids of the retina. Invest Ophthalmol Vis Sci 51(9): 4351–4357
38. Keilhauer CN, Delori FC (2006) Near-infrared autofluorescence imaging of the fundus: visualization of ocular melanin. Invest Ophthalmol Vis Sci 47(8):3556–3564
39. Kellner U, Kellner S, Weber BH, Fiebig B, Weinitz S, Ruether K (2009) Lipofuscin- and melanin-related fundus autofluorescence visualize different retinal pigment epithelial alterations in patients with retinitis pigmentosa. Eye (Lond) 23(6):1349–1359
40. Robson AG, El-Amir A, Bailey C et al (2003) Pattern ERG correlates of abnormal fundus autofluorescence in patients with retinitis pigmentosa and normal visual acuity. Invest Ophthalmol Vis Sci 44(8):3544–3550
41. Hood DC, Lazow MA, Locke KG, Greenstein VC, Birch DG (2011) The transition zone between healthy and diseased retina in patients with retinitis pigmentosa. Invest Ophthalmol Vis Sci 52(1):101–108
42. Sujirakul T, Lin MK, Duong J, Wei Y, Lopez-Pintado S, Tsang SH (2015) Multimodal imaging of central retinal disease progression in a 2-year mean follow-up of retinitis Pigmentosa. Am J Ophthalmol 160(4):786–98.e4. https://doi.org/10.1016/j.ajo.2015.06.032
43. Fakin A, Jarc-Vidmar M, Glavac D, Bonnet C, Petit C, Hawlina M (2012) Fundus autofluorescence and optical coherence tomography in relation to visual function in usher syndrome type 1 and 2. Vis Res 75:60–70
44. Lenassi E, Troeger E, Wilke R, Hawlina M (2012) Correlation between macular morphology and sensitivity in patients with retinitis pigmentosa and hyperautofluorescent ring. Invest Ophthalmol Vis Sci 53(1):47–52
45. Robson AG, Saihan Z, Jenkins SA et al (2006) Functional characterisation and serial imaging of abnormal fundus autofluorescence in patients with retinitis pigmentosa and normal visual acuity. Br J Ophthalmol 90(4):472–479. https://doi.org/10.1136/bjo.2005.082487
46. Jauregui R, Takahashi VKL, Park KS et al (2019) Multimodal structural disease progression of retinitis pigmentosa according to mode of inheritance. Sci Rep 9(1):10712

47. Sandberg MA, Rosner B, Weigel-DiFranco C, Dryja TP, Berson EL (2007) Disease course of patients with X-linked retinitis pigmentosa due to RPGR gene mutations. Invest Ophthalmol Vis Sci 48:1298–1304
48. Hamel C (2006) Retinitis pigmentosa. Orphanet J Rare Dis 1:40
49. Delori F, Greenberg JP, Woods RL et al (2011) Quantitative measurements of autofluorescence with the scanning laser ophthalmoscope. Invest Ophthalmol Vis Sci 52(13):9379–9390
50. Sparrow JR, Duncker T, Schuerch K, Paavo M, de Carvalho JRL Jr (2019) Lessons learned from quantitative fundus autofluorescence. Prog Retin Eye Res 74:100774
51. Greenberg JP, Duncker T, Woods RL, Smith RT, Sparrow JR, Delori FC (2013) Quantitative fundus autofluorescence in healthy eyes. Invest Ophthalmol Vis Sci 54(8):5684–5693
52. Duncker T, Greenberg JP, Ramachandran R et al (2014) Quantitative fundus autofluorescence and optical coherence tomography in best vitelliform macular dystrophy. Invest Ophthalmol Vis Sci 55(3):1471–1482
53. Schuerch K, Woods RL, Lee W et al (2017) Quantifying fundus autofluorescence in patients with retinitis pigmentosa. Invest Ophthalmol Vis Sci 58(3):1843–1855
54. Lorenz B, Wabbels B, Wegscheider E, Hamel CP, Drexler W, Preising MN (2004) Lack of fundus autofluorescence to 488 nanometers from childhood on in patients with early-onset severe retinal dystrophy associated with mutations in RPE65. Ophthalmology 111(8): 1585–1594
55. Duncker T, Tabacaru MR, Lee W, Tsang SH, Sparrow JR, Greenstein VC (2013) Comparison of near-infrared and short-wavelength autofluorescence in retinitis pigmentosa. Invest Ophthalmol Vis Sci 54(1):585–591
56. Jauregui R, Park KS, Duong JK, Sparrow JR, Tsang SH (2018) Quantitative comparison of near-infrared versus short-wave autofluorescence imaging in monitoring progression of retinitis pigmentosa. Am J Ophthalmol 194: 120–125

Chapter 8

The Use of Optical Coherence Tomography in Evaluation of Retinitis Pigmentosa

Ha Min Kim, Jin Kyun Oh, and Stephen H. Tsang

Abstract

Optical coherence tomography (OCT) is a noninvasive imaging technology that has gained widespread use in the evaluation of multiple retinal pathologies, including retinitis pigmentosa (RP). OCT allows for visualization of distinct retinal layers and the choroid and facilitates study of morphological features associated with RP. OCT can be used to detect and to track progression of RP, as well as to correlate structural findings with functional manifestations of the disease. This chapter provides a basic overview of OCT technology and details elements of importance in the use of OCT for diagnosis and assessment of progression of RP.

Key words Choroid, Genetic mutation, Optical coherence tomography, Photoreceptors, Retinal dystrophy, Retinal pigment epithelium (RPE), Retina, Retinitis pigmentosa

1 Introduction

Optical coherence tomography (OCT), which is likened to ultrasound in ophthalmology, is a relatively new technology which uses low-coherence interference properties of light and reflective properties of tissue to generate three-dimensional images of superficial tissues such as the retina. OCT was developed in 1991 when Fujimoto, Swanson, and Huang at Massachusetts Institute of Technology showed that multiple A-scan images generated from continuous-wave light low-coherence interferometry could be combined into 2D grayscale (B-scan) images [1]. David Huang described the first OCT image of the in vitro human retina after removal of the cornea and lens and showed that OCT could be applied to create noninvasive cross-sectional images of tissue in both transparent and turbid media, namely, the peripapillary retina and coronary artery [2].

Stephen H. Tsang and Peter M. J. Quinn (eds.), *Retinitis Pigmentosa*,
Methods in Molecular Biology, vol. 2560, https://doi.org/10.1007/978-1-0716-2651-1_8,

Continued technological advancements led to the development of time-domain OCT (TD-OCT) and Fourier-domain OCT (FD-OCT). The original technology of TD-OCT captures the depth of tissue and generates retinal images by changing the length of the reference arm [3], which results in slower scanning speed and susceptibility to increased noise-to-signal ratio secondary to eye movement. In contrast, FD-OCT utilizes a stationary reference arm and provides depth-resolved, ultra-high-speed, and high-resolution images, with increased sensitivity over TD-OCT [4]. There are two ways of implementing an FD-OCT system: the spectral domain OCT (SD-OCT) and swept source OCT (ss-OCT). SD-OCT uses a spectrometer to detect interference patterns from a broadband light source (superluminescent diode or mode-locked ultra-fast laser source) with large spectral width and small coherence length to achieve high spatial resolution [5]. Figure 1 shows a basic schematic of the SD-OCT system [6]. ss-OCT or optical frequency domain imaging (OFDI) uses a single balanced detector and a rapidly tunable laser source which oscillates over a broad optical spectrum. Both implementations acquire multiple simultaneous tissue depth measurements and obtain a depth profile via Fourier transformation of multiple

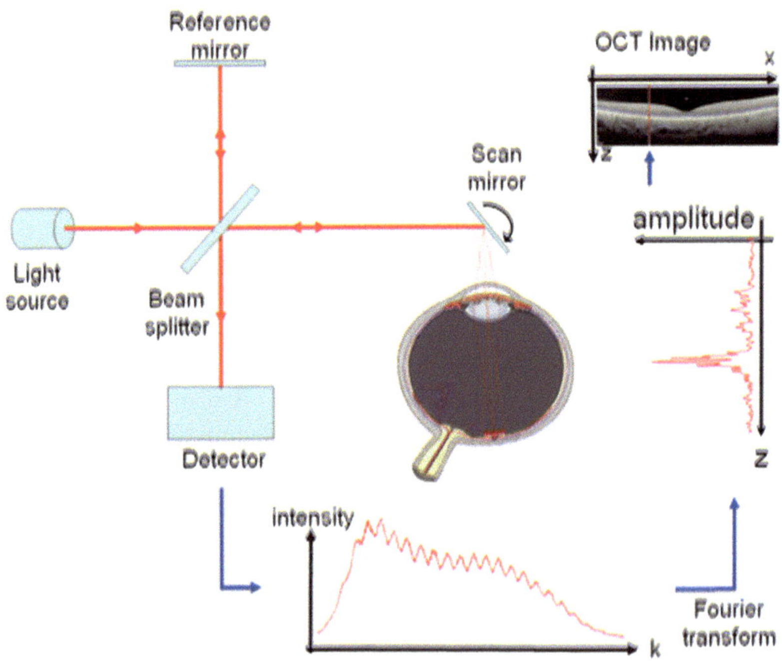

Fig. 1 Schematic of the spectral domain optical coherence tomography (SD-OCT) system. SD-OCT is produced via a single balanced detector that captures the interference pattern created from a stationary reference mirror and a rapidly tunable laser (light) source that oscillates over a broad optical spectrum. In turn, this system allows for the simultaneous acquisition of multiple tissue depth measurements as well as a depth profile via Fourier transformation of multiple wavelengths detected from tissue, finally producing the delineated layers seen in a SD-OCT image

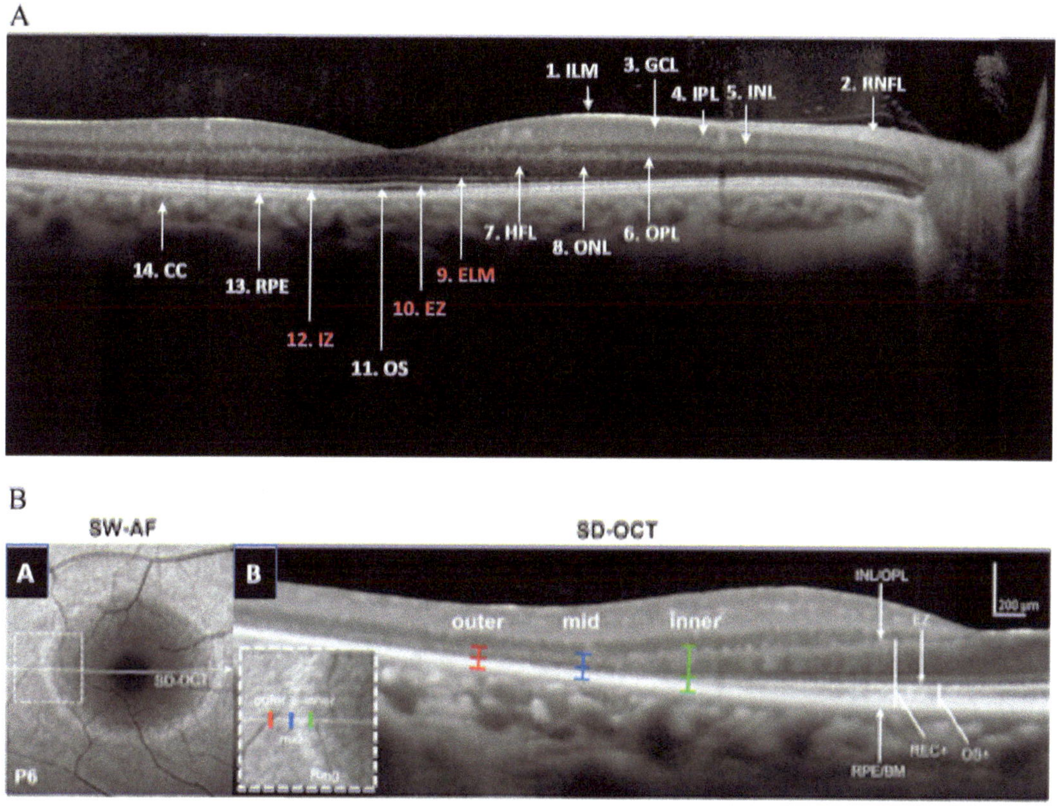

Fig. 2 Basic spectral domain OCT system schematic and processing workflow [6]. (Used with Permission from Theelan and Teussink (2018)). (**a**) Spectral domain optical coherence tomography horizontal macula line scan image of retinal layers: (1) ILM = inner limiting membrane; (2) RNFL= retinal nerve fiber layer; (3) GCL= ganglion cell layer; (4) IPL = inner plexiform layer; (5) INL= inner nuclear layer; (6) OPL= outer plexiform layer; (7) HFL = Henle's fiber layer; (8) ONL= outer nuclear layer; (9) ELM= external limiting membrane; (10) EZ= ellipsoid zone (previously called photoreceptor IS/OS junction or IS/OS line); (11) OS= outer segment of photoreceptors; (12) IZ = interdigitation zone; (13) RPE= retinal pigment epithelium; (14) CC = choriocapillaris. (**b**) SD-OCT image of the RP ring, showing photoreceptor death and transition zone near the fovea. Panel (**a**) shows a short-wavelength fundus autofluorescence image (SW-AF) of the RP ring. Outside of the hyperautofluorescent ring (red line in figure, labeled "outer" in panel **b**), the ONL, ELM, and the IS/OS junction (EZ band) have completely disappeared. Inside the RP ring (blue line, "mid"), the ONL is severely thinned, ELM barely visible, and the IS/OS junction not present. Inside the ring (green line, "inner"), all layers of the retina have maintained full thickness, and the ELM and IS/OS junction are visible

wavelengths detected from tissue. These have allowed for the acquisition of 2-D and 3-D retinal images at a clinically applicable speed, resolution, and retinal coverage [1], as well as for applications in many other disciplines such as cardiology, dermatology, and oncology [7].

OCT has become an important part of the diagnosis and monitoring of progression of many ophthalmological diseases including retinitis pigmentosa (RP). B-scans of the macula have proven to be especially important for monitoring disease progression associated with visual fixation. Figure 2a shows a SD-OCT horizontal macula line scan of a healthy eye with each layer of the retina labeled, and Fig. 2b shows a close-up of the fovea and parafoveal area which contains the transition zone, a structural marker which approximates the extent of retinal damage secondary to RP [8]. Outside of the hyperautofluorescent ring (red line in Fig. 2b, labeled "outer" in panel B), the outer nuclear layer (ONL), external limiting membrane (ELM), and the inner segment/outer segment (IS/OS) junction (ellipsoid zone [EZ] band) have completely disappeared. Inside the RP ring (blue line, "mid"), the ONL is severely thinned, the ELM barely visible, and the IS/OS junction not present. Inside the ring (green line, "inner"), all layers of the retina have maintained full thickness, and the ELM and IS/OS junction are visible.

2 Materials

- Clinical diagnosis of RP: fundus examination by inherited retinal dystrophy (IRD) specialist.
- OCT machine: confocal laser scanning ophthalmoscope; Spectralis HRA + OCT, (Heidelberg Engineering).

3 Methods

OCT in the diagnosis and management of RP uses the following guidelines:

3.1 Clinical Diagnosis

The clinical diagnosis of RP can be made by the presence of nyctalopia, progressive loss of visual acuity, centripetal loss of visual fields, progressive dysfunction of first rod, and then cone photoreceptors as assessed through electroretinogram testing [3, 4]. Fundus examination shows characteristic waxy pallor of the optic disc, arterial attenuation, and mid-peripheral retinal degeneration ranging from "carpet-like" changes to intraretinal "bone spicule" pigmentation. Although OCT is not necessary for the diagnosis of RP [9], it is a well-established, noninvasive imaging modality that is valuable in the evaluation and monitoring of structural changes due to disease progression.

3.2 OCT and Outer Retina

RP is primarily a disease of the outer retina, which affects the photoreceptor and retinal pigment epithelial (RPE) complex, leaving the inner retina relatively intact [10]. Studies have shown good evidence for evaluation of the ellipsoid zone width using horizontal or vertical OCT macular line scans [11] or EZ area using OCT en face images [12]. The change in length of the EZ (also known as the photoreceptor IS/OS junction) has been demonstrated to be a reliable indicator of disease progression and is well correlated with functional tests, such as visual field and full-field electroretinogram, as well as structural measurements such as the diameters of the hyperautofluorescent ring seen on short-wavelength autofluorescence (SW-AF) imaging [13, 14, 15]. However, unlike other functional testing, measurements of the EZ line benefit from low test–retest variability and are sensitive to smaller changes over shorter periods of time [15].

Research suggests a simple linear relationship between the loss of local photoreceptor thickness (product of OS and ONL thickness, proxy for number of photoreceptors) and visual field (VF) loss in patients with good foveal sensitivity, and VF sensitivity of −10 dB or worse is correlated with disappearance of the outer segment [10]. Thus, tracking the location of where the EZ line disappears (i.e., where the OS disappears and the ellipsoid zone becomes indistinguishable from the RPE, also known as IS/OS junction) is a good structural marker of disease progression, which accompanies the functional marker of progressive VF loss [15, 16], and is a better marker of disease progression and photoreceptor loss than OS thickness measurements [11].

A study by Jauregui et al. has also demonstrated that changes in EZ width vary by pattern of inheritance in RP, with the fastest progression observed in patients with X-linked RP (XLRP) and the slowest progression seen in patients with autosomal dominant RP [17]. These findings corroborate prior studies that have suggested that disease progression and severity differ among inheritance patterns [13, 18, 19]. Figure 3 shows a SD-OCT imaging displaying horizontal macular b-scans of a 12-year-old patient with a known compound heterozygous frameshift mutation in the *PROM1* gene causing Leber congenital amaurosis, as reported by Ragi et al. [20]. The blurred EZ line is present at the fovea and absent at the periphery (yellow arrows in Fig. 3), indicating progressive degeneration of photoreceptors and movement of the IS/OS junction towards the fovea. Figure 4 shows progressive

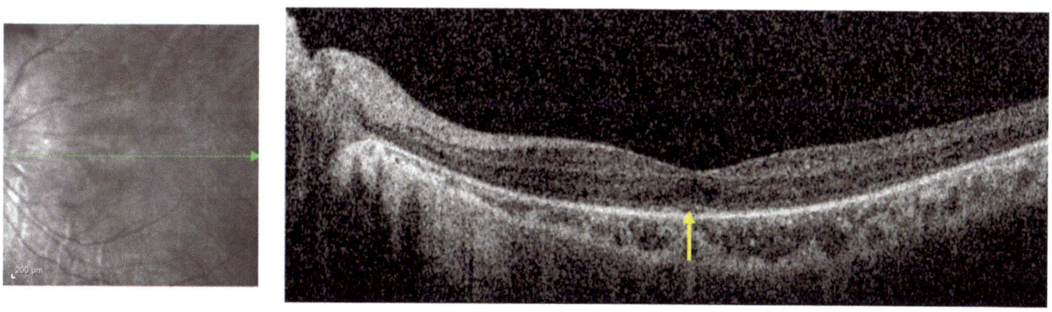

Fig. 3 Horizontal macula scans obtained with SD-OCT (confocal scanning laser ophthalmoscope; Spectralis HRA + OCT, Heidelberg Engineering). Yellow arrow points to blurred ellipsoid zone line at the fovea that is absent on the periphery. The internal layers are well delineated [20]

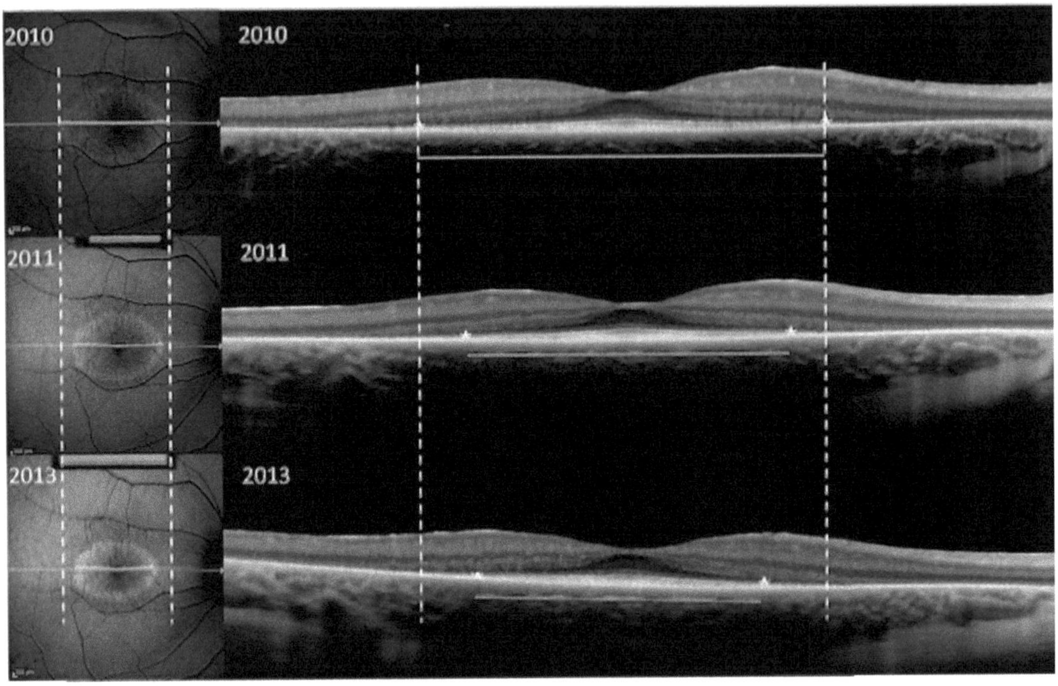

Fig. 4 Representative scans from a RP patient with progressive shortening of the EZ band from 2010 to 2013. Stars (*) indicate transition zone, and the width of the line between the two stars represents EZ width

shortening of the EZ band from 2010 to 2013 secondary to RP, as evidenced by the decreasing width between the transition zones (* in figure) on either side of the fovea.

Similarly, Hariri et al. have described the use of en face SD-OCT to evaluate changes of EZ area and found it to be a robust and precise method to evaluate disease progression. Benefits of this method include that the EZ band can be assessed across the entire retina as opposed to only at the fovea and may therefore be a more complete measure of disease progression. This is especially important as RP is known to progress at different rates across different axes [13].

In addition to the EZ line, two additional hyperreflective lines in the OCT b-scan of the outer retina (Fig. 2a, in red) are useful in the evaluation of photoreceptor segments affected by RP, from the inner to the outer retina: ELM, which marks the beginning of the IS of photoreceptors, and the interdigitation zone (IZ), which represents the apices of RPE cells encasing the tips of cells in the OS [21]. In RP, degeneration of photoreceptors leads to shortening of these hyperreflective photoreceptor lines as well [21].

Once degenerative changes to the RPE have been noted, disease progression and response to treatment can be followed with in vivo OCT studies of the transition zone from healthy RPE to diseased retina, which is the border between thinned and healthy photoreceptor/pigment epithelial complex [22] around the central retina. Transition zones demonstrate orderly progression from initial decrease in photoreceptor OS thickness, followed by thinning of the ONL plus outer plexiform layer (ONL+: receptor cell bodies, receptor fibers, OPL connection to cells of the INL), to disappearance of the OS layer, to near complete loss of IS layer (ELM disappears), to near complete loss of cell bodies in ONL to an asymptotic level, and to disruption of the RPE region [22, 23].

OCT can also be used to track overall thinning of the outer segment secondary to RP. In a study examining obligate female carriers of a mutation for XLRP, a condition that accounts for nearly 20% of all cases of RP, SD-OCT scans showed thinning of the outer retina (OS+: receptor outer segment + RPE; REC+ thickness: distance from INL/OPL line to BM/choroid line) within the central 30° in all carriers, which is consistent with other reports of outer retinal thinning in RP [24].

Complications of RP can also be diagnosed and followed with OCT, as well as response to treatment of these complications. Figure 5 shows a SD-OCT horizontal macular line scan from a patient with cystoid macular edema secondary to autosomal recessive RP. Panel A shows the initial exam before treatment, and panel B shows the macula after treatment with the topical carbonic anhydrase inhibitor dorzolamide hydrochloride ophthalmic solution (Trusopt). The marked improvement after treatment can be assessed through OCT and can guide further clinical interventions.

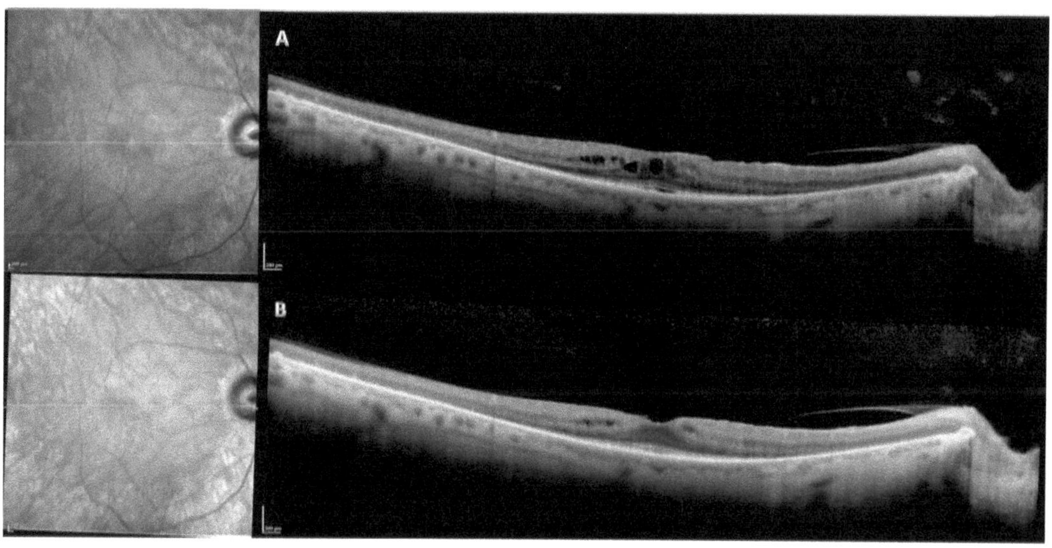

Fig. 5 SD-OCT of 65-year-old man with cystoid macular edema secondary to autosomal dominant retinitis pigmentosa due to a heterozygous variant in RP1. Panel (**a**) shows the macula before treatment (visual acuity (VA) 20/40 OD). Panel (**b**) shows post 9 months of treatment with the topical carbonic anhydrase inhibitor dorzolamide hydrochloride ophthalmic solution (Trusopt) (VA 20/30 OD)

3.3 OCT and Inner Retina

Despite progressive outer retinal thinning, most studies have shown that the inner retinal thickness remains normal, including the inner nuclear layer (INL), ganglion cell layer (RGC), and retinal nerve fiber layer (RNFL). A few studies have also demonstrated inner retinal thickening [21] especially along the horizontal meridian, which may be due to proliferation of glial cells within the RNFL, and RNFL and RGC "stretching" to fill the space evacuated by degenerated receptor cells [22]. These findings are consistent with histopathological evaluation of postmortem eyes from patients with RP, which demonstrate that while all layers of the retina are affected in severe RP, both the RGC and the INL are the most preserved [25]. As therapies are often targeted towards electrical stimulation of RGC or restoration of photoreceptors, determining the integrity of post-receptor cells of the inner nuclear and RGC layers is essential to evaluating clinical outcomes; moreover, measurements of macular RGCs may be a better method to determine and follow visual function in RP [22].

In RP, hyperreflective foci (HF), thought to be composed of macrophages, extravasated lipoproteins, and migrating RPE cells, have been observed in the inner nuclear layer, outer nuclear layer, and subretinal space [21]. Such HF have also been observed in other complex retinal degenerations such as age-related macular degeneration (AMD), where they are hypothesized to be microglia activated in response to inflammation [26]. Similarly, in RP, the location of hyperreflective foci is correlated with the extent of photoreceptor damage. Unlike in AMD, in early stages of RP, HF are seen in the INL near intact IS/OS junction or the area where IS/OS border junction. HF in the ONL are seen in more advanced RP patients with no or disrupted IS/OS junction, which is thought to be a result of photoreceptor cell death and resultant RPE migration. In very advanced stages of RP, HF may no longer be distinct [27].

3.4 Summary

Since its conception by Huang et al., the OCT has drastically improved the diagnosis and understanding of complex retinal degenerations, such as RP, by providing an accurate and reliable method to visualize retinal architecture. This has not only allowed for the characterization of natural history and numerous potential outcome measurements in future therapies of RP, such as shortening of the EZ width and retinal thinning, but has also refined the routine management of complications of RP such as cystoid macular edema. Future development of OCT technology and improvements to existing modalities will further enhance our understanding of RP and play a crucial role in therapeutic endeavors.

Conflicts of Interest

Stephen H. Tsang receives financial support from Abeona Therapeutics, Inc and Emendo. He is also the founder of Rejuvitas and is on the scientific and clinical advisory board for Nanoscope Therapeutics.

References

1. Fujimoto J, Swanson E (2016) The development, commercialization, and impact of optical coherence tomography. Investig Ophthalmol Vis Sci 57:OCT1–OCT13
2. Huang D, Swanson EA, Lin CP et al (1991) Optical coherence tomography. Science 254: 1178–1181
3. Leitgeb R, Hitzenberger C, Fercher A (2003) Performance of fourier domain vs time domain optical coherence tomography. Opt Express 11:889
4. Wojtkowski M, Leitgeb R, Kowalczyk A et al (2002) In vivo human retinal imaging by Fourier domain optical coherence tomography. J Biomed Opt 7:457
5. Yaqoob Z, Wu J, Yang C (2005) Spectral domain optical coherence tomography: a better OCT imaging strategy. BioTechniques 39: S6–S13
6. Theelen T, Teussink MM (2018) Inspection of the human retina by optical coherence tomography. In: Boon C, Wijnholds J (eds) Retinal gene therapy. Methods in Molecular Biology, vol 1715. Humana Press, New York, NY. https://doi.org/10.1007/978-1-4939-7522-8_26
7. Zysk AM, Nguyen FT, Oldenburg AL et al (2007) Optical coherence tomography: a review of clinical development from bench to bedside. J Biomed Opt 12:051403
8. Tsang SH and Sharma T (2018) Optical coherence tomography BT - atlas of inherited retinal diseases, presented at the
9. Zhang Q (2016) Retinitis pigmentosa. Asia-Pacific J Ophthalmol 5:265–271
10. Rangaswamy NV, Patel HM, Locke KG et al (2010) A comparison of visual field sensitivity to photoreceptor thickness in retinitis pigmentosa. Invest Opthalmol Vis Sci 51:4213
11. Ramachandran R, Zhou L, Locke KG et al (2013) A comparison of methods for tracking progression in X-linked retinitis pigmentosa using frequency domain OCT. Transl Vis Sci Technol 2:5
12. Hariri AH, Zhang HY, Ho A et al (2016) Quantification of ellipsoid zone changes in retinitis pigmentosa using en face spectral domain-optical coherence tomography. JAMA Ophthalmol 134:628–635
13. Sujirakul T, Lin MK, Duong J, Wei Y, Lopez-Pintado S, Tsang SH (2015) Multimodal imaging of central retinal disease progression in a 2-year mean follow-up of retinitis pigmentosa. Am J Ophthalmol 160(4):786–798 e784
14. Cabral T, Lima de Carvalho JR Jr, Kim J, Oh JK, Levi SR, Park KS, Duong JK, Park J, Boudreault K, Belfort R Jr, Tsang SH (2020) Comparative analysis of functional and structural decline in retinitis pigmentosas. Int J Mol Sci 21(8)
15. Birch DG, Locke KG, Wen Y, Locke KI, Hoffman DR, Hood DC (2013) Spectral-domain optical coherence tomography measures of outer segment layer progression in patients with X-linked retinitis pigmentosa. JAMA Ophthalmol 131(9):1143–1150
16. Hood DC, Ramachandran R, Holopigian K et al (2011) Method for deriving visual field boundaries from OCT scans of patients with retinitis pigmentosa. Biomed Opt Express 2: 1106
17. Jauregui R, Takahashi VKL, Park KS, Cui X, Takiuti JT, Lima de Carvalho JR Jr, Tsang SH (2019) Multimodal structural disease progression of retinitis pigmentosa according to mode of inheritance. Sci Rep 9(1):10712
18. Fishman GA (1978) Retinitis pigmentosa. Visual loss. Arch Ophthalmol 96(7): 1185–1188
19. Fishman GA, Farber MD, Derlacki DJ (1988) X-linked retinitis pigmentosa. Profile of clinical findings. Arch Ophthalmol 106(3):369–375
20. Ragi SD, De Carvalho JRL, Tanaka AJ et al (2019) Compound heterozygous novel frameshift variants in the PROM1 gene result in Leber congenital amaurosis. Cold Spring Harb Mol Case Stud 5:a004481
21. Liu G, Liu X, Li H et al (2016) Optical coherence tomographic analysis of retina in retinitis pigmentosa patients. Ophthalmic Res 56: 111–122

22. Hood DC, Lin CE, Lazow MA et al (2009) Thickness of receptor and post-receptor retinal layers in patients with retinitis pigmentosa measured with frequency-domain optical coherence tomography. Investig Ophthalmol Vis Sci 50:2328–2336
23. Hood DC, Lazow MA, Locke KG et al (2011) The transition zone between healthy and diseased retina in patients with retinitis pigmentosa. Invest Ophthalmol Vis Sci 52:101
24. Acton JH, Greenberg JP, Greenstein VC et al (2013) Evaluation of multimodal imaging in carriers of X-linked retinitis pigmentosa. Exp Eye Res 113:41–48
25. Santos A, Humayun MS, de Juan E Jr, Greenburg RJ, Marsh MJ, Klock IB, Milam AH (1997) Preservation of the inner retina in retinitis pigmentosa. A morphometric analysis. Arch Ophthalmol 115(4):511–515
26. Coscas G, De Benedetto U, Coscas F, Li Calzi CI, Vismara S, Roudot-Thoraval F, Bandello F, Souied E (2013) Hyperreflective dots: a new spectral-domain optical coherence tomography entity for follow-up and prognosis in exudative age-related macular degeneration. Ophthalmologica 229(1):32–37
27. Kuroda M, Hirami Y, Hata M et al (2014) Intraretinal hyperreflective foci on spectral-domain optical coherence tomographic images of patients with retinitis pigmentosa. Clin Ophthalmol 8:435–440

Chapter 9

Optical Coherence Tomography Angiography (OCTA) Findings in Retinitis Pigmentosa

Vlad Diaconita, Alexis Kassotis, and Wei Kiong Ngo

Abstract

Optical coherence tomography angiography (OCTA) is a noninvasive new imaging modality that can be used to diagnose and monitor progression of retinitis pigmentosa (RP). Cohorts and case series have shown correlation between OCTA findings and visual function and disease severity. Although an early use of the technology is promising, there are concerns about segmentation errors and artifacts. There is also a paucity of data on genotype and how that correlates with OCTA findings. Despite its limitations, OCTA remains a useful tool for clinicians managing retinitis pigmentosa patients.

Key words Optical coherence tomography angiography, Retinitis pigmentosa, Traditional intravenous fluorescein angiography, Indocyanine green angiography, Vasculature, Choriocapillaris

1 Introduction

Optical coherence tomography angiography (OCTA) is a noninvasive, in vivo, optical imaging system that combines traditional OCT-generated volumetric representations of b-scans taken through the retina with computer-generated retinal and choroidal blood flow images. The details of the design and background of OCTA are beyond the scope of this chapter. However, it is important to know that this is achieved with the use of phase-variance or amplitude/intensity-variance, both of which use contrast based on motion of blood erythrocytes observed over time and space in the OCT b-scan data. Newer methods combine multiple signals of variance and amplitude and are more accurate with fewer artifacts. Using the acquired data, two-dimensional perfusion map scans of the retina are created. Multiple maps can be combined to create a three-dimensional representation of the retinal layers and are superimposed on cross-sectional angiographic images of the retina and choroid. This process is heavily reliant on segmentation software,

Stephen H. Tsang and Peter M. J. Quinn (eds.), *Retinitis Pigmentosa*,
Methods in Molecular Biology, vol. 2560, https://doi.org/10.1007/978-1-0716-2651-1_9,

which can cause errors [1–3]. Recent innovations in the technology allowed for better quality renderings of multiple layers including the choriocapillaris and an increase in window imaging size [4].

2 Comparison to Traditional Intravenous Fluorescein Angiography and Indocyanine Green Angiography

As opposed to traditional intravenous fluorescein angiography (IVFA) and indocyanine green angiography (ICG), OCTA is noninvasive and dye-free and allows faster image acquisition and segmentation of blood flow through individual retinal layers and choriocapillaris. This allows OCTA to be used in situations that do not warrant injection. As a noninvasive tool, it allows for frequent testing and imaging to track progression, as it is often paired with a traditional OCT scan. Since it can image the retinal vasculature and choroidal vasculature at once, it may be preferred in situations where both structures are important to visualize, without the need of multiple injections. Disadvantages include increase blink and projection artifacts, segmentation artifacts, reliance of software optimization, and a small scanning area (traditionally 3 × 3 mm, 6 × 6 mm, or 15 × 9 mm, but newer machines are able to scan much larger windows). More importantly, there is no functional information about leakage, making OCTA unable to provide information about active inflammation, particularly in the setting of retinal vasculitis or uveitis [5, 6].

Multiple companies have OCTA systems, and their offerings are changing at a rapid pace. The first OCTA was made commercially available only in 2016, and since then a steady increase in innovation has led to multiple machines from different industry partners. Each of their systems is able to deliver quality information of retinal and choroidal vasculature, but each differ slightly in the hardware and software that provides clinicians with such data. In particular, the use of wide-field OCTA allows for visualization of retinitis pigmentosa (RP) pathology which extends outside the posterior pole [7].

For the purposes of RP, no system has been found superior to another, although larger scanning windows, better resolution, and decrease in artifact are preferred in an OCTA system for all its intended clinical uses. RP is no different.

3 Changes in Microvasculature of Retina, Choroid, and Optic Nerve Head in RP

Murakami et al. originally used laser speckle flowgraph to show that decreased blood flow in the macula was associated with decreased function in RP patients [8]. Since then, a number of studies have used OCTA to find microvasculature changes in patients with RP. Results have shown that retinal and choriocapillaris microvasculature is affected in RP [9–13].

3.1 RP in the Superficial and Deep Capillary Plexus of the Retina

RP progression impairs the retinal vasculature. Toto et al. found that vascular changes were related to the macular function, as well as to ganglion cell complex thickness. They reported that superficial and deep capillary plexus and choriocapillaris density was reduced in RP patients. Additionally, the deep and superficial capillary plexus density was correlated with ganglion cell complex thickness and multifocal ERG [14].

Battaglia et al. reported on a cross-sectional case series of 16 Italian RP patients which revealed that the deep capillary plexus had a reduction in mean vessel density compared to the superficial capillary plexus reduction. Both were significantly reduced compared to healthy controls. They also showed foveal avascular zone (FAZ) was significantly larger in the deep capillary plexus of RP patients, but the superficial capillary plexus was not statistically different from controls. They could not show a significant difference in the choriocapillaris [15].

Sughara et al. found that both superficial and deep capillary plexuses in retinal vasculature were decreased in flow density in Japanese RP eyes as compared to healthy eyes. The foveal avascular zone (FAZ) was also significantly increased in size in RP eyes. This was associated with a decrease in outer, inner, and total parafoveal retinal thickness, showing that there are changes in retinal flow density and anatomy of the foveal and parafoveal retina [13].

Alnawaiseh et al. showed an increase of two times in the superficial capillary plexus (SCP) foveal avascular zone and 40% in the deep capillary plexus (DCP) foveal avascular zone in 20 RP patients as compared to 21 controls in a prospective cohort study. Their findings correlated visual acuity with flow density in the superficial retinal plexus. Specifically, visual field was correlated with parafoveal flow density in the SCP and DCP and peripapillary flow density [9].

Inooka et al., in a study of 53 RP patients and 46 controls, showed an increase in FAZ and decrease in perfusion density in the retina and in each of the segmented superficial and deep retinal layers [10]. A prospective case-control study of 12 patients with moderate to severe RP conducted in Italy showed a significant reduction in perfusion density (PD) in foveal and parafoveal regions of the deep capillary plexus [16]. Another case-control study of 37 eyes with RP showed a decrease in microvascular density in RP patients as compared to age-matched controls. Furthermore, RP eyes had decreased retinal flow as compared to controls, with severe RP eyes having more vascular loss in the deep capillary plexus as compared to superficial capillary plexus [17]. Lastly, Hagag et al. found that the deep capillary plexus was more affected than the superficial capillary plexus [18].

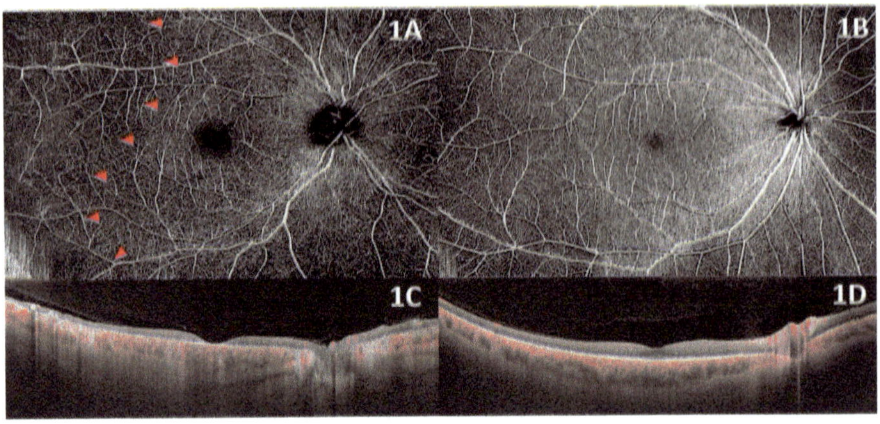

Fig. 1 (**a**) OCTA (superficial capillary plexus) of a 65-year-old female with USH2A retinitis pigmentosa showing enlarged FAZ and temporal areas of decreased capillary density (red arrowheads) corresponding to temporal inner and outer retinal atrophy. (**b**) OCTA (superficial capillary plexus) of a 36-year-old normal control for comparison. (**c**) OCT B-scan with flow overlay showing decreased flow signal in the inner retinal layers and optic nerve head compared to normal control. (**d**) OCT B-scan with flow overlay in normal control

Overall, RP is associated with increase in foveal avascular zone (FAZ) as well as hypoperfusion (Fig. 1). Reduction in perfusion density has been documented in the superficial and deep capillary plexuses. Some studies have suggested that the deep capillary plexus is more affected than the superficial retinal vasculature. This could be due to the DCP's proximity to the cones and choroidal vessels.

3.2 Choriocapillaris

Initial studies on RP and OCTA did not find that the choriocapillaris was significantly affected. Since then, innovation in the quality of image acquisition and wide-field OCTA has allowed for higher resolution and larger scanning windows, which is perhaps why more recent studies showed a significant decrease in choriocapillaris flow deficit and vessel density. Toto et al. originally reported in 2016 that choriocapillaris density was reduced in RP patients [14]. Mastropasqua et al. showed a reduction in perfusion density in foveal and parafoveal regions of the choriocapillaris. They also described a lower vessel length density (VLD) in the choriocapillaris [16]. This is in keeping with previous work by Alnawaiseh et al. who also found a correlation between flow density in the choriocapillaris [9]. Rezaei et al. used OMAG algorithm to show choriocapillaris flow voids in 25 RP patients [12].

Guduru et al. studied 54 patients and found an increase in number of choriocapillaris flow voids as well as increase in average hypoperfusion area [19]. Miyata et al. showed that 43 eyes of RP patients showed flow deficits on wide-field 12 × 12 mm OCTA in the choriocapillaris layers as compared to healthy controls [20], while Liu et al. compared 53 patients with RP and 53 controls to also find significant decrease in choroidal vessel density

[21]. Original data was unclear, but there are multiple studies that now show that the choriocapillaris is affected in RP and can be followed with OCTA [9, 12, 14, 16, 19–21].

3.3 Optic Nerve Head Perfusion in RP

Optic nerve perfusion has also been studied in RP patients. Arrigo et al. showed a decreased perfusion in the peripapillary region in RP patients of various genotypes as compared to controls, mostly in the deep capillary plexus and radial peripapillary capillaries [22]. These patients had decrease in retinal nerve fiber layer (RNFL) thickness. Mastropasqua et al. showed in a case-control study of 11 RP patients and 16 control subjects that the vessel density in the peripapillary area was significantly reduced in the 19 RP eyes [16]. Furthermore, RNFL thickness was significantly reduced, on average 85.9 ± 20.4 μm vs 104.0 ± 6.4 μm. This shows that there is significant variation in RNFL thickness in RP patients, which may be correlated with severity of disease. Finally, Alnawaiseh et al. showed a decrease in perfusion of the optic nerve head in RP patients which was (along with parafoveal flow density in the SCP and DCP) correlated with visual field [9]. It is likely that visual field progression in RP patients is at least in part due to changes in perfusion of the RNFL.

4 Neovascularization

Cases of choroidal neovascularization in the setting of RP have been described. OCTA is helpful in the diagnosis and long-term management of these lesions in other diseases and may be of use in RP [23–27].

5 RP with Macular Edema

Cystoid macular edema (CME) as seen by OCT occurs in 10–50% of RP patients [28]. Only a few studies, however, have examined CME and RP [15, 18, 29]. One study in particular, a larger retrospective chart review of 132 consecutive RP patients, found 35 patients to have CME in at least 1 eye. A case-control comparison of 42 eyes in patients with RP (of which 35 eyes had CME) and 42 normal control eyes showed that OCTA could identify decrease in parafoveal flow density (PFD) between RP eyes and non-RP eyes. However, in comparing patients with RP and CME and those RP patients without CME, there was no statistically significant difference in OCTA-measured microvascular disruption or capillary dropout, even in areas of CME. RP-CME eyes had significantly higher central macular thickness (CMT) and lower PFD in choriocapillaris, but not in the superficial or deep capillary plexus when compared to RP non-CME eyes [29, 30]. In a similar cohort,

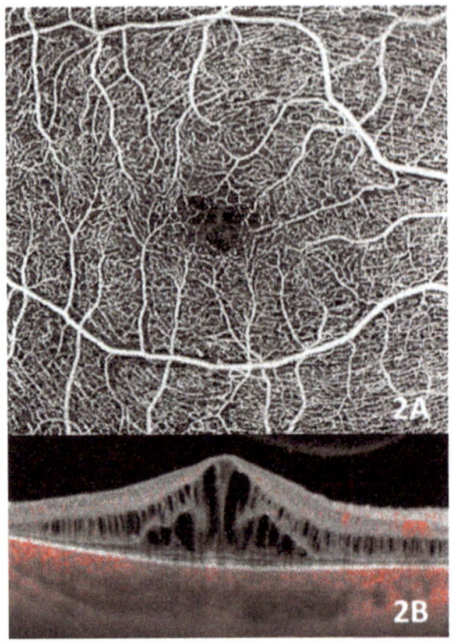

Fig. 2 (**a**) OCTA focusing on the fovea of a 20-year-old female with retinitis pigmentosa and cystoid macular edema showing FAZ irregularity and capillary fallout surrounding it. (**b**) Corresponding B-scan with flow overlay shows cystoid macular edema

Hagag et al. conducted a cross-sectional study of 44 eyes with RP and showed that eyes with RP and CME had more severe hypoperfusion than eyes without CME [18, 30]. We present a 20-year-old female with RP whose OCTA (Fig. 2) shows irregular foveal avascular zone and microvascular disruption surrounding the fovea. Whether this finding is a result of CME or RP, or both, remains uncertain, and we await more information from future studies.

6 Correlation with Function and Progression of Disease

OCTA has not been in use long enough to provide large and robust datasets on correlation with function and progression. A number of case reports, small studies, and case series have shown that OCTA findings can correlate with vision, visual field, and ERG. One cohort of 73 RP patients showed a correlation between decrease parafoveal flow density, increase in FAZ, and decrease in central visual acuity [11].

Furthermore, some with longer follow-up have described changes in OCTA over time as RP disease severity increases. Takagi et al. described results from a case-control study comparing RP patients with 20/20 vision or better with age and refraction-matched healthy controls. In 50 eyes, the authors described changes in retinal vasculature despite good central visual acuity, hinting perhaps that OCTA may be a good early maker for disease progression. Similar findings were reported by Koyanagi et al. and Mastropasqua et al. showing that a decrease in microperimetry in RP patients was correlated to their PD and VLD values, while Lin et al. showed in 37 eyes that the decreases in microvascular density were correlated with a decrease in cone density, which was more pronounced in severe RP. Liu et al. compared 53 patients with RP and 53 controls to also find significant decrease in choroidal vessel density which was associated with ellipsoid zone (EZ) line, visual acuity, visual field, and ERG b-wave amplitude. These findings show that OCTA can be a useful marker not only for structure in RP but also function [11, 16, 17, 21, 31].

Jauregui et al. presented an unmatched case series of 28 eyes with RP which were followed for over 1 year [32]. They were able to show that the perfusion density decreased over time at a rate of $2.42 \pm 0.62\%$ per year in the superficial capillary plexus and $2.41 \pm 0.76\%$ per year in the deep capillary plexus. Furthermore, they confirmed that the foveal avascular zone increases in RP and that the size of the FAZ increases yearly at a rate of 0.078 ± 0.021 mm^2 in the SCP and 1.52 ± 0.039 mm^2 in the DCP. The choriocapillaris flow was also not found to change over time. Changes on OCTA correlated with a visual acuity decrease at a LOGMAR rate of 0.049 ± 0.021 per year. Long-term follow-up of RP patients in a clinical setting may help provide more information on progression and more importantly function in these patients [10, 21, 32–34].

7 Future Directions

Recent studies suggest that OCTA measurements can be good markers for function in RP eyes. This provides another tool in the armamentarium available to the ophthalmologist who manages inherited retinal disease patients. There are knowledge gaps that the literature has not yet addressed with regard to OCTA and RP. First of all, RP is a multigenetic disease. Large prospective studies of RP progression on OCTA should be coupled with genetic data so that accurate models can be used by clinicians. As OCTA becomes more readily available, that may change. Secondly, what makes the use of OCTA more challenging in a clinical setting is segmentation errors and artifacts, both of which are common. That is especially true in the setting of retinal disease like RP. For now, clinicians should closely review all RP OCTA images and have repeat studies performed if they encounter possible artifacts. Only in that way can disease progression be followed accurately. Despite these limitations, OCTA provides a rapid and valuable solution to image RP patients [35].

References

1. Kim DY et al (2013) Optical imaging of the chorioretinal vasculature in the living human eye. Proc Natl Acad Sci U S A 110(35): 14354–14359
2. Ferrara D, Waheed NK, Duker JS (2016) Investigating the choriocapillaris and choroidal vasculature with new optical coherence tomography technologies. Prog Retin Eye Res 52: 130–155
3. Kashani AH et al (2017) Optical coherence tomography angiography: a comprehensive review of current methods and clinical applications. Prog Retin Eye Res 60:66–100
4. Jia Y et al (2015) Quantitative optical coherence tomography angiography of vascular abnormalities in the living human eye. Proc Natl Acad Sci U S A 112(18):E2395–E2402
5. Spaide RF et al (2018) Optical coherence tomography angiography. Prog Retin Eye Res 64:1–55
6. Huang D et al (2016) Optical coherence tomography angiography using the optovue device. Dev Ophthalmol 56:6–12
7. Liu G et al (2017) Extended axial imaging range, widefield swept source optical coherence tomography angiography. J Biophotonics 10(11):1464–1472
8. Murakami Y et al (2015) Correlation between macular blood flow and central visual sensitivity in retinitis pigmentosa. Acta Ophthalmol 93(8):e644–e648
9. Alnawaiseh M et al (2019) Optical coherence tomography angiography in patients with retinitis pigmentosa. Retina 39(1):210–217
10. Inooka D et al (2018) Quantification of macular microvascular changes in patients with retinitis pigmentosa using optical coherence tomography angiography. Invest Ophthalmol Vis Sci 59(1):433–438
11. Koyanagi Y et al (2018) Optical coherence tomography angiography of the macular microvasculature changes in retinitis pigmentosa. Acta Ophthalmol 96(1):e59–e67
12. Rezaei KA et al (2017) Retinal and choroidal vascular features in patients with retinitis pigmentosa imaged by OCT based microangiography. Graefes Arch Clin Exp Ophthalmol 255(7):1287–1295
13. Sugahara M et al (2017) Optical coherence tomography angiography to estimate retinal blood flow in eyes with retinitis pigmentosa. Sci Rep 7:46396
14. Toto L et al (2016) Macular features in retinitis pigmentosa: correlations among ganglion cell complex thickness, capillary density, and macular function. Invest Ophthalmol Vis Sci 57(14):6360–6366
15. Battaglia Parodi M et al (2017) Vessel density analysis in patients with retinitis pigmentosa by means of optical coherence tomography angiography. Br J Ophthalmol 101(4):428–432
16. Mastropasqua R et al (2020) Widefield swept source OCTA in retinitis pigmentosa. Diagnostics (Basel) 10(1):50
17. Lin R et al (2019) Relationship between cone loss and microvasculature change in retinitis pigmentosa. Invest Ophthalmol Vis Sci 60(14):4520–4531
18. Hagag AM et al (2019) Projection-resolved optical coherence tomographic angiography of retinal plexuses in retinitis pigmentosa. Am J Ophthalmol 204:70–79
19. Guduru A et al (2018) Quantitative assessment of the choriocapillaris in patients with retinitis pigmentosa and in healthy individuals using OCT angiography. Ophthalmic Surg Lasers Imaging Retina 49(10):e122–e128
20. Miyata M et al (2019) Concentric choriocapillaris flow deficits in retinitis pigmentosa detected using wide-angle swept-source optical coherence tomography angiography. Invest Ophthalmol Vis Sci 60(4):1044–1049
21. Liu R et al (2019) Effect of choroidal vessel density on the ellipsoid zone and visual function in retinitis pigmentosa using optical coherence tomography angiography. Invest Ophthalmol Vis Sci 60(13):4328–4335
22. Arrigo A et al (2019) Vascular patterns in retinitis pigmentosa on swept-source optical coherence tomography angiography. J Clin Med 8(9):1425
23. Sayadi J et al (2017) Type 3 neovascularization associated with retinitis pigmentosa. Case Rep Ophthalmol 8(1):245–249
24. Attanasio M et al (2020) Swept-source optical coherence tomography angiography findings in a case of Pachychoroid Neovasculopathy in retinitis pigmentosa. Retin Cases Brief Rep 16(3): 300–304
25. Aloe G et al (2019) Bilateral retinal angiomatous proliferation in a variant of retinitis pigmentosa. Case Rep Ophthalmol Med 2019: 8547962
26. Marano F et al (2000) Hereditary retinal dystrophies and choroidal neovascularization. Graefes Arch Clin Exp Ophthalmol 238(9): 760–764
27. Cheng JY, Adrian KH (2009) Photodynamic therapy for choroidal neovascularization in

stargardt disease and retinitis pigmentosa. Retin Cases Brief Rep 3(4):388–390
28. Hajali M, Fishman GA, Anderson RJ (2008) The prevalence of cystoid macular oedema in retinitis pigmentosa patients determined by optical coherence tomography. Br J Ophthalmol 92(8):1065–1068
29. de Carlo TE et al (2016) Analysis of choroidal and retinal vasculature in inherited retinal degenerations using optical coherence tomography angiography. Ophthalmic Surg Lasers Imaging Retina 47(2):120–127
30. Yeo JH, Kim YJ, Yoon YH (2020) Optical coherence tomography angiography in patients with retinitis pigmentosa-associated cystoid macular edema. Retina 40(12):2385–2395
31. Takagi S et al (2018) Optical coherence tomography angiography in patients with retinitis pigmentosa who have normal visual acuity. Acta Ophthalmol 96(5):e636–e642
32. Jauregui R et al (2018) Quantitative comparison of near-infrared versus short-wave autofluorescence imaging in monitoring progression of retinitis pigmentosa. Am J Ophthalmol 194:120–125
33. Tang PH et al (2019) Optical coherence tomography angiography of RPGR-associated retinitis pigmentosa suggests foveal avascular zone is a biomarker for vision loss. Ophthalmic Surg Lasers Imaging Retina 50(2):e44–e48
34. Wang XN et al (2019) Quantitative evaluation of primary retinitis pigmentosa patients using colour Doppler flow imaging and optical coherence tomography angiography. Acta Ophthalmol 97(7):e993–e997
35. Lauermann JL et al (2018) Prevalences of segmentation errors and motion artifacts in OCT-angiography differ among retinal diseases. Graefes Arch Clin Exp Ophthalmol 256(10):1807–1816

Chapter 10

Electroretinogram (ERG) to Evaluate the Retina in Cases of Retinitis Pigmentosa (RP)

Wan-Chun Huang, Pei-Kang Liu, and Nan-Kai Wang

Abstract

Electroretinogram (ERG) captures the electrical responses of photoreceptors, the summation of action potentials from all neurons in the retina elicited by illumination. ERG testing is an incredibly useful tool in obtaining more specific information regarding a retinal dystrophy. Specifically, ERGs are typically used to test photoreceptors and inner retinal function in humans and animals, to diagnose retinal dystrophies, and to monitor disease progression. In this chapter, we will introduce the components of ERGs and the standard ERG protocols for clinical examination. We will also introduce the various specialized ERG tests, which can help to differentiate retinitis pigmentosa (RP) from other retinal disorders. Lastly, we will elaborate on how to use ERGs to predict visual prognosis in RP.

Key words Electroretinogram (ERG), The International Society for Clinical Electrophysiology of Vision (ISCEV), Full-field ERG, a-wave, b-wave, Retinitis pigmentosa (RP)

1 Introduction

1.1 Overview of the Visual System

The visual system is comprised of the retina, visual pathways from the retina via the lateral geniculate nucleus (LGN) to the primary visual cortex, and other brain areas involved in visual information processing. First, light signals are converted into electrical signals in the photoreceptors of the retina. These signals are sent to interneurons, such as bipolar cells, horizontal cells, and amacrine cells, and then to ganglion cells. Transmitted down the axons of the ganglion cells through the optic nerves, the signals travel down the optic tracts, across the optic chiasm, until they reach the LGN. The primary visual cortex receives signals from the LGN, and those signals are further processed in the visual associative cortex.

1.2 Historical Perspective

Dewar (1877) was the first to successfully perform an ERG on humans [1]. However, using Dewar's design, it was impossible to derive quantitative measurements because eye movements resulted

Stephen H. Tsang and Peter M. J. Quinn (eds.), *Retinitis Pigmentosa*,
Methods in Molecular Biology, vol. 2560, https://doi.org/10.1007/978-1-0716-2651-1_10,

in baseline disturbances. Therefore, these difficulties limited the demand for this test in the clinical setting. Kahn and Löwenstein (1924) recorded the ERG by placing a string galvanometer and leads over an anesthetized eyeball; however, this was fraught with difficulties [2]. Granit (1934) initially examined the ERG waveforms in detail and correlated each component of the ERG (P-I, P-II, and P-III) to individual cells in the retina. Today, a-wave (the large negative component PIII), b-wave (the development of positive component PII followed by the resulting PIII and PII), and c-wave (the summation of P-I and P-III) have long been used in ERG interpretation, which are still based on Granit's analysis. Granit was awarded the Nobel Prize in Physiology or Medicine in 1967 for his discoveries of the primary physiological and chemical visual processes in the eye [3]. With advances in technology, Lorrin Riggs (1941) introduced the design of the contact lens electrode, which made it possible to employ the ERG as part of a routine examination in a clinical setting [4]. Moreover, a better understanding of the components of the ERG facilitated its use in clinical applications.

1.3 The Components of ERG

ERG responses represent a mass response generated from all types of cells in the retina. In other words, all retinal cell types can contribute to the responses of ERGs. While some cells make a large contribution to the ERG waveforms, others have a negligible effect. Different orientations of these cells might result in different responses to a change in illumination [5]. For example, radial voltage current flow in extracellular media from radially oriented cells will sum up, while lateral currents will be offset by each other because of the incredible symmetry in retinal lateral arrangement [6]. Photoreceptors are the first in the retina to be activated by light and together with bipolar cells are major contributors to major waves in ERG responses. Therefore, an initial negative a-wave is mainly generated by photoreceptors and followed by a positive b-wave, produced from the OFF- and ON-bipolar cells, respectively. Compared to photoreceptors and bipolar cells, horizontal and amacrine cells make fewer contributions to the waveforms captured by ERG as a result of their lateral orientation [5].

1.3.1 The Origin of a-Wave

The a-wave is mainly generated by photoreceptors, but it also relates to the post-receptoral pathway. The dark-adapted a-wave, an initial cornea-negative deflection that occurs in response to light stimuli after dark adaptation, is primarily driven by rods (with or without cones depends on the light intensities). The light-adapted a-wave, an initial negative wave in response to a flash of light after light adaptation, is generated mainly by the cone photoreceptors since the activity of rod photoreceptors is inhibited [7].

1.3.2 The Origin of b-Wave

After the first negative deflection, the ensuing positive deflection is b-wave. The major generators are ON-bipolar cells and Muller cells. On the one hand, the b-wave is generated from the voltage drop of extracellular current resulting from radial current flow through the ON-bipolar cells. On the other hand, a release of potassium produced by the depolarizing ON-bipolar cells causes depolarization of Muller cells, resulting in a cornea-positive deflection [8–12]. In clinical application, the b-wave is an indicator to assess inner retinal function or signal from photoreceptors.

1.3.3 The Origin of c-Wave

In the subretinal space, a reduction in the concentration of potassium ion results in the generation of the c-wave, the process that leads to apical polarization of the retinal pigment epithelium (RPE) [3]. Also, normal c-wave relies on the unimpaired photoreceptors, which trigger a reaction chain to decrease in the extracellular concentration of potassium ions when they respond to light. The ERG c-wave can be used as a tool to assess the RPE function, the integrity of the photoreceptors, and the interactions between them [6].

1.3.4 The Origin of d-Wave

In the retina, not only the onset of light but also the cessation of light elicits the responses, which are called ON-response and OFF-response, respectively. The d-wave is a positive-going deflection in the photopic ERG, derived from strong hyperpolarizing (OFF) cone bipolar cells at light offset [7].

2 Materials

2.1 Types of Recording Electrodes

2.1.1 Recording Electrodes

Active ERG electrodes are connected to the positive input for ERG recording, and all of them can be placed on the cornea, bulbar conjunctiva, or skin of the lower eyelid. These include Burian–Allen electrode (contact lens electrode, bipolar electrode), Henkes Lovac (contact lens electrode), Goldlens (contact lens electrode), ERG Jet (contact lens electrode), gold foil electrode (lid-hook electrode), C-glide (lid-hook electrode), HK loop (lid-hook electrode), Dason–Trick–Litzkow (DTL) electrode, and skin electrodes [13].

Contact lens electrodes give more reliable and reproducible recordings and provide the highest amplitudes compared to other skin or lid electrodes. The Burian–Allen electrode is most commonly used because it holds the lid apart to prevent blinking and lid closure [14], and it has different sizes for premature infants, children, and adults. However, it also has some disadvantages, such as low tolerance in some people due to irritation and risk of corneal or conjunctival abrasions. In such cases, it is usually necessary to use topical anesthetic eye drops and 0.5 or 1% methylcellulose solution over the corneal surface to protect cornea before the insertion of Burian–Allen electrode [13, 15, 16].

The Dawson–Trick–Litzkow (DTL) electrode is the second most popular electrode after the Burian–Allen type. The design of the DTL electrode is based on a nylon thread whose individual fiber is silver-impregnated, and the conductive thread is placed in the inferior fornix for ERG recording. Compared to contact lens electrodes, the DTL electrode provides better patient tolerance. If the wrong placement of the thread occurs, the recording might fail because of induced eye movements, such as blinking and eyelid closure. In general, the amplitudes recorded using the DTL electrode are about 10% lower compared to the amplitudes recorded using contact lens electrodes [15, 16].

Skin electrodes are usually not recommended as standard recording electrodes for adults but may be considered in infants and young children who cannot tolerate irritation from contact lens electrodes. The signals recorded using skin electrodes are usually smaller, more variable, and much noisier than signals recorded using corneal contacting electrodes [16].

2.1.2 Reference Electrodes

Reference electrodes are connected to the negative input of the system. In bipolar electrodes, the lid speculum covered by conductive material over its outer surface serves as a built-in reference electrode. The contact lens–speculum assembly provides a more stable signal in recording than monopolar contact lens electrodes with a separate reference [17]. Alternatively, skin electrodes are placed temporally near the orbital rim or on the forehead. Moreover, it should be noted that electrical activity produced by skeletal muscles might interfere with ERG recordings if the reference electrodes are placed over muscle masses.

2.1.3 Common Electrode

The common electrode type is connected to the common input of the recording system. Typical locations for common electrodes are the earlobe, mastoid, and forehead.

3 Methods

3.1 The Clinical ERG Procedures

The human ERG recorded at the cornea and elicited by a full-field stimulus is a mass response generated by cells across the entire retina. To get reproducible amplitudes and implicit times in the ERGs, the flash stimuli and background light should be homogeneous, and all reach over around the entire retina. Therefore, all of the receptors are stimulated or adapted in the same condition.

Clinical electrophysiology tests include ffERG, electrooculogram (EOG), multifocal ERG (mfERG), pattern ERG (pERG), and visual evoked potential (VEP). Each test is intended to test specific cell function in the visual system and provides information to support clinical diagnosis or function to predict prognosis. Correlation between each test and function is summarized in Table 1.

The International Society for Clinical Electrophysiology of Vision (ISCEV) proposed several standard settings for these tests

Table 1
Clinical use of the various electrophysiological tests

Type of test	Clinical use of the various electrophysiological tests
ERG	Assess the functions of photoreceptors and neurons in the inner nuclear layer
EOG	Assess generalized retinal pigment epithelium (RPE) function
mfERG	Reflect macular and central cone function
Pattern ERG	Reflect retinal ganglion cell function in macula
VEP	Quantify nerve function from retina to visual cortex, such as optic nerve, optic chiasm, and retrochiasmal pathways

[15, 18, 19], which allow physicians and scientists to communicate and discuss the visual electrophysiological function using the same settings.

3.2 The ISCEV Standard for Clinical ERG

The ISCEV Standard is reviewed regularly. In this chapter, we used the most recently published versions of the ISCEV Standard protocols (2015, 2018). The ISCEV Standard ERG includes six steps for ffERG, which are named after the adaptation state and the flash intensities (stimulus calibrations in cd·s/m^2) [20].

1. Dark-adapted 0.01 ERG (rod ERG).
2. Dark-adapted 3 ERG (combined rod-cone standard flash ERG).
3. Dark-adapted oscillatory potentials.
4. Dark-adapted 10 ERG (strong flash ERG).
5. Light-adapted 3 ERG (standard flash "cone" ERG).
6. Light-adapted 30 Hz flicker ERG.

3.3 The Standard Procedure for Performing ERGs on Patients

1. Pupillary dilatation. To get fully dilated pupils, both tropicamide (relaxes the circular muscles of the iris) and phenylephrine (contracts radial muscles of the iris) are used for mydriasis. According to the ISCEV Standard, the sizes of the pupils should be measured before and after the ERG recordings.
2. Dark adaptation. Dark adaptation for at least 20 minutes is necessary before this first step in ERG examination.
3. Insertion of corneal contact electrodes after dark adaptation. Electrodes are inserted under dim red light rather than strong red light, and then an additional 5 minutes recovery time is recommended. (*see* **Note 1**).
4. Fixation for ERG recording. Patients should be instructed to look at a target point and avoid eye movements. Eye movements might change the positions of the electrodes on the eye, and blinking or closing the eyelids might cause large artifacts.

5. Dark-adapted 0.01 ERG (rod ERG). This is the first step after dark adaption, and the weak flashes should be tested before the strong flashes. The a-wave is not detected because the signal from the rod photoreceptors is too small under the dim stimuli, but the b-wave is elicited when the signals are amplified by around 100-fold through the rod-initiated pathways [15, 21].
6. Dark-adapted 3 ERG (combined rod-cone standard flash ERG). The dark-adapted 3 ERG is the second step after the dark-adapted 0.01 ERG. Under these stimuli (3 cd·s/m^2), the a-wave and b-wave can be recorded by activation of photoreceptors and by ON- and OFF-bipolar cells, respectively.
7. Dark-adapted oscillatory potentials. After dark adaptation, the dark-adapted oscillatory potentials (OP) are recorded with the flash strength of 3.0 cd·s/m^2. The extraction of the OPs might be from an intact ERG. Amacrine cells (or inner retina, such as bipolar cells) are involved in the generation of the OPs [15, 22].
8. Dark-adapted 10 ERG (strong flash ERG). Compared to the dark-adapted 3 ERG, the dark-adapted 10 ERG features the increase in the amplitudes of a-wave and b-wave, the shortening peaking time (greater distinction of negative ERG waveforms, when b-wave amplitudes are reduced), and the emerging of oscillatory potentials at the ascending phase of the b-wave. These brighter flashes might give more reliable responses in patients with opaque media or immature retinae.
9. Light-adapted 3 ERG (standard flash "cone" ERG). Light adaptation for at least 10 minutes is required to maximize cone response and minimize rod activity. The a-wave in the light-adapted 3 ERG arises from the cone photoreceptors and OFF-bipolar cells and the b-wave from cone ON- and OFF-bipolar cells.
10. Light-adapted 30-Hz flicker ERG. The light-adapted 30-Hz flicker ERG is recorded with a flash strength of 3 cd·s/m^2. The 30-Hz flash stimulus reflects cone systems with post-receptoral ON- and OFF-pathways [15, 18].

See ISCEV Standard ERGs for details of stimulus strength, inter-stimulus time (rate), and recording bandpass (Hz) in the six steps.

3.4 ERG in Infants

It is challenging to record ERG responses from infants or young children because of the short attention span and poor cooperation. To alleviate their stress in the process, they need a quiet and calm environment accompanied by their primary caregiver [16]. Sometimes, it would be helpful to use sedation agents for noncompliant children, but the level of sedation might affect ERG responses.

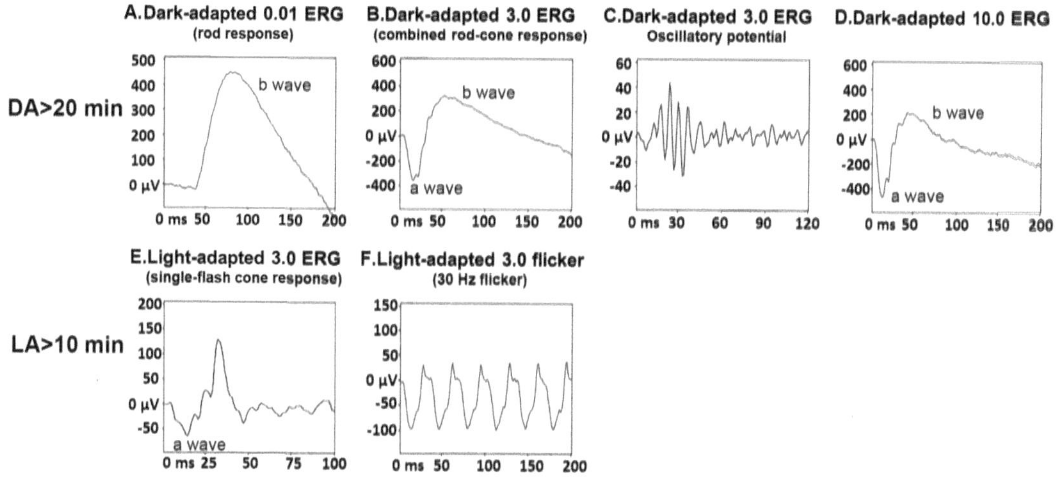

Fig. 1 Normal full-field electroretinogram (ffERG) responses. ffERG is recorded according to ISCEV standards. After a dark adaptation for at least 20 minutes, scotopic ffERG responses are elicited with different flash strength for dark-adapted 0.01 ffERG (**a**), dark-adapted 3 ffERG (**b**), dark-adapted 3 oscillatory potentials (**c**), and dark-adapted 10 ffERG (**d**). Following light adaptation for at least 10 minutes, photopic ffERG responses are elicited with certain flash strength for light-adapted 3 ffERG (**e**) and 30-Hz flicker stimuli for light-adapted 3.0 flicker ffERG (**f**)

3.5 Interpretation of ERG Responses

The amplitude and implicit time (or called peak time) of the a-wave and b-wave, as well as the latency of response, are important information for ERG analysis. The amplitude of the a-wave is a measure of the displacement from the baseline to the a-wave negative trough and that of the b-wave is from the a-wave negative trough to the b-wave positive peak. The implicit time is the time interval from the onset of the stimulus to its peak. The recording duration for single flash in a protocol is in the range of 250 millisecond (mS) [16] (*see* Fig. 1 for normal ERG responses).

To evaluate ERG responses, we should check for a change in amplitude (decreased) and implicit time (delay). The amplitudes of a-wave and b-wave correspond to the numbers of functional photoreceptors. The extent of retinal damage correlates to the degree of amplitude decrease. If some photoreceptors are damaged from focal lesions, such as retinal detachment, this might result in amplitude decrease without significant implicit time delayed in ERG responses. If the functions of photoreceptors are impaired in general, such as in rod-cone or cone-rod dystrophy, the amplitudes are usually decreased together with significant implicit time delayed.

Clinically, the ERG results using different equipment or from different labs/institutes might not be the same, even in a normal subject. Therefore, institutes/centers are suggested to establish their normative data for further ERG analysis. Clinicians can interpret the ERG results based on the electrode-specific and age-matched normative data. Also, test-retest reproducibility is important if clinicians plan to use ERG to monitor disease progression or test safety and efficacy after treatments [15, 16, 18].

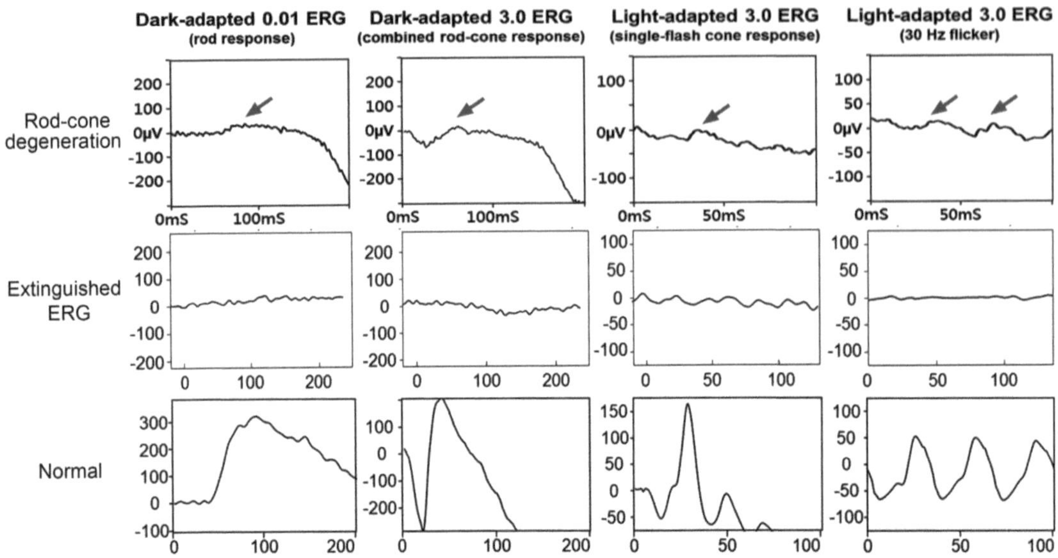

Fig. 2 Abnormal full-field electroretinogram (ffERG) responses for retinitis pigmentosa (RP). A patient in the early stages of rod-cone degeneration is illustrated by a decreased b-wave amplitudes in scotopic and photopic ffERGs (arrow) as well as delayed implicit times of the b-wave. In moderate to severe stages of degeneration, the responses are small or extinguished

3.6 The Typical ERG Findings in Patients with RP

In RP patients, their symptoms and clinical findings vary, even in those patients carrying the same gene variants or from the same family. RP falls into the category of "rod-cone dystrophy," which means the rod function is affected more than cone function. Generally, RP is characterized by rod photoreceptor dysfunction in the early stage and progressive rod and cone dysfunction in more advanced stages [16]. Typically, the dark-adapted 0.01 ERG (rod responses) shows the reduced amplitude and delayed implicit time of b-wave. The dark-adapted 3.0 ERG and dark-adapted 10.0 ERGs (combined rod-cone response) show reduced a-wave amplitude, which indicates impaired rod photoreceptor function. The b-wave amplitude is reduced because it is derived from ON-bipolar cells, which are connected to the abnormal rod photoreceptors. The light-adapted 30-Hz and light-adapted 3.0 ERGs (cone response) are typically delayed and/or reduced, but cone function is less affected than rod function (Fig. 2). With progression of the disease, the responses could be small or even nondetectable in severe or end-stage RP patients [16].

3.7 The Specialized Protocols for Differential Diagnosis

Although ffERG is used to evaluate the whole retinal function, ISCEV encourages more extensive protocols for a specific clinical condition. Clinicians should be familiar with these protocols and select suitable protocols based on patients' clinical presentation. In clinical practice, some diseases present with similar symptoms and

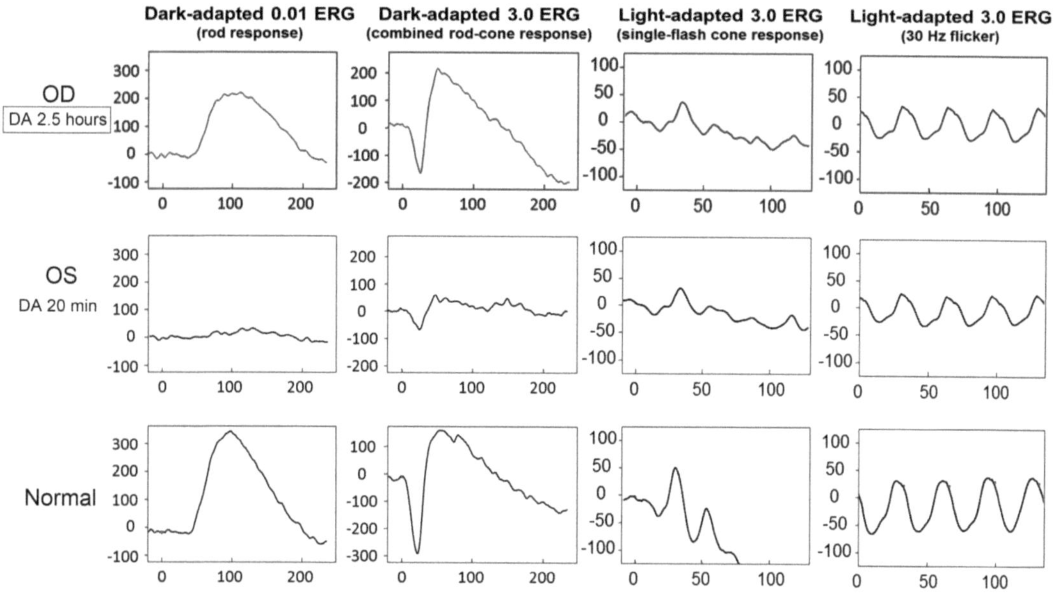

Fig. 3 Full-field electroretinogram (ffERG) recovery in fundus albipunctatus (FA) after prolonged dark adaptation. This FA patient underwent ffERG testing, revealing responses that are representative to those of a typical RP patient in the left eye, following impaired rod function in the left eye. The rod response of right eye recovered after prolonged dark adaptation (2.5 hours)

signs as RP; however, the information from ffERG is not sufficient to make the correct diagnosis, which will require specialized protocols. In this section, some specialized ERG protocols will be introduced.

3.8 Prolonged Dark Adaption

Patients with some hereditary retinal dystrophies, such as fundus albipunctatus and retinitis punctata albescens, present with retinal white dots and night blindness. Using ISCEV Standard ERG, we cannot distinguish between these two diseases. Fundus albipunctatus is characterized by multiple yellowish white dots with sparing of the macula. Compared to RP, fundus albipunctatus is stationary or relatively slowly progressive. A prolonged 2.5-hour dark adaptation can improve rod response in fundus albipunctatus (Fig. 3) [18, 23], while there is still abnormal (no change) in retinitis punctata albescens.

3.9 S-Cone ERG

Patients with enhanced S-cone syndrome (ESCS) present with night blindness and retinal pigmentation, which can resemble RP. However, there are three unique features of ESCS in full-field ERG, which could be helpful to differentiate ESCS from RP. First, extinguished rod responses in dark-adapted 0.01 ERG. Second, the waveforms in dark-adapted 3 ERG are similar to those in light-adapted 3 ERG except the amplitudes, which indicate a cone cell dominant retina. Third, the amplitude of a-wave in light-adapted

3 ERG is larger than the amplitude in light-adapted 30-Hz flicker ERG [24]. Although genetic testing of the *NR2E7* gene remains the gold standard for diagnosis of ESCS, clinicians could further test patients with the S-cone ERG, which show "enhanced" S-cone response compared to the normal population, thereby making a diagnosis before screening *NR2E3* gene [24]. S-cone ERG is an additional ERG protocol to assess short-wavelength cone response. ISCEV provides an extended protocol for the S-cone ERG by Perlman et al. [25]. For more information on this protocol, refer to https://iscev.wildapricot.org/standards/.

3.10 Predict Visual Prognosis in Patients with Retinitis Pigmentosa

ERG can be used to evaluate the photoreceptor function in patients with RP and can identify early stages of RP by detecting a delay in implicit times of b-wave [20, 26]. Moreover, ERG can be used to predict visual prognosis. Berson (2007) proposed to use a 30-Hz cone ERG amplitude to predict the remaining visual function in RP patients. His technique includes using computer averaged consecutive narrow bandpassed (electronically filtered) cone responses to improve the signal-to-noise ratio, which allows to record down to 0.05 μV. A cone ERG actuarial table, based on 6553 visits of 1039 patients, showed an estimated number of years for RP patients with their 30-Hz cone ERG amplitude to decline to 0.05 μV (i.e., virtual blindness) [27].

ERG is useful in predicting visual prognosis when patients are anxious about how RP would develop or what should be expected for their future. However, there are some limitations. For example, different ERG recording settings, such as stimulus strength range, inter-stimulus time, or recording bandpass, might result in the variability of ERG responses in RP. Caution is needed when evaluating the remaining visual function and prognosis from ERG responses of RP patients.

4 Notes

1. It should be noted that proper placement of the electrodes is essential to get accurate and reliable ERG recordings and proper electrode cleaning is also required to prevent transmission of infectious agents [15].
2. Although the ISCEV recommends a minimum of 30-minute recovery time after fundus photography, optical coherence tomography, fluorescein angiography, and retinal imaging for ERG testing, it would be better to avoid using strong light for retinal imaging before ERG testing.
3. Many factors might account for the variabilities in ERG responses, such as age, gender, refractive error, pupil size, clarity of cornea or lens, depth of anesthesia, body temperature,

duration of stimulus, time of dark adaptation or light adaptation, inter-stimulus time, systemic circulation, medication, and maturation of retina. All of these procedures should be standardized to minimize the artifacts [28].

References

1. Dewar J (1877) The physiological action of Light1. Nature 15(385):433–435
2. Kahn RH, Löwenstein A (1924) Das Elektroretinogramm. Albrecht von Graefes Archiv für Ophthalmologie 114(2):304–331
3. de-Rouck AF (2006) History of the electroretinogram. In: Heckenlively JR, Arden GB (eds) Principles and practice of clinical electrophysiology of vision. MIT Press, Cambridges, pp 3–10
4. Riggs LA (1941) Continuous and reproducible records of the electrical activity of the human retina. Proc Soc Exp Biol Med 48(1):204–207
5. Frishman LJ, Wang MH (2011) Electroretinogram of human, monkey and mouse. In: Levin LA et al (eds) Adler's physiology of the eye. Elsevier Health Sciences, pp 480–501
6. Perlman I (2007) The electroretinogram: ERG. In: Kolb H, Fernandez E, Nelson R (eds) Webvision: the organization of the retina and visual system [Internet]. University of Utah Health Sciences Center, pp 1323–1364
7. Frishman LJ (2006) Origins of the electroretinogram. In: Heckenlively JR, Arden GB (eds) Principles and practice of clinical electrophysiology of vision. MIT Press, Cambridges, pp 139–184
8. Falk G, Shiells R (2006) Synaptic transmission: sensitivity control mechanisms. In: Heckenlively JR, Arden GB (eds) Principles and practice of clinical electrophysiology of vision. MIT Press, Cambridges, pp 79–92
9. Gurevich L, Slaughter MM (1993) Comparison of the waveforms of the ON bipolar neuron and the b-wave of the electroretinogram. Vis Res 33(17):2431–2435
10. Miller RF, Dowling JE (1970) Intracellular responses of the Muller (glial) cells of mudpuppy retina: their relation to b-wave of the electroretinogram. J Neurophysiol 33(3): 323–341
11. Newman EA, Odette LL (1984) Model of electroretinogram b-wave generation: a test of the K+ hypothesis. J Neurophysiol 51(1):164–182
12. Stockton RA, Slaughter MM (1989) B-wave of the electroretinogram. A reflection of ON bipolar cell activity. J Gen Physiol 93(1): 101–122
13. Coupland SG (2006) Electrodes for visual testing. In: Heckenlively JR, Arden GB (eds) Principles and practice of clinical electrophysiology of vision. MIT Press, Cambridges, pp 245–254
14. Burian HM, Allen L (1954) A speculum contact lens electrode for electroretinography. Electroencephalogr Clin Neurophysiol 6(3): 509–511
15. McCulloch DL et al (2015) ISCEV standard for full-field clinical electroretinography (2015 update). Doc Ophthalmol 130(1):1–12
16. Lam BL (2005) Electrophysiology of vision: clinical testing and applications. CRC Press
17. Lawwill T, Burian HM (1966) A modification of the Burian-Allen contact-lens electrode for human electroretinography. Am J Ophthalmol 61(6):1506–1509
18. Robson AG et al (2018) ISCEV guide to visual electrodiagnostic procedures. Doc Ophthalmol 136(1):1–26
19. Marmor MF et al (2009) ISCEV standard for full-field clinical electroretinography (2008 update). Doc Ophthalmol 118(1):69–77
20. Berson EL (1981) Retinitis pigmentosa and allied diseases: applications of electroretinographic testing. Int Ophthalmol 4(1–2):7–22
21. Falk G (1988) Signal transmission from rods to bipolar and horizontal cells: a synthesis. Prog Retin Res 8:255–279
22. Wachtmeister L (1998) Oscillatory potentials in the retina: what do they reveal. Prog Retin Eye Res 17(4):485–521
23. Wang NK et al (2012) Multimodal fundus imaging in fundus albipunctatus with RDH5 mutation: a newly identified compound heterozygous mutation and review of the literature. Doc Ophthalmol 125(1):51–62
24. Wang NK et al (2009) Cellular origin of fundus autofluorescence in patients and mice with a defective NR2E3 gene. Br J Ophthalmol 93(9):1234–1240
25. Perlman I et al (2019) ISCEV extended protocol for the S-cone ERG. Doc Ophthalmol 140: 95–101
26. Berson EL (1993) Retinitis pigmentosa. The Friedenwald Lecture. Invest Ophthalmol Vis Sci 34(5):1659–1676

27. Berson EL (2007) Long-term visual prognoses in patients with retinitis pigmentosa: the Ludwig von Sallmann lecture. Exp Eye Res 85(1): 7–14
28. Nusinowitz S, Heckenlively JR (2006) Evaluating retinal function in the mouse retina with the electroretinogram. In: Heckenlively JR, Arden GB (eds) Principles and practice of clinical electrophysiology of vision. MIT Press, Cambridges, pp 899–910

Chapter 11

Visual Function Tests: Visual Fields

Angela Y. Chang

Abstract

Visual field tests, also known as perimetry tests, are used to assess progression of ophthalmic diseases such as retinitis pigmentosa (RP) by monitoring changes in a patient's visual field (VF). VF loss corresponds to damage at any point in the visual pathway, including the retina, such as in RP. Damage to different parts of this pathway corresponds to characteristic VF defects. Perimetry tests are subjective, as they are functional tests that help physicians identify abnormal fields as well as quantitatively assess VF sensitivity. The results may also be informative of a patient's visual function crucial for performing day-to-day activities. Automated perimetry tests are among the most commonly used, with the most common being automated static perimetry.

Key words Interpreting visual fields, Perimetry, Retinitis pigmentosa, Scotoma, Visual field

1 Introduction

Retinitis pigmentosa (RP) results in progressive peripheral visual field (VF) loss, leading to tunnel vision in end stages in which only the central VF is preserved. VF defects in RP frequently present with a partial or complete ring scotoma, a concentric area of field loss in the midperiphery, the area of the retina that contains the highest density of rod photoreceptors [1, 2]. These initial changes typically manifest as nyctalopia, or night blindness [1]. Subsequent VF loss can occur toward the periphery or toward the center from the ring scotoma and affect the cone photoreceptors. As the cones undergo degeneration in advanced stages of RP, the macular region of the retina may become affected [1, 2].

The etiology of VF loss may show characteristic changes in the VF. In addition to the aforementioned pattern typically seen in RP, cataracts may lead to global attenuation in VF sensitivity. In glaucoma, an arcuate defect following the pattern of the retinal nerve fibers or a nasal step is often observed in early stages. Later stages of glaucomatous damage result in loss of peripheral VF [3]. Macular degeneration, in contrast, leads to VF defects in the central field.

Stephen H. Tsang and Peter M. J. Quinn (eds.), *Retinitis Pigmentosa*,
Methods in Molecular Biology, vol. 2560, https://doi.org/10.1007/978-1-0716-2651-1_11,

Given the specificity of VF defects to each respective retinal dystrophy, VF tests serve as essential tools used in the diagnosis and clinical management of ophthalmic or neurologic disorders.

Perimetry is the clinical measurement of the VF, and it typically assesses the monocular field of vision when the eye is fixated on a central point. With central fixation, a normal VF extends 90° temporally, 50° superiorly and nasally, and 60° inferiorly [4]. The physiologic scotoma lays within the temporal hemifield 12–17° from fixation and 1.5° below the horizontal meridian [4]. This blind spot corresponds to the location where the retinal ganglion cell axons that comprise the optic nerve exit the retina. Thus, there are no photoreceptors in this region.

The VF varies along the *island of vision*, which is a reflection of the distribution of the rod and cone photoreceptors in the retina. The visual acuity in a specific area of the VF is a reflection of the distribution of these photoreceptors. Rod photoreceptors are concentrated in the periphery and are more responsible for night vision. Ninety-five percent of the photoreceptors in human eyes are rods, and they have their maximum density 20° outside the fovea [1]. The remaining 5% of photoreceptors are cones, most densely concentrated in the fovea, and they are responsible for color vision [1]. Additionally, the fovea is a depression in the retina that is responsible for the highest degree of visual acuity. The macular region at the center of the retina encompasses the fovea and is critical for acuity-related vision. This region, encompassing ±8° surrounding the fovea, contains the highest density of retinal ganglion cells (RGCs) [5]. Thus, the macula is a particular area of interest in the retina given its importance in determining visual function, quality of life, and ability to perform day-to-day activities [6].

Given that each dystrophy involves progressive degeneration of various regions of the retina, changes to visual acuity may not always adequately assess progression. VF tests that focus on measuring the central VF may be more sensitive to changes in visual functioning, while those that encompass a more comprehensive measure of the VF can uncover scotomas in the periphery of which a patient may not immediately be aware. Thus, perimetry tests may be useful in evaluating different types and stages of disease. Changes in and presence of scotomas in the VF do not necessarily indicate early disease—these changes in the VF may indicate that substantial structural damage has already occurred. In diseases such as RP, which begins with progressive loss in the peripheral VF, even with extensive loss of peripheral vision, patients may still retain their visual acuity. In more advanced stages, when the macula becomes affected, there are often more significant changes in visual acuity.

2 Materials

1. *Confrontation VF testing* is commonly used to screen for VF defects. The patient is asked to fixate at a point straight ahead, such as the evaluator's nose, and state how many fingers they see the evaluator holding up without shifting gaze. The examiner covers their eye that is on the opposite side of the VF being tested to ensure appropriate assessment of the patient's VF. During the test, the examiner holds up different numbers of fingers midway between the examiner and the patient in the four quadrants of the VF. Confrontation testing is a method to screen for any gross scotomas that may be present. It is also used when the patient is unable to take an automated perimetry test, which may be due to physical limitations or ability to concentrate for the full length of the test.
2. An *Amsler grid* is used to assess changes in the central VF, and it is a measurement of macular function. The grid is composed of intersecting black vertical and horizontal lines, as shown in Fig. 1. The patient holds the grid 14–16 inches away from their eye and focuses one eye on the dot at the center of the grid at a time. If any of the vertical or horizontal lines appear wavy, blurry, or blank to the patient, there may be changes in the

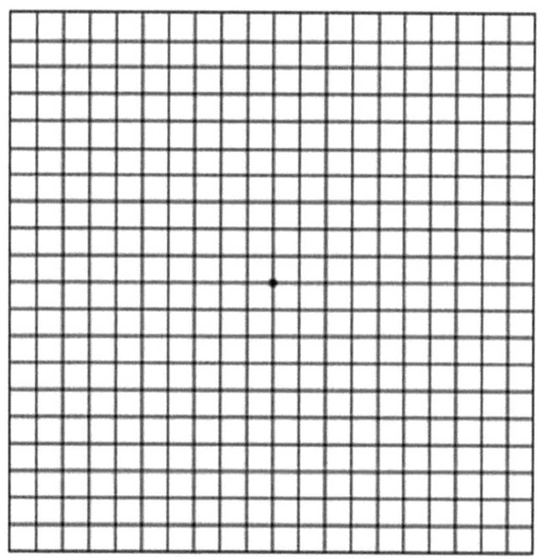

Fig. 1 Amsler grid [17]. An Amsler grid provides a means to assess changes in the central visual field (VF)/macular function. The grid is composed of intersecting black vertical and horizontal lines. The patient holds the grid 14–16 inches away from their eye and focuses one eye on the dot at the center of the grid at a time. If any of the vertical or horizontal lines appear wavy, blurry, or blank to the patient, there may be changes in the patient's central VF. These signs may also indicate disease progression

patient's central VF. These signs may also indicate disease progression. The Amsler grid is often used to monitor VF changes in patients with age-related macular degeneration and can indicate the transition from dry to wet macular degeneration, where fluid accumulation under the retina may make the straight lines appear different [7].

3. In *kinetic perimetry*, moving light stimuli of constant intensity are used to map out the borders of the VF. An example is Goldmann perimetry, where the stimuli are moved from areas outside the VF into the VF.
4. In *static automated perimetry*, stationary light stimuli of different intensities are shown to map out the patient's VF, typically for 200 ms. The stimuli are presented at predetermined locations by the perimeter. The intensities may change throughout the test, depending on the patient's response. Intensity refers to the size, luminance, and intensity of the light stimulus [8]. An example of automated perimetry is the Humphrey Field Analzyer. Automated perimetry tests are typically static and are used to obtain a detailed map of VF that is more sensitive and specific to VF defects. Using lights of different intensities and sizes, the machine maps out the patient's field of vision.

   Among the most commonly used automated static perimetry tests are the Humphrey VF 10-2, 24-2, and 30-2 tests. They differ in the size of the VF that is tested and the number of points tested. These tests measure the central 10° (10-2), 24° (24-2), or 30° (30-2) of the VF. The 30-2 tests the central 30° of the VF with 76 points each spaced 6° apart. The 24-2 tests the central 24° of the VF with 54 points each spaced 6° apart. Importantly, only four of these points are in the macular region. The large spacing between these points means that changes in the macula affecting the central vision may be missed. The 10-2 test tests the central 10° field with 68 points each spaced 2° apart. Thus, VF testing using 24-2 or 30-2 may miss damage within the central 10° of the VF, the region that corresponds to the macula. In contrast, the 10-2 test is more sensitive to central defects and changes in the macular region. Especially toward end stages of RP, evaluating VF changes in the central, macular region is crucial.

   The second parameter outlined in the test name, such as the 2 in 24-2, indicates the alignment of the tested VF grid is aligned to the visual axis [9]. The 2 indicates that the points being tested straddle the horizontal and vertical meridians [9]. A parameter of 1 would indicate that the points overlay the horizontal and vertical meridian. The parameters in the most commonly used tests, such as the 30-2 and 24-2, are chosen to maximize speed of test and, thus, patient compliance. Additionally, they were chosen to maximize the amount of the visual cortex that is measured. The 24-2 and 30-2 tests examine 80% and 83% of the visual cortex, respectively [10, 11].

3 Methods

3.1 Taking a VF Test

When taking the VF test, the patient looks into a dome-shaped VF machine and fixates their eye at a specific point. Each eye is tested individually, and the one not being tested is covered. If the patient has a refractive error in the tested eye, a prescription lens is placed in front of that eye during the test to ensure that the visual stimuli presented during the test appear in focus. This type of refractive correction is done for tests measuring up to 30° of the central field [8]. It is important that the technician running the VF test ensures proper alignment of the test subject's eye and the lens. The examiner should also examine the patient's eyelids for evidence of ptosis, which may interfere with evaluation of the VF. In this case, taping of the eyelids can rid potential visual obstruction and result in a more accurate assessment of the VF [8]. To ensure integrity of the test, the ambient lighting in the room of test administration should be set at the level recommended by the manufacturer to ensure test validity [8]. During the test, light stimuli of different sizes and intensities appear at different locations on the perimeter encompassing a 180° space to map out the patient's field of vision. Each time the patient sees a light stimulus, they are told to press a button.

3.1.1 Testing Stimuli

Stimulus sizes range from I to V from smallest to largest (1/4–64 mm^2) [12]. Most commonly, a size III (2.26 mm diameter, 4 mm^2), white stimulus is used. Red and blue stimuli projected on the white background can also be used. Background luminance typically ranges from 1 to 10 cd/m^2 [8]. In static automated perimetry, the intensity of a stimulus depends on luminance, size, and contrast [8]. The value is expressed in decibels (dB) on a logarithmic scale.

3.1.2 Testing Algorithms to Estimate Threshold Intensities

The full threshold algorithm determines the lowest intensity stimulus that can be visualized at each of the tested points 50% of the time. To determine the threshold at each point, the stimulus intensity is decreased until it is no longer detected. The intensity is then increased until it is visualized again. While this method allows for careful determination of the sensitivities at each point, the testing duration may be very long, extending up to 20 min for patient with glaucoma [13]. Thus, patients may lose focus during the exam and decrease the reliability of the results. While abbreviated full threshold tests such as the Fastpac are available, they are not as reliable as the full threshold test [13]. A newer algorithm, the Swedish

Interactive Testing Algorithm (SITA), maintains the same or even greater testing reliability as the full threshold algorithm while shortening test times by up to 50% [13]. Full threshold values, as described above, are determined for the first four points in each quadrant of the VF. Subsequent threshold values are determined by estimating threshold values based on stimuli presented at that location as well as adjacent locations.

3.2 Interpreting the VF Test Printout

The top of the printout from the VF test is divided into two sections: Test Parameters and Reliability Indices. The *Test Parameters* section highlights demographic information including patient name, date of birth, eye that was tested, whether a trial lens was used, and test parameters (e.g., 24-2). In addition to correctly identifying the patient, having the correct date of birth is crucial because threshold values from the test are compared to values from age-adjusted normal controls. Since different test programs are used to evaluate and follow different diseases, noting that the correct test program was used is essential. Additionally, a pupillary diameter of at least 2.5 mm should be noted; miosis can result in an erroneously depressed or constricted VF [10].

The *Reliability Indices* section includes fixation losses, false positives, false negatives, and the gaze tracking monitor, all of which help assess the reliability of a test. According to the Humphrey VF manufacturer, a reliable field meets the following standards: less than 33% false positives, 33% false negatives, and less than 20% fixation losses [14].

The gaze tracking monitor records the movement of the tested eye and is a subjective tool that allows clinicians to evaluate fixation during the VF test. It is particularly useful if scotomas surround the physiological blind spot [15].

The Heijl–Krakau method is employed by many automated perimeters to monitor fixation losses. This method involves the VF machine first determining the patient's physiologic blind spot and then periodically presenting stimuli into the physiologic blind spot throughout the test. Any stimuli presented to the patient's blind spot that the patient indicates as perceived signifies fixation loss. For example, if the patient looks around during the test, stimuli projected at the location of the predetermined physiologic blind spot may be perceived. High rates of fixation losses may mask underlying VF defects, especially those in early stages [16].

False negatives occur when the patient does not detect a stimulus at a higher intensity, usually 9 dB, at the same location a previous lower intensity stimulus was perceived. False negatives may be due to testing fatigue or lapses in attention. False positives occur when the patient indicates perception of a stimulus when none is present. False positive responses are recorded when there is a response sooner than the minimum reaction time of 180 ms or when there is a recorded response between the presentation of two stimuli [14]. High rates of false positives may occur when the patient is "trigger happy" and eager not to miss any presented stimuli. Of all the reliability indices, a high false positive rate is the most detrimental to the integrity and reliability of the test, since it can mask scotomas, especially those in early stages. Additionally, false positives may be a good indicator of patient alertness throughout the duration of the test, since false negatives could be a reflection of a true VF defect [14].

Below the reliability indices are a series of graphs, including the visual sensitivity map and its corresponding gray scale, the total deviation, and pattern deviation. At the top is the *visual sensitivity map* that measures the threshold of stimulus activity at all the tested points recorded as decibels (dB) of attenuation. The threshold is defined as the lowest intensity stimulus that is seen 50% of the time at each location [11]. Higher sensitivity values correlate with being able to visualize a lower intensity stimulus. A sensitivity of 0 dB correlates with the brightest, nonattenuated stimulus shown. In total, 51 dB corresponds to the dimmest stimulus. The sensitivity at each location tested is plotted on the map.

The gray scale is a visual representation of the sensitivity values from the visual sensitivity map. Darker regions indicate poorer sensitivity to the stimuli, while lighter regions indicate higher sensitivity. The gray scale is useful for quickly identifying any gross scotomas and patterns of field loss. However, it only indicates depressions in the visual with respect to the patient's baseline in other areas of the field.

The *total deviation* plot compares the sensitivity values at each point in the patient's VF with those of an age-matched control. It allows for visualization of abnormal points in a VF that are more likely to be statistically significant. A value of 0 dB indicates that there is no difference in sensitivity at that location compared to the control. Negative values in this plot indicate decreased visual sensitivity with respect to the mean population. Larger negative values correlate with a greater depression in sensitivity. The numeric total deviation plot also has a corresponding visual plot, which indicates the probability that each of the tested points is normal [10]. The scale ranges from <5% to <0.5%. The lower the probability that a point is normal, the darker the point appears on the graph [10]. Darker regions are more likely to correlate with statistically significant points of VF depression. It should be noted that any processes that lead to a global attenuation in sensitivity, such as a cataract, would be reflected as a generalized depression in sensitivity in the total deviation plot. To assess for any focal areas of depression in visual sensitivity, the *pattern deviation* plot should be used. The plot accounts for any overall depression in sensitivity with respect to the eye's island of vision by subtracting the TD values in the upper 85th percentile, highlighting underlying focal scotomas.

The global indices section summarizes quantitatively the patient's VF loss and includes the mean deviation, pattern standard deviation, and VF index. The *mean deviation* is the average of all the values from the total deviation plot. It highlights the overall depression in a patient's VF with respect to a normal patient. Normal values are typically 0–2 dB. The values become more negative as the overall field worsens. Since the mean deviation is an average of field changes at all the tested points, it is more useful for monitoring global changes in VF loss than focal changes. The pattern standard deviation reflects the standard deviation of all points in the pattern deviation graph and compares the shape of the VF with that of a control. Large values correlate with increased abnormalities in the patient's hill of vision [10].

3.3 Challenges and Limitations with VF Testing

While automated perimetry is useful for gaining a comprehensive evaluation of the VF, the testing conditions and requirements may be impractical for certain patients or in certain situations [4]. Patients with physical limitations or short attention spans, particularly those at the extremes of age, may not be able to complete the test, reducing reliability. Patients also need to understand a complex set of directions to accurately take the test.

Additionally, VF exams are subjective tests based on patient perception. Thus, they should be paired with anatomic structural tests such as optical coherence tomography (OCT) to monitor progression. The development of optical coherence tomography (OCT) has revolutionized how physicians are able to detect changes in the retina. OCT is a noninvasive imaging test that takes cross-sections of the retina and allows for visualization of the different layers of the retina and the optic nerve. Regions of structural changes in the retina can correspond to abnormal regions on the VF, but OCT is also sensitive to regions of thinning on patients who have VF determined to be within normal limits [5]. Theoretically, there should be correlation in the patterns of change on the VF and OCT, but patient subjectivity may influence the degree of correlation.

VF tests measure a patient's subjective visual function and are informative for assessing their ability to carry out activities of daily living. These tests are valuable tools for diagnosis and monitoring of disease progression. There are many types of VF tests used to assess different types of vision loss, and they may be useful for differentiating between ophthalmic and neurologic processes. Among them, automated perimetry tests are some of the most commonly used VF tests to map VFs and assess ophthalmic disease processes. These subjective tests can be paired with structural anatomical tests such as OCT to monitor ophthalmic disease progression.

References

1. Liu G, Liu X, Li H et al (2016) Optical coherence tomographic analysis of retina in retinitis pigmentosa patients. Ophthalmic Res 56(3): 111–122. https://doi.org/10.1159/000445063
2. Vamos R, Tatrai E, Nemeth J et al (2011) The structure and function of the macula in patients with advanced retinitis pigmentosa. Invest Ophthalmol Vis Sci 52(11):8425–8432. https://doi.org/10.1167/iovs.11-7780
3. Broadway DC (2012) Visual field testing for glaucoma - a practical guide. Community Eye Health 25(79–80):66–70
4. Spector R (1990) Chapter 116 Visual fields. In: Clinical methods: the history, physical, and laboratory examinations, 3rd edn. Butterworths, Boston
5. Hood DC, Raza AS, de Moraes CG et al (2013) Glaucomatous damage of the macula. Prog Retin Eye Res 32:1–21. https://doi.org/10.1016/j.preteyeres.2012.08.003
6. De Moraes CG, Sun A, Jarukasetphon R et al (2019) Association of macular visual field measurements with glaucoma staging systems. JAMA Ophthalmol 137(2):139–145. https://doi.org/10.1001/jamaophthalmol.2018.5398
7. Boyd K (2016) Have AMD? Save your sight with an Amsler grid. https://www.aao.org/eye-health/tips-prevention/facts-about-amsler-grid-daily-vision-test
8. Sample PA, Dannheim F, Artes PH et al (2011) Imaging and Perimetry Society standards and guidelines. Optom Vis Sci 88(1):4–7. https://doi.org/10.1097/OPX.0b013e3181fc3735
9. Carroll JN, Johnson CA (2013) Visual field testing: from one medical student to another. http://EyeRounds.org/tutorials/VF-testing/
10. Yaqub M (2012) Visual fields interpretation in glaucoma: a focus on static automated perimetry. Community Eye Health 25(79–80):1–8
11. American Academy of Ophthalmology. Automated static perimetry. https://www.aao.org/bcscsnippetdetail.aspx?id=7d681413-674c-4f69-a630-12ee8d82da35
12. Humphrey Field Analyzer (2010) Humphrey Field Analyzer II-i series User Manual
13. Bengtsson B, Heijl A, Olsson J (1998) Evaluation of a new threshold visual field strategy, SITA, in normal subjects. Swedish Interactive Thresholding Algorithm. Acta Ophthalmol Scand 76(2):165–169. https://doi.org/10.1034/j.1600-0420.1998.760208.x
14. Katz J, Sommer A, Witt K (1991) Reliability of visual field results over repeated testing. Ophthalmology 98(1):70–75. https://doi.org/10.1016/s0161-6420(91)32339-x
15. Kunimatsu S, Suzuki Y, Shirato S et al (2000) Usefulness of gaze tracking during perimetry in glaucomatous eyes. Jpn J Ophthalmol 44(2): 190–191
16. Ishiyama Y, Murata H, Asaoka R (2015) The usefulness of gaze tracking as an index of visual field reliability in glaucoma patients. Invest Ophthalmol Vis Sci 56(11):6233–6236. https://doi.org/10.1167/iovs.15-17661
17. Macular Edema (2019) National Institutes of Health. https://www.nei.nih.gov/learn-about-eye-health/eye-conditions-and-diseases/macular-edema

Chapter 12

Visual Function Tests

Ritah Chumdermpadetsuk, Sara D. Ragi, and Stephen H. Tsang

Abstract

Inherited retinal diseases (IRDs), including retinitis pigmentosa, have devastating consequences for the visual function of affected individuals. Chief among these are a gradual loss of visual field, visual acuity, and night vision (otherwise known as nyctalopia). These changes often occur slowly, over a course of decades. Objective modalities for assessing these many aspects of visual function are crucial, not only to the monitoring of disease progression but, in recent years, also to evaluating the efficacy or lack thereof of new therapeutic interventions in the setting of clinical trials. This chapter will provide descriptions of these valuable assessment modalities, alongside discussions of their advantages and limitations in the context of serving those afflicted by IRDs.

Key words Inherited retinal disease, Retinitis pigmentosa, Visual field, Visual acuity, Nyctalopia, Visual function

1 Introduction

1.1 Visual Acuity

Visual acuity (VA) refers to the sharpness or clarity of vision and the ability of eyes to perceive fine details. It is required in detail-oriented tasks such as reading and facial recognition. It is dependent on (1) how accurately the cornea and lens focus light on the retina, (2) the health and functioning of the photoreceptors of the retina and retinal pigment epithelium (RPE), and (3) the ability of the brain to interpret information received from the eyes [1]. VA is lost in advanced stages of retinitis pigmentosa (RP), as a result of the degeneration of cone photoreceptors in the macula [2]. The measurement of VA allows clinicians and researchers to follow the progression and/or improvement of disease and to assess the efficacy of various therapeutic interventions.

VA is the most common measure of visual function in both clinical practice and in clinical trials. It is often tested using high-contrast charts with standardized letters of graded sizes to determine the smallest object which may be seen at a specified distance [3]. The gold standard for VA measurements in clinical studies is

Stephen H. Tsang and Peter M. J. Quinn (eds.), *Retinitis Pigmentosa*,
Methods in Molecular Biology, vol. 2560, https://doi.org/10.1007/978-1-0716-2651-1_12,

the Early Treatment of Diabetic Retinopathy Study (ETDRS) best-corrected VA (BCVA) test chart [3]. Subjects are tested, one eye at a time, at three distances (4 m, 2 m, and 0.5 m), under optimal conditions (namely, using best correction either with the patient's own glasses or contact lenses and conducting the test within a well-illuminated setting) [3]. Within each eye, and at each distance, VA is determined based on the lowest lines (sporting the smallest letters) on which the letters were correctly identified. An equivalent test for children is the HOTV chart, which includes only the letters H, O, T, and V, all of which are centered around a vertical axis and could be easily identified by children [3]. VA is reported as one distance over another, for example 20/400. This denotes that the patient can see at 20 feet what someone with normal vision can see at 400 feet. In some cases of severe disease, subjects are unable to identify even the largest lines of the letters on the chart. In these cases, off-chart VA measurements can be collected. These refer to a gradation of counting fingers, hand motion perception, light perception, and no light perception [3].

The letter size on each successive line of the ETDRS chart follows a geometric progression, such that BCVA can be converted to a visual angle score (LogMAR, or Logarithm of the Minimum Angle of Resolution) allowing for comparison analyses where smaller LogMAR values correlate with VA loss [3]. For these analyses, a 0.1 change in LogMAR corresponds to a five-letter (one line) change on the ETDRS chart [3]. Off-chart VA measurements, on the other hand, are analyzed by assigning LogMAR values using a scale adapted from Lange et al., in which there is a 0.3-log-unit step in between two successive grades of VA (e.g., counting fingers and hand motion perception) [4].

1.2 Visual Field (VF)

The VF is the spatial array of visual sensation that is available to an individual while their eye is focused on a central point [5]. In normal individuals, the monocular VF consists of central vision, which includes the inner 30° of vision and central fixation, and the peripheral VF, which extends approximately 60° nasally and 100° temporally from the vertical meridian and 60° above and 75° below the horizontal meridian [5]. The binocular VF results from the superimposition of the two monocular fields.

VF loss of a certain severity may have a significant impact on the quality of life, independence, and mobility of patients [6]. It results in the reduced ability of patients to detect peripheral objects and to avoid obstacles, which, in turn, negatively impacts their performance of tasks requiring ambulation in challenging settings (e.g., along crowded city streets, negotiating stairwells) and driving [6]. For example, many countries and states have set legal limits for VF in order for an individual to qualify for a driver's license.

In RP, there is generally a pattern of progressive concentric VF loss [2]. Changes usually begin with asymmetric VF loss and/or scotomas in the mid-peripheral regions, which, over many years, can progress to an end stage in which only the central VF remains [2]. For this reason, VF testing is another important modality in following the progression of RP.

VFs can be assessed by kinetic and/or static techniques, by instruments that are operated either manually or automatically (computerized) [3]. All methods follow the same basic setup first developed by Hans Goldmann, which comprises an apparatus where a patient is seated with their chin in a chin rest and a dome-shaped screen [3]. The patient is asked to focus the eye being tested on a central point on the dome-shaped screen, while the contralateral eye is patched. In kinetic perimetry, the test stimulus (most often, a bright light superimposed on a white background) is moved from the non-seeing to the seeing area (in other words, from beyond the edge of the VF into the field), and the boundary at which the test stimuli are first perceived is mapped out; this boundary constitutes the limits of the patient's VF [3]. On the other hand, static perimetry involves the measurement of the relative intensity thresholds of individual points in the VF [3]. In reaching these measurements, the size and location of the target stimulus is kept constant, while the brightness is incrementally diminished until a threshold level is identified for each specified test location [3].

2 Materials

1. Goldmann visual field.
2. Humphrey visual field.
3. Full-field stimulus (FST) testing.
4. Visual Function Questionnaire (VFQ-25).

3 Methods

3.1 Goldmann Visual Field

The Goldmann VF test remains the gold standard and most often used method for kinetic perimetry [3]. In this manual test, the patient fixates upon the central target, situated 33 cm away, while the technician, who sits opposite the patient, views them through an eyepiece and ensures good fixation. The technician moves the light from the far periphery centrally into the patient's VF, as the patient indicates when they can first detect the light by pressing a button. The technician manually plots the patient's responses on a standardized graphic display form representing the VF. The test is repeated using a variety of sizes (graded I through V) and intensities of the target light stimuli. Finally, the isopters (a contour line connecting all the points of detection in the VF for stimuli of the same size and intensity) are drawn, demonstrating the boundaries of the patient's VF otherwise known as the "hill of vision" [5].

While in clinical practice, Goldmann VF tests are usually assessed qualitatively, by subjective comparison of shape, size, and area of the fields, in order to gain an impression of any changes over time, a more rigorous, numerically based method of assessment has been developed for use in research and clinical trials. In this approach, Goldmann VFs are reported as a sum total number of degrees that patients are able to perceive across all 24 meridians [3]. The extent of the VF is measured along each of the 24 meridians from the central fixation point to the boundary of the detected VF [3]. Then, the measure from each of the 24 meridian measurements is added together, representing the sum total for that eye [3]. Higher sum total degrees demonstrate a greater area of functional and light-sensitive retina, in other words, a less limited VF in the tested eye [3]. In this approach, the maximal VF is approximately 1200–1400 sum total degrees in individuals without VF defects [3].

3.2 Humphrey Visual Field

The Humphrey VF Analyzer is a computerized system, first introduced in the 1970s, which is an excellent modality for the measurement of static fields [3]. It involves the same basic setup as the Goldmann test, in which the patient sits in front of a dome-shaped white screen, with their chin stabilized by a chin rest [3]. Like in the Goldmann test, the tested eye is fixed on a central target, while the contralateral eye is patched; the patient indicates by pressing a button when a light stimulus is detected [3]. The key difference between the Goldmann perimetry and Humphrey VF is that in the Humphrey test, the test stimulus is stationary rather than moving across the VF [3]. The automated machine displays test stimuli of pre-determined size and location, each for a duration of 200 ms, in incrementally reduced intensities until the dimmest stimulus which can be detected by the patient 50% of the time is reached. Unlike Goldmann, the Humphrey VF test only utilizes target stimuli of one size, with the default being size V.

This process is repeated at multiple locations across the VF. Generally, the most common setup is the "24-2" setting, which tests 54 locations across the central 24°. Smaller and wider visual angle setups are also available and include, for example, the 10-2 which assesses the central 10° with a 68-point grid or the 30-2 which assesses the central 30° with a 76-point grid. In addition, the mean macula threshold may be calculated by deriving the mean of 16 points tested within the central 4° of vision, which correspond anatomically to the macular region of the retina [3], while the foveal threshold (which measures the function of the central cone-rich area of the macula, where VA is highest) is measured directly by the computerized analyzer [3]. Wider visual angles, on the other hand, come with the trade-off of poorer grid resolutions and, hence, a greater probability of missing small scotomas.

The Goldmann and Humphrey VF tests each have their own limitations and advantages. For one, the Goldmann test allows for maximal engagement of patient cooperation and for patient fixation to be monitored by the technician. Hence, it is more frequently used in patients with poor vision or nystagmus. On the other hand, this is a test which is limited by the availability of skilled personnel and is more vulnerable to human fatigue and bias, while the Humphrey test, through being based in computerized algorithms, is both more convenient and allows for automatic comparison of each patient's result to age-matched normative data [3]. Furthermore, while Goldmann perimetry more sensitively identifies peripheral scotomas, the Humphrey Analyzer is more sensitive to slight changes in the central field (the macula and fovea) [3]. All in all, the two tests are complementary of one another and are often best employed simultaneously in clinical and research settings.

3.3 Full-Field Stimulus (FST) Testing

The FST test is a modality for assessing light sensitivity of the entire retina by measuring the patient's perception of different light intensities [3]. It is an especially valuable test for nyctalopia, or an insufficient capacity to adapt to darkness, which is commonly experienced by patients with RP as they lose the function of their rod photoreceptors [3]. Patients not only see more poorly in darkness but also require a greater period of adjustment from brightly lit areas to dim ones. Nyctalopia becomes progressively more severe over the natural course of the disease; the use of the FST test allows for these changes to be monitored over time [2].

To conduct this test, the patient's eye is first dilated and double-patched in a dark room for a duration of 40 min, allowing for dark adaptation to occur [3]. After this period, each eye is tested individually (keeping the contralateral eye patched). The patient is brought before a Ganzfeld dome (a 40-cm diameter dome-shaped white screen), where a light flashes inside the entire dome accompanied by a beeping sound [3]. Each time a beep sounds, the patient indicates whether or not they had perceived a light via pressing a button [3]. The test is often repeated, for each eye, using different-colored stimuli [3]. A computerized algorithm then identifies the minimal luminous intensity at which the light was reliably perceived and converts the measurement from the relative unit (decibels) to the absolute unit (candela second per square meter) [3]. The light sensitivity of the retina is computed based on its inverse relationship with the recorded threshold luminous intensity [3].

The advantages of FST for IRDs are many-fold. For one, as mentioned above, it is an excellent means of assessing nyctalopia. In addition, unlike many other tests of visual function, its reliability is not affected by the condition of nystagmus [3], which, although rare in RP, is often seen in Leber congenital amaurosis. Moreover, it covers a broad spectrum of visual function and is therefore a useful tool for the assessment of patients at various stages of the disease course, ranging from those with normal vision to those with profound impairment [3]. Furthermore, this test measures the overall visual function of the eye being tested and does not rely on extrapolation of findings in specific areas of the retina, thus eliminating the inherent sampling bias of many other tests.

3.4 Visual Function Questionnaire (VFQ-25)

Last but not least, visual function may be assessed by patient-reported outcome, which, although far less objective than all the aforementioned modalities, has the unique advantage of providing a holistic picture of the patient's overall performance and disease narrative. There have been various attempts to standardize and quantify the patient narrative aspect of visual function assessment, for example, the 25-item Visual Function Questionnaire (VFQ-25) [7], whose development was sponsored by the National Eye Institute. The survey was created for general use in all patients with chronic eye diseases and measures the impact of visual impairment on activities of daily living which are dependent on vision, as well as generic health domains such as emotional well-being and social functioning.

The VFQ-25 consists of a base set of 25 vision-related questions spanning 11 domains, plus an additional single-item general health rating question [7]. These 11 domains include global vision rating (1 question), difficulty with near vision activities (3 questions), difficulty with distance vision activities (3 questions), limitations in social functioning due to vision (2 questions), role limitations due to vision (2 questions), dependency on others due to vision [3], mental health symptoms due to vision (4 questions), driving difficulties (3 questions), limitations with peripheral (1 question) and color vision (1 question), and ocular pain (2 questions) [7].

Each question is accompanied by a scale of numerical answers, in which higher scores correspond to greater perceived degree of difficulty (and thus, greater vision loss). For example, one question asks, "Because of your eyesight, how much difficulty do you have going down steps, stairs, or curbs in dim light or at night?" In response, patients must choose a number on a 1–6 scale in which 1 corresponded to "No difficulty at all," 5 corresponded to "Stopped doing this because of my eyesight," and 6 corresponded to "Stopped doing this for other reasons." The patient's responses are then re-coded on a scale of 0–100, following a standardized algorithm, so that a high score represents better functioning

[7]. Finally, the average of the all 25 numerical responses is reported as the patient's final score [7]. Increases in this score over time represent an alleviation of the patient's perceived difficulty in their activities of daily living and, potentially, improvements in their visual function [7].

Of all the tests mentioned above, this is one which is most vulnerable to inherent bias. Disease trajectories revealed by this method should undergo correlation and/or confirmation with other visual function assessment modalities.

3.5 Summary

In RP, the degeneration of RPE and photoreceptors leads to many modalities of vision loss. In the early stages of the disease, the loss of rod photoreceptors often manifests as nyctalopia and mid-peripheral scotomata (areas of partial alteration in the VF consisting of a partially diminished or entirely degenerated VA surrounded by a field of relatively well-preserved vision) that expand over time to involve the entire periphery. In advanced disease, loss of cone photoreceptors in the macula leads to progressive constriction of the central VF and worsening VA.

The gold standard for VA assessment in clinical trials is the ETDRS BCVA test chart, which may be applied to other patients, including those with RP. The assessment of VF is best conducted with both the kinetic and static techniques, which have complementary sets of advantages and limitations. The Goldmann test remains the gold standard method of kinetic perimetry, while the Humphrey VF Analyzer is a computerized system that has demonstrated its excellent utility in the measurement of a static field. Moreover, the FST test, which assesses the light sensitivity of the entire retina, is relatively new but also proven method, which is particularly useful for the detection of nyctalopia. Using a combined approach to these modalities, the progression or improvement of RP may be accurately followed over time.

Conflicts of Interest

Stephen H. Tsang receives financial support from Abeona Therapeutics, Inc and Emendo. He is also the founder of Rejuvitas and is on the scientific and clinical advisory board for Nanoscope Therapeutics.

References

1. Levenson JH, Kozarsky A (1990) Visual acuity. In: Walker HK, Hall WD, Hurst JW (eds) Clinical methods: the history, physical, and laboratory examinations, 3rd edn. Butterworths, Boston. Chapter 115. Available from: https://www.ncbi.nlm.nih.gov/books/NBK219/
2. Roberta A (1988) Pagon, retinitis pigmentosa. Surv Ophthalmol 33(3):137–177. ISSN 0039-6257, https://doi.org/10.1016/0039-6257(88)90085-9
3. Spark Therapeutics Briefing Document: October 12, 2017

4. Lange C, Feltgen N, Junker B, Schulze-Bonsel-K, Bach M (2009) Resolving the clinical acuity categories "hand motion" and "counting fingers" using the Freiburg Visual Acuity Test (FrACT). Graefes Arch Clin Exp Ophthalmol 247(1):137–142
5. Levenson JH, Kozarsky A (1990) Visual fields. In: Walker HK, Hall WD, Hurst JW (eds) Clinical methods: the history, physical, and laboratory examinations, 3rd edn. Butterworths, Boston. Chapter 116. Available from: https://www.ncbi.nlm.nih.gov/books/NBK219/
6. National Academies of Sciences, Engineering, and Medicine; Health and Medicine Division; Board on Population Health and Public Health Practice; Committee on Public Health Approaches to Reduce Vision Impairment and Promote Eye Health (2016) In: Welp A, Woodbury RB, McCoy MA et al (eds) Making eye health a population health imperative. National Academies Press (US), Washington, DC
7. National Eye Institute (August 2000) Version 2000 The National Eye Institute 25-item visual function questionnaire. https://nei.nih.gov/sites/default/files/nei-pdfs/manual_cm2000.pdf

Chapter 13

Visual Acuity as a Measurement of Visual Function

Zachary E. Snow

Abstract

Visual acuity (VA) is a traditional measure of central visual function, particularly the ability of the eye to perceive details. In a clinical setting, standardized charts are commonly used to quickly assess VA. Namely, the Early Treatment of Diabetic Retinopathy Study (ETDRS) VA test chart is the gold standard for VA testing in the clinical setting. This chapter outlines the standard procedures associated with measuring VA.

Key words Early Treatment of Diabetic Retinopathy Study (ETDRS), HOTV chart, Visual acuity, VA testing, Visual impairment

1 Introduction

Retinitis pigmentosa (RP) is an inherited retinal dystrophy (IRD) defined by the loss of photoreceptors and characterized by retinal pigment deposits visible on fundus examination. The most common form of RP is a rod-cone dystrophy in which the first symptom is night blindness, followed by the progressive loss in the peripheral visual field in daylight, and eventually leading to complete loss of central and peripheral vision after several decades [1]. Because of this pathogenesis, consistent visual acuity (VA) testing can be used to track the course of the disease. In this chapter, we outline the common techniques used to assess VA.

VA is a traditional measure of central visual function, particularly the ability of the eye to perceive details. VA is the most common measure of visual function both in clinical practice and in clinical trials. Loss of acuity manifests as a decrease in the ability to perform detail-oriented tasks, such as reading and face recognition. In the patient population with infantile Refsum disease due to biallelic *RPE65* mutations, VA is often severely impaired early in life.

In a clinical setting, standardized charts are commonly used to quickly assess VA. Using standardized charts, physicians are able to

Stephen H. Tsang and Peter M. J. Quinn (eds.), *Retinitis Pigmentosa*,
Methods in Molecular Biology, vol. 2560, https://doi.org/10.1007/978-1-0716-2651-1_13,

accurately mark patients' VA on a normal distribution. For patients whose VA lie outside of this normal curve, VAs can also be measured using off-chart methods.

2 Materials

Early Treatment of Diabetic Retinopathy Study (ETDRS) VA test chart or analogous HOTV chart.

3 Methods

In the voretigene neparvovec clinical program, VA testing used high-contrast charts with standardized letters of graded sizes to determine the smallest object seen at a specified distance. Early Treatment of Diabetic Retinopathy Study (ETDRS) VA test charts (Fig. 1), the gold standard for VA measurements in clinical studies,

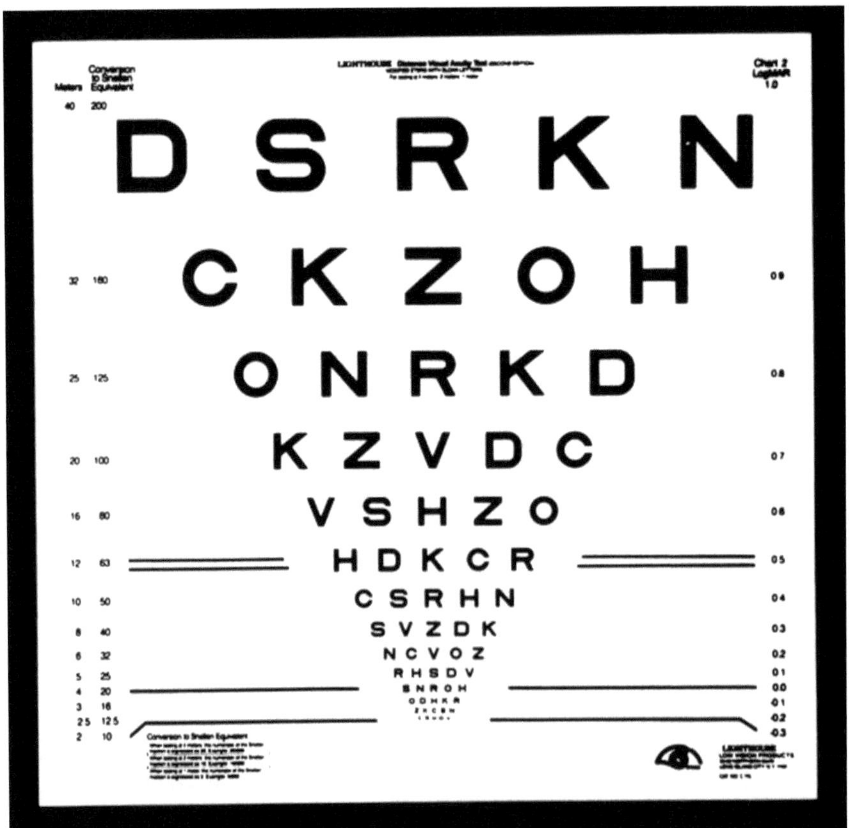

Fig. 1 Early Treatment of Diabetic Retinopathy Study (ETDRS) visual acuity (VA) test chart. The current gold standard of VA measurement in clinical practice and clinical research is the retro-illuminated logarithm of the minimum angle of resolution (logMAR) chart that was used in the ETDRS [4]. Each line of the chart contains five optotypes, and the optotype size is changed on each line by a constant proportion

were used for most subjects in the clinical studies [1]. For some young children, an analogous HOTV chart was used. HOTV charts include only the letters H, O, T and V, all of which center around a vertical axis and can be identified verbally by young children or shown to the test-taker on a matching HOTV card.

Subjects were tested (using best correction [with optimal glasses/contact lens prescription] and well-illuminated charts) with each eye individually at three distances: 4 m, 2 m, and 0.5 m (*see* **Note 1**). VA was determined based on the lowest lines (smallest letters) on which letters were correctly identified at each distance. The ETDRS chart includes letter sizes on each line following a geometric progression, such that VA can be converted to a visual angle score (LogMAR, or Logarithm of the Minimum Angle of Resolution) allowing for comparison analyses, where smaller LogMAR values indicate better acuity (i.e., less VA loss). For the VA analyses, a 0.1 change in LogMAR corresponds to a five-letter (equivalent to one line) change on the ETDRS chart (*see* **Note 2**).

For subjects unable to correctly identify the largest line of letters on the chart, off-chart VA measurements were collected (i.e., counting fingers, hand motion perception, light perception, no light perception) and then were assigned a LogMAR value using the scale adapted from Holladay [2] (*see* **Note 3**). Counting fingers at a given distance can be converted to a Snellen equivalent by assuming that the fingers are approximately the size of the elements of a 200 letter. Therefore, a person who can count fingers at 20 feet would have approximately 20/200 vision. A person able to count fingers at 2 feet would have 2/200 vision or the equivalent of 20/2000. This scale utilizes a 1-log-unit step between, for example, counting fingers and hand motion perception. Given this large step, this scale is conservative with respect to quantifying VA in assessment of safety, as it assigns worse acuity to off-chart VA than other scales. Based on recommendations from regulators and the Data Safety Monitoring Board overseeing the clinical program, a scale with a reduced 0.3-log-unit step between counting fingers and hand motion was used for sensitivity analyses beginning in 2013. This scale, adapted from Lange et al. (2009), was recommended given concerns with overestimating any treatment effect (improvement or reduction in LogMAR) for subjects with off-chart vision measurements at baseline; this same scale is associated with Freiburg vision testing, or FrACT, though this testing method itself (developed by Professor Michael Bach [senior author on the Lange et al. (2009) publication] and colleagues for patients with very low vision) was not used in the clinical program [3].

4 Notes

1. A standardized chart is a wonderfully simple tool in the measurement of VA, but as with every tool, the human element brings with it an opportunity for mistakes. The most common of which being inconsistent distance between test subject and ETDRS VA test chart. Naturally, if each VA assessment done over time is with the subject at a varied distance from the chart, the assessment has no validity, and the outcome means nothing. It's imperative to have consistency in this aspect.
2. Other common inconsistencies come when a subject or patient can get through part of a line in the chart but not the entire thing. One must have consistency here, as well whether you count this as partial credit or no credit at all.
3. Also, one must keep in mind that VA tested in this way is effort dependent. The patient's will to participate affects the outcome. Thus, there must be consistency in how much you push patients to strain and read difficult lines. The theme here is consistency. As long as that is accounted for, it's difficult to go wrong.

References

1. Hamel C (2006) Retinitis pigmentosa. Orphanet J Rare Dis 1(1):1–12. https://doi.org/10.1186/1750-1172-1-40
2. Holladay JT (2004) Visual acuity measurements. J Cataract Refract Surg 30(2):287–290
3. Lange C, Feltgen N, Junker B, Schulze-Bonsel-K, Bach M (2009) Resolving the clinical acuity categories "hand motion" and "counting fingers" using the Freiburg Visual Acuity Test (FrACT). Graefes Arch Clin Exp Ophthalmol 247(1):137–142
4. Laidlaw DAH, Abbott A, Rosser DA (2003) Development of a clinically feasible logMAR alternative to the Snellen chart: performance of the "compact reduced logMAR" visual acuity chart in amblyopic children. Br J Ophthalmol 87:1232–1234

Chapter 14

Measure of Visual Function

Sitara H. Hirji

Abstract

This chapter describes various methods of the assessment of visual function used for assessing disease progression and treatment response in patients with retinitis pigmentosa (RP). These methods include full-field stimulus testing (FST), near-infrared autofluorescence (NIR-AF), quantitative fundus autofluorescence (qAF), and quantitative near-infrared autofluorescence (qNIR-AF). This chapter will also outline the protocol for adaptive optics (AO) imaging of RP patients and cover how each of these methods is used for RP patients, with details including the expected findings, as evidenced by recent literature.

Key words Retinitis pigmentosa, Visual function, Genetic retinopathy, Pigment epithelium, Autofluorescence, FST, NIR-AF, qAF

1 Introduction

Retinitis pigmentosa (RP) is characterized by a progressive loss of photoreceptors, leading to a progressive decline in visual function. There have been various methods of visual function tested established for RP patients. These methods include full-field stimulus (FST) testing, several modalities based on fundus autofluorescence (AF), and adaptive optics imaging. As RP is defined as a classical degeneration of rods prior to cone degeneration, FST testing is especially useful as it is a rod-based visual function test [1]. Alternatively, the AF-based imaging takes advantage of the fluorophores of the normal fundus, lipofuscin and melanin, to evaluate changes in the retinal pigment epithelium (RPE) [2]. Analysis of the AF may be qualitative or quantitative. Research studies in RP patients aim to standardize the quantification of these analyses [3]. Adaptive optics (AO) imaging is used to assess retinal structure in the living human eyes, with the capability of achieving optical resolutions of 2 μm or less in order to visualize cellular structures [4]. Regular measurement of visual function is necessary to track progression of disease and level of visual impairment in RP patients.

Stephen H. Tsang and Peter M. J. Quinn (eds.), *Retinitis Pigmentosa*,
Methods in Molecular Biology, vol. 2560, https://doi.org/10.1007/978-1-0716-2651-1_14,

1.1 Full-Field Stimulus Testing (FST)

FST measures the light sensitivity of a patient's visual field by estimating the lowest luminance of a flash that elicits a visual sensation. Patients are exposed to flashes of varying luminance. For each visible flash, the patient will press a response button. Based on the response or lack thereof, a different luminance is presented according to a predetermined algorithm. The FST test is a method of assessing retinal function with higher sensitivity than electroretinography (ERG) [1]. Additionally, it is a rod-specific test of visual function, which is useful for RP patients as a majority of patients exhibit rod degeneration primarily until late stage disease. FST does not require fixation and is able to capture a wide range of luminance [1]. It is therefore a useful method of assessing visual function in low vision patients, such as those with RP. Low vision patients often have trouble with fixation, which skews other visual function tests such as standard visual field testing. In a study performed to quantify rod-mediated vision in retinal degenerations, such as RP, FST was analyzed as an outcome measure compared to dark-adapted perimetry and was found to be both accurate and reproducible in all patients studied, including those with severe retinal degeneration [5]. This study identified FST as a suitable method of quantifying response to rod-specific treatments that are on the horizon in RP research. This is important as RP patients have historically been evaluated with cone function tests in studies assessing the efficacy of nutrition therapies [6–8]. While the rod-ERG is a rod-specific quantitative visual function test, there is often no measurable rod activity on ERG early on in disease as patients lose peripheral vision. In a study examining 25 eyes of patients with retinal dystrophies—including RP patients—who had non-detectable vision on ERG, a light threshold was determined in eight of the nine eyes that had reported visual acuity of light perception. A light threshold was also determined in all eyes with counting fingers capability. The eye with no light perception and one of the nine eyes capable of light perception did not produce a light threshold on FST [9]. This study demonstrated an ability of FST to measure light thresholds beyond that of ERG measurements. A larger study of 94 eyes of patients with RP specifically also identified FST as a reliable alternative to VF or ERG in patients with trouble fixating or with non-detectable ERGs; FST showed a stronger correlation to full-field ERG amplitude than with sensitivity measured using standard visual field testing [10].

1.2 Near-Infrared Autofluorescence (NIR-AF) (HRA2 Heidelberg)

NIR-AF uses short-wavelength excitation to generate intrinsic fluorescence of the retina. Fundus fluorescence exhibits a band of emission between 500 and 750 nm with optimal excitation of 510 nm. Fluorescence is highest at 7–15° from the fovea, while the center of the fovea exhibits a well-defined minimum [11]. Fluorescence also decreases towards the periphery of the retina. The dominant fluorophore of the retina is lipofuscin, which accumulates as a byproduct of the phagocytosis of photoreceptors within the

RPE. It has been demonstrated that elevated levels of lipofuscin are associated with high turnover of photoreceptors in patients with macular degeneration as well as the two inherited retinal dystrophies, Stargardt disease and ceroid lipofuscinosis [12, 13]. Beyond accumulating within the RPE, it has been postulated that lipofuscin also inhibits the function of the RPE and may actually contribute to the pathogenesis of AMD [14, 15]. In patients with RP, NIR-AF is used to identify both melanin-related AF as well as lipofuscin-related fundus AF. It is used as a noninvasive technique to visualize RPE alterations and delineate progression of disease. In a study of NIR-AF patterns in RP patients, absence of AF was found to indicate photoreceptor cell death and nonviable RPE. Increased autofluorescence is seen in areas of higher metabolic demand and photoreceptor loss or dysfunction [2]. Patients with RP exhibit a characteristic parafoveal ring of high density, regardless of genetic subtype [16]. There was a strong correlation between the size of the parafoveal ring and the degree of macular damage in RP patients; the smaller the diameter of the ring, the more extensive the damage. The high-density area of the ring represents the demarcation between normal and degenerated retina; normal tissue is found within the ring and degenerated tissue outside the ring as demonstrated by ERG values. The size of the ring was found to be more indicative of extent of damage than both ERG and visual acuity [16]. Therefore, NIR-AF is another noninvasive measure of retinal degeneration that may be especially useful for monitoring treatment efficacy as new therapies surface for RP patients. It may be the preferred method as compared to the previously used short-wave AF (SW-AF) as the two modalities have been shown to demonstrate similar rates of progression, but NIR-AF is associated with higher patient comfort and cooperation as it has the advantage of being low-luminance [17].

1.3 Quantitative Fundus Autofluorescence (qAF) Heidelberg HRA2, qAF Module

As mentioned above, AF imaging of patient with RP often shows a parafoveal ring of hyperautofluorescence relative to its surrounding. Over time, the diameter of this ring constricts, indicating progressive damage to the photoreceptors. qAF is a modification of AF imaging that allows for the quantification of AF intensities of the retinal as a surrogate for the amount of lipofuscin in the RPE. This is superior to qualitative analysis as it allows for AF to be compared among patients and/or among different images of the same patient. AF intensities are calibrated to an internal reference to compensate for variations in detectors. qAF was used to analyze the parafoveal rings in RP patients to better understand its relation to disease progression. Measurements taken internal to the inner borders of the rings in the eyes with RP generally demonstrated qAF values that fell within the 95% confidence interval of healthy eyes. Measurements taken external to the outer borders of the rings in eyes with RP generally demonstrated qAF values that were lower than that taken from healthy eyes [18]. However, some patients exhibited increased qAF values both within and external to the ring, and some patients did not exhibit increased qAF levels at any point on the fundus. This suggests that qAF may vary with disease progression. Increased qAF correlated to thinning on SD-OCT and functional studies that indicated the degeneration of photoreceptors. This has been postulated to be due to disabled photoreceptors being incapable of detoxifying excess retinaldehyde of the visual cycle, leading to accelerated lipofuscin accumulation [19, 20]. Further studies may be helpful in determining expected qAF values at progressive stages of disease.

1.4 Quantitative Near-Infrared Autofluorescence (qNIR-AF) Heidelberg HRA2

As mentioned above, NIR-AF is used to identify both melanin-related AF and lipofuscin-related AF. It is used as a noninvasive technique to visualize RPE alterations and delineate progression of disease. NIR-AF of patients with RP often demonstrates a parafoveal ring of elevated AF relative to its surrounding. Over time, the diameter of the hyperfluorescent ring constricts, indicating progressive damage to the photoreceptors. qNIR-AF is a modification of NIR-AF imaging that allows for the quantification of AF intensities of the retinal as a surrogate for the amount of lipofuscin in the RPE. This is superior to qualitative analysis as it allows for AF to be compared among patients and/or among different images of the same patient. A large portion of studies using AF imaging are still employing qualitative analysis; the few studies reporting quantitative results do so by the use of an internal reference or by keeping system parameters constant between scans. However, there are unknown individual differences in the transmission of light prior to retinal excitation. Additionally, upon atrophy of the RPE cells, remnant signals are still captured in some patients from the choroid, which leads to difficulty interpreting and comparing results [3]. While there is limited literature about qNIR-AF in patients with RP, the imaging modality has been studied in patients with diabetic macular edema; average fluorescence intensity was quantified and correlated to SD-OCT imaging and specific pathological patterns of damage to elucidate pathogenesis of the condition [21]. In patients with retinal dystrophies including RP, Cideciyan et al. suggest a method of differentiating melanin-based fluorophores that are in the RPE versus in the choroid, which allows for better quantification of retinal atrophy and pigmentation as well as a partial compensation for differences in preretinal light transmission [3]. Further studies in RP patients will better be able to assess the value in qNIR-AF versus other imaging modalities in this patient population.

1.5 Adaptive Optics (AO) Imaging

AO imaging is a noninvasive method of retinal imaging that has allowed for exquisite detailing of retinal structure and function in the living eye. With a resolution capable of identifying microscopic structures on the retina, clinicians are able to distinguish photoreceptors, which is a level of detail previously only seen in postmortem tissue [22].

AO imaging uses a scanning focused beam source of light across the retina and confocal pinhole to restrict illumination to a single retinal region, thus giving more control over scattering light. It takes advantage of highly sensitive detectors called photomultiplier tubes. AO uses a wavefront sensor and a deformable mirror that can change the shape of the beam of light entering the eyes; this technique allows for the compensation of chromatic aberrations of the eye caused by the different indices of refraction for different wavelengths of light. It also allows for the compensation of monochromatic aberrations of the eye that arise from variations in tear films, cornea, and lens [4].

Many different wavefront sensors are commercially available, as is new technology in which AO may be performed without a sensor, termed sensorless AO (SAO). The following protocol delineates the steps for traditional hardware AO (HAO) which uses the wavefront sensor and deformable mirrors to maximize spatial resolution.

2 Materials

1. *Dilation chemical.*
   - Tropicamide Ophthalmic Solution, USP 1% from Akorn, Inc.
   - Phenylephrine Hydrochloride Ophthalmic Solution, USP 2.5% from BioTeck, Inc.
2. *Instrument.*
   - AO scanning laser ophthalmoscope.

3 Methods

1. Patients were administered topical 1% tropicamide and 2.5% phenylephrine to dilate the pupil and minimize accommodative fluctuations.
2. Room lights were dimmed (monitor glow only) to reduce possible effects on the test and to minimize distraction of the subjects.
3. The subject's head was secured in the chin-head-rest to set and maintain eye alignment during the wavefront correction and imaging.

4. The retinal location of wavefront correction and imaging was controlled by having the subject view a fixation target.
5. The imaging sequence began with wavefront sensing and correction.
6. The wave aberration is measured with the same light that is used to form the image, which reduces non-common aberrations. A 37-channel deformable mirror (Xinetics, Andover, MA) is placed in the path conjugate to the entrance pupil of the eye. Aberrations are corrected on both the ingoing and outgoing light paths.
7. The light originates from a diode laser and is coupled into a single-mode optical fiber. The tip of the fiber provides a point source, which is collimated by a 100-mm achromatic lens. An aperture placed after the system sets the entrance pupil diameter.
8. The entrance pupil is relayed by mirror telescopes to the deformable mirror, the horizontal scanner, the vertical scanner, and finally to the eye.
9. Light scanning and AO correction are done in planes that are conjugate to the entrance pupil plane.
10. The beam is scanned on the retina with a galvanometric scanner combination (Electro-Optics Products Corp, Flushing Meadows, NY). The resonant scanner scans the beam horizontally in a sinusoidal pattern. The galvanometric scanner coupled to the resonant scanner operates in a saw-tooth pattern at a fraction of the horizontal scan frequency.
11. This configuration provides 525 lines per frame at about 30 frames per second. Both scanners are placed optically conjugate to the entrance pupil.
12. The light from the retina is de-scanned and is focused onto a confocal pinhole in the detection arm and is then detected with a photomultiplier tube. Signals are converted to voltage and amplified before being fed to a frame grabbing board (GenesisLC, Matrox, Montreal, Canada).
13. Images were acquired and stored uncompressed in a digital format.

Protocol adapted from: Roorda A, Romero-Borja F, Donnelly III WJ, Queener H, Hebert TJ, Campbell MCW (2002) Adaptive optics scanning laser ophthalmoscopy. Opt Express 10:405–412

References

1. Klein M, Birch DG (2009) Psychophysical assessment of low visual function in patients with retinal degenerative diseases (RDDs) with the Diagnosys full-field stimulus threshold (D-FST). Doc Ophthalmol 119(3):217–224
2. Popović P, Jarc-Vidmar M, Hawlina M (2005) Abnormal fundus autofluorescence in relation to retinal function in patients with retinitis pigmentosa. Graefes Arch Clin Exp Ophthalmol 243(10):1018–1027
3. Cideciyan AV, Swider M, Jacobson SG (2015) Autofluorescence imaging with near-infrared excitation:normalization by reflectance to reduce signal from choroidal fluorophores. Invest Ophthalmol Vis Sci 56(5):3393–3406
4. Roorda A, Romero-Borja F, Donnelly WJ III, Queener H, Hebert TJ, Campbell MCW (2002) Adaptive optics scanning laser ophthalmoscopy. Opt Express 10:405–412
5. Roman AJ, Schwartz SB, Aleman TS, Cideciyan AV, Chico JD, Windsor EA, Jacobson SG (2005) Quantifying rod photoreceptor-mediated vision in retinal degenerations: dark-adapted thresholds as outcome measures. Exp Eye Res 80(2):259–272
6. Berson EL, Rosner B, Sandberg MA, Hayes KC, Nicholson BW, Weigel-DiFranco C, Willett W (1993) A randomized trial of vitamin A and vitamin E supplementation for retinitis pigmentosa. Arch Ophthalmol 111:761–772
7. Berson EL, Rosner B, Sandberg MA, Weigel-DiFranco C, Moser A, Brockhurst RJ, Hayes KC, Johnson CA, Anderson EJ, Gaudio AR, Willett WC, Schaefer EJ (2004) Clinical trial of docosahexaenoic acid in patients with retinitis pigmentosa receiving vitamin A treatment. Arch Ophthalmol 122:1297–1305
8. Hoffman DR, Locke KG, Wheaton DH, Fish GE, Spencer R, Birch DG (2004) A randomized, placebo-controlled clinical trial of docosahexaenoic acid supplementation for X-linked retinitis pigmentosa. Am J Ophthalmol 137:704–718
9. Klein M, Birch D (2009) The Diagnosis full-field stimulus threshold (D-FST) is a useful tool to assess visual function in low vision subjects December 2008. In: Conference: Association for Research in Vision and Ophthalmology meeting. At: Fort Lauderdale, Florida
10. Messias K, Jägle H, Saran R, Ruppert ADP, Siqueira R, Jorge R, Messias A (2013) Psychophysically determined full-field stimulus thresholds (FST) in retinitis pigmentosa: relationships with electroretinography and visual field outcomes. Doc Ophthalmol 127(2): 123–129
11. Delori FC, Dorey CK, Staurenghi G, Arend O, Goger DG, Weiter JJ (1995) In vivo fluorescence of the ocular fundus exhibits retinal pigment epithelium lipofuscin characteristics. Invest Ophthalmol Vis Sci 36(3):718–729
12. Dorey CK, Wu G, Ebenstein D, Garsd A, Weiter JJ (1989) Cell loss in the aging retina: relationship to lipofuscin accumulation and macular degeneration. Invest Ophthalmol Vis Sci 30:1691–1699
13. Eagle RC, Lucier AC, Bernadino VB, Janoff M (1980) Retinal pigment epithelial abnormalities in fundus flavimaculatus: a light and electron microscopic study. Ophthalmology 87: 1189–1200
14. Dorey K, Staurenghi G, Delori FC (1993) Lipofuscin in aged and ARMD eyes. In: Hollyfield JG et al (eds) Retinal degeneration. Plenum Press, New York, pp 3–14
15. Young RW (1987) Pathophysiology of age-related macular degeneration. Surv Ophthalmol 31:291–306
16. Robson AG, El-Amir A, Bailey C, Egan CA, Fitzke FW, Webster AR, Holder GE (2003) Pattern ERG correlates of abnormal fundus autofluorescence in patients with retinitis pigmentosa and normal visual acuity. Invest Ophthalmol Vis Sci 44(8):3544–3550
17. Jauregui R, Park KS, Duong JK, Sparrow JR, Tsang SH (2018) Quantitative comparison of near-infrared versus short-wave autofluorescence imaging in monitoring progression of retinitis pigmentosa. Am J Ophthalmol 194: 120–125
18. Schuerch K, Woods RL, Lee W, Duncker T, Delori FC, Allikmets R et al (2017) Quantifying fundus autofluorescence in patients with retinitis pigmentosa. Invest Ophthalmol Vis Sci 58(3):1843–1855
19. Sparrow JR, Yoon KD, Wu Y, Yamamoto K (2010) Interpretations of fundus autofluorescence from studies of the bisretinoids of the retina. Invest Ophthalmol Vis Sci 51:4351–4357
20. Gelman R, Chen R, Blonska A, Barile G, Sparrow JR (2012) Fundus autofluorescence imaging in a patient with rapidly developing scotoma. Retin Cases Brief Rep 6:345–348
21. Yoshitake S, Murakami T, Horii T, Uji A, Ogino K, Unoki N, Yoshimura N (2014) Qualitative and quantitative characteristics of near-infrared autofluorescence in diabetic macular edema. Ophthalmology 121(5):1036–1044
22. Burns SA, Elsner AE, Sapoznik KA, Warner RL, Gast TJ (2019) Adaptive optics imaging of the human retina. Prog Retin Eye Res 68:1–30

Chapter 15

Ophthalmic Fluorescein Angiography

Divin O. Baddam, Sara D. Ragi, Stephen H. Tsang, and Wei Kiong Ngo

Abstract

Following its implementation in the 1960s, fluorescein angiography (FA) has become a widely used and reliable tool in the diagnosis of retinal and choroidal disorders. FA is an imaging modality utilized to examine the circulation of the retina and choroid. Here, we describe the process of obtaining fundus images with sodium fluorescein dye as a contrast agent. Using this methodology, ophthalmologists may examine the retinal and choroidal vasculature to diagnose a wide scope of retinal and choroidal diseases.

Key words Fluorescein angiography, Ophthalmic imaging, Macular degeneration, Choroid, Invasive procedure

1 Introduction

The basic principle of fluorescein angiography (FA) is the concept of sodium fluorescein absorbing excitation light of wavelengths between 465 and 490 nm (blue) and spontaneously emitting light at wavelengths between 520 and 530 nm (yellow). This emitted fluorescent light is picked up by a specialized camera fitted with a green-yellow filter and allows evaluation of the retinal and, to a lesser extent, the choroidal vasculature.

FA is used as an adjunct in the diagnosis of retinal and choroidal diseases. Sodium fluorescein dye is mostly injected venously in the arm, or some centers may administer it orally, especially in pediatric populations averse to needles. When the dye reaches the retinal and choroidal circulation, a specialized camera is then used to capture emitted fluorescent light from the fundus while filtering out the reflected blue excitation light. The resultant image is therefore an anatomical map of the fundus composed of bright (hyperfluorescent) and dark (hypofluorescent) areas. Careful interpretation of these areas allows for the diagnosis and evaluation of the condition.

FA is extensively used in the evaluation of diseases such as age-related macular degeneration, diabetic retinopathy, retinal

Stephen H. Tsang and Peter M. J. Quinn (eds.), *Retinitis Pigmentosa*,
Methods in Molecular Biology, vol. 2560, https://doi.org/10.1007/978-1-0716-2651-1_15,

vascular occlusive diseases, and inflammatory and infective diseases of the retina and choroid.

1.1 History of FA

In 1871, a German scientist by the name of Adolf Von Baeyer discovered the utility of sodium fluorescein dye. By dissolving it in the current of the Danube River and detecting it in the Rhine River approximately 300 miles away, Baeyer was able to prove its usefulness in monitoring circulation [1]. Paul Ehrlich was able to build on these findings 10 years later, when he applied the dye to assess circulatory properties in a living organism [2]. He was able to successfully detect the presence of sodium fluorescein after administration in a rabbit's eye. These techniques were implemented in the field of ophthalmology by Burke, who used the dye to study the optic nerve and chorioretinal inflammatory disorders [3]. These studies, having demonstrated the non-toxicity of the dye to living tissues, helped prove the safety of FA. The use of FA was popularized by Dr. John Donald McIntyre Gass in the 1960s [4]. Today, FA is a standard technique utilized by ophthalmologists.

2 Materials

Providers should ensure that prior to a test all mechanical equipment is properly functioning and calibrated to produce accurate, high-quality images. Unless indicated otherwise, prepare and store all solutions mentioned below in a setting of room temperature. After completing the use of solutions or other medical equipment in the procedure, ensure that all waste disposal regulations are followed to prevent future contamination.

2.1 Sodium Fluorescein Dye

*Sodium Fluorescein can be bought in solution form from many chemical suppliers; in the event that only crude sodium fluorescein is available, follow the below steps to produce sodium fluorescein dye.

*It is recommended that the solution be stored in a temperature of 4 °C when not in use.

2.1.1 Preparation

1. Obtain the required amount of saline solution required to reconstitute the sodium fluorescein powder. Administer the solution into the required amount of Sodium Fluorescein stock solution (dye). Put the mixture in a container suitable for vortexing.
2. Vortex stock solution at high speed for 5 min. Store solution in a suitable container while not in use. Ensure that the storage container is sterile in order to prevent the contamination of the dye.

2.1.2 Working Solution of Fluorescein 102 Preparation

1. Check the concentration of the solution and make appropriate dilutions with sterile saline.
2. Filter final solution* with a syringe filter into a syringe or a suitable container for later use.

*If not immediately used, keep storing the solution in a temperature of 4 °C.

*The dye is typically administered in 5 mL of 10% solution or 3 mL of 25% solution.

2.2 Other Required Materials

1. Digital fundus camera or SLO-based systems*.
2. Exciter filter.
3. Barrier filter.
4. Digital photo processing software.
5. 5-mL Syringe.
6. 21- to 25-gauge butterfly catheter.
7. Armrest for injection.
8. Tourniquet.
9. Alcohol swabs.
10. Bandages.
11. Standard dilation eye drops.
12. Standard first response emergency equipment.

*Modern digital fundus camera have a field of view ranging from 35° to 200°. Some camera systems also allow for video angiography to allow real-time examination of the precise filling of the vasculature.

3 Methods

During and after the test, ensure all waste disposal regulations are met. It is the doctors' responsibility to inform the patient of what the process will entail and any potential side effects (*see* **Notes 1** and **2**). Informing the patient of what to expect during the procedure may alleviate any anxiety or concerns experienced by the patient. It is recommended that a clinician or trained personnel be present together with the photographer during the test so that an anaphylactic reaction to the sodium fluorescein can be recognized early and managed.

3.1 Performing FA

1. Administer the dilation eye drops to the patient 30–45 min prior to the procedure. Ensure adequate dilation before proceeding.

2. Ensure that the camera is fully functioning and the lens is free of any dust or dirt that may obscure images (*see* **Notes 3** and **4**).
3. Position the patient's chin and forehead in line with the chin-rest and headrest, respectively, in order to ensure that the head remains still throughout the test.
4. Ask the patient to blink a few times to help moisten the cornea and to produce clearer images.
5. A baseline red-free photograph is usually taken at the start of the examination.
6. Draw the prepared sodium fluorescein dye into a sterile syringe.
7. Ensure all air is removed from the syringe in order to prevent potential air embolism.
8. Locate a visible vein on the arm/hand (if no vein is clearly visible, tying rubber strips around selected areas of the arm may help increase the visibility of a vein).
9. The injecting doctor may now insert the needle into the selected vein and give verbal confirmation to the photographer manning the camera that venous access has been successful and injection will commence (*see* **Note 5**).
10. After venous access is successful, a doctor may now request that the lights be turned off (however, it is important to have enough light to monitor the infusion until it is complete, in order to prevent extravasation).
11. The injecting clinician may now begin the bolus injection of the fluorescein dye.
12. A control photograph is taken at the start of the injection of fluorescein dye, and the timer is started to document the timing of the subsequent photographs.
13. In order to not miss the fluorescein entering the fundus, images should start being taken 8–12 s following the commencement of bolus injection.
14. For the first 45 s, focus on the macula (and/or area of interest) of the eye with pathology (or the eye which is chosen by the clinician as the study eye of choice). Images should be taken rapidly at intervals of 1–2 s.
15. After 45 s, the photographer then starts to take composite images of the peripheral retina (unless an ultrawide field imaging system is used). The photographer also starts to take images of the fellow eye. Additional images of both eyes are taken at 3, 5, and 10 min.
16. Inform the patient of side effects, such as discoloration of urine and the potential discoloration of vision which are temporary.
17. Inform the patient to drink lots of water to help flush out the remaining dye.

3.2 Interpretation of FA

In a normal angiogram, the sodium fluorescein dye reaches the eye typically 10–15 s after injection in the arm. The fluorescence appears first in the choroid (choroidal phase) and initially fills in a patchy, irregular manner. The central retinal artery and arterioles (arterial phase) start to fill 1–2 s after the choroidal phase. The time taken from injection of the dye in the arm to the first appearance of the dye in the retinal arterial system is described as the arm-retina time. The retinal veins start to fill 1–2 s after the arterial phase, and lamellar flow is seen in the larger retinal veins (arteriovenous phase). The veins fill up completely over the next 5–10 s (venous phase). Around 2 min after the injection of the dye, the vascular fluorescence in the fundus starts to decrease in the recirculation phase due to the first pass effect of the dye through the kidneys. In the late phase (10 min), there is gradual complete removal of the dye from the retinal and choroidal circulation, and there is late staining of the optic disc.

The identification of areas of abnormal fluorescence deviating from the normal angiogram is key to its interpretation. The causes of hyper- and hypofluorescent areas on the angiogram are listed below.

3.2.1 Hyperfluorescence

Hyperfluorescence occurs when there is greater than the normal expected level of fluorescence; it can be seen in several distinct patterns:

1. Autofluorescence: Occurs when hyperfluorescence is detected before the injection of fluorescein dye. It occurs due to the innate fluorescent ability of certain ocular structures such as optic nerve head drusen and lipofuscin or vitelliform material deposition. In fleck retinal dystrophies such as Stargardt disease, the flecks will appear hyperfluorescent on the autofluorescence image.
2. Pseudo-autofluorescence: Occurs due to overlap of excitation and barrier filters resulting in the reflected blue excitation light passing through the entire camera system and registering a false signal.
3. Leakage: Occurs due to the extravasation of dye into an anatomical space or into surrounding tissue. Characteristically, the hyperfluorescence increases in both size and intensity with time. Examples include leakage from retinal neovascularisation, choroidal neovascularisation, and vasculitis. In the study of inherited retinal dystrophies, FA may be used to examine secondary neovascular membranes or Coat's-like changes associated with the dystrophy.

4. Pooling: Occurs when the dye extravasates into an anatomical space and collects within it. Characteristically, the hyperfluorescence gradually takes up the shape and size of the anatomical space and then increases in intensity without increase in size beyond that of the anatomical space. Examples include subretinal or sub-RPE fluid collections in central serous chorioretinopathy and age-related macular degeneration. When evaluating patients with retinitis pigmentosa and cystoid macular edema, petaloid hyperfluorescence resulting from the pooling of dye into the cystoid spaces at the macula can be appreciated on FA.
5. Staining: Occurs when the dye diffusely extravasates into surrounding tissue. Examples of tissues that stain include scars, sclera, and optic nerve head. In fleck retinal dystrophies (i.e., Stargardt disease), flecks appear as hyperfluorescent staining on FA with a dark choroidal background accentuating it.
6. Transmission defect: Due to the loss of pigmentation of the retinal pigment epithelium (i.e., in atrophy), the choroidal fluorescence is unmasked and appears hyperfluorescent. Hyperfluorescence due to transmission defect occurs early in the choroidal phase and increases in intensity over the early phases. It does not, however, change in shape and size over time and starts to fade due the recirculation and late phases. FA may show hyperfluorescent window defects corresponding to atrophic retinal areas in patients with inherited retinal dystrophies.

3.2.2 Hypofluorescence

1. Hypofluorescence occurs when fluorescence is lower than the expected level. Similar to hyperfluorescence, it is seen in distinct patterns:
2. Vascular filling defect: Occurs when the retinal or choroidal vasculature fails to fill with blood properly. Examples include capillary fallout secondary to ischemia from diabetes, occlusive vasculitis, and retinal vascular occlusions.
3. Blocked fluorescence: Occurs when the fluorescence from the retinal or choroidal vasculature is blocked by overlying lesions. Examples include hemorrhage (pre-retinal, retinal, subretinal, or sub-RPE), scars, pigmentation, or depository material.

3.3 Safety of FA

FA is regarded as one of the safest diagnostic procedures in medicine, with a low complication rate of 5% [5]. However, like other procedures, this technique may cause adverse reactions which have been well-documented [6–9]. Adverse reactions include nausea (most common), emesis, and pruritus. These minor reactions typically resolve in approximately 1.5 h [5]. Additionally, more severe reactions have been seen in tests and thus warrant extreme caution and the availability of emergency response equipment [7]. These severe reactions involve shock and toxicity that could lead to death. While the chance of death is quite low (1 in 200,000), precaution is needed in order to prevent such an occurrence [8, 9].

4 Notes

1. All allergies must be documented prior to the procedure. Any renal impairment or renal dialysis should also be documented, and the dose of fluorescein may need to be adjusted according to drug label. The procedure is contraindicated in patients who have known allergies to the component ingredients of sodium fluorescein.
2. If a patient is pregnant, it is current practice to avoid undergoing FA [10].
3. It is vital that the camera lens be inspected and if necessary be cleaned prior to the taking of any photos. Blow any loose impurities off with an air bulb. Moisten a lens tissue with lens cleaning fluid, and clean the lens surface with small circular motions staring in the center. If needed, remove any remaining film with a dry lens tissue.
4. A soft cloth and water should be used to clean the body of the camera, and ensure that no water comes in direct contact with the electrical components of the camera. The headrest may be cleaned with alcohol as it comes in direct contact with patients. The camera back should be cleaned with compressed air.
5. In the event that there is extravasation of the fluorescein dye, immediately stop the infusion and apply cold compression to the area. Explain to the patient that there may be temporary discoloration of the surrounding skin. Advise patient to watch for increasing pain, redness, or swelling over the next few days and to seek appropriate medical attention if worsening of symptoms.

Conflicts of Interest

Stephen H. Tsang receives financial support from Abeona Therapeutics, Inc and Emendo. He is also the founder of Rejuvitas and is on the scientific and clinical advisory board for Nanoscope Therapeutics.

References

1. Baeyer A (1871) Uber ein neue Klasse van farbstoffen. Der Deutschen Chem Ges 4:555
2. Ehrlich P (1882) Uber provilirte fluoresceinzerscheinungen. Am Aug Dtsch Med Wochenschr:8–21
3. Burke A (1910) Die klinische physiologische und pathologie bedeuting der fluorescein im auge nach darrerching von-uranin. Klin Monatsbl Augenheilkd 48:445–454
4. Gass JDM, Sever RJ, Sparks D et al (1967) A combined technique of fluorescein fundoscopy and angiography of the eye. Arch Ophthalmol 78:455–461
5. Arevalo JF (2009) Retinal angiography and optical coherence tomography. Springer, pp 1–471
6. Bloome MA (1980) Fluorescein angiography: risks. Vis Res 20:1083–1097

7. Kelley JS (1977) Fluorescein angiography: techniques and toxicity. Int Ophthalmol Clin 17:25–33
8. Jennings BJ, Mathews DE (1994) Adverse reactions during retinal fluorescein angiography. J Am Optom Assoc 65:465–471
9. Yannuzzi LA, Rohrer KT, Tindel LJ et al (1986) Fluorescein angiography complication survey. Ophthalmology 93:611–617
10. Halperin LS, Olk J, Soubrane G et al (1990) Safety of fluorescein angiography during pregnancy. Am J Ophthalmol 109:563–566

Chapter 16

Protocol for Indocyanine Green Angiography

Divin O. Baddam, Sara D. Ragi, Stephen H. Tsang, and Wei Kiong Ngo

Abstract

Indocyanine green (ICG) angiography was first approved by the Food and Drug Administration for human use in the 1956. Prior to its use in chorioretinal angiograms, ICG was used to measure blood flow and track cardiac output. It was only in 1969 when two researchers, Kyuga Kogure and Earl Choromokos from the University of Miami, first used ICG to create more accurate angiograms. In the following years, researchers were able to hone the underlying science of this new form of angiography. As time passed and technology advanced, the application of ICG in clinical practice became widespread. Today ICG is used to diagnose and monitor the progression of retinal and choroidal diseases affecting millions of individuals across the globe. ICG utilizes the injection of indocyanine green dye into a patient's bloodstream to visualize abnormalities of the choroid and retina by evaluating choroidal circulation. ICG angiography is useful in the diagnosis and management of occult choroidal neovascularization in age-related macular degeneration and may be used in other inflammatory conditions with central serous chorioretinopathy. ICG angiography offers advanced imaging for improved monitoring and treatment of a wide variety of choroidal and retinal diseases.

Key words Angiography, Blood flow, Choroid, ICG, Indocyanine green angiography, Macular degeneration, Retina

1 Introduction

Fluorescein angiography (FA) has limitations in the visualization of the choroidal circulation due to its lesser ability to penetrate the retinal pigmentation such as melanin and xanthophyll. It is also lesser bound (~70–80%) to plasma proteins such as albumin, and the unbound portion readily diffuses out of the choriocapillaris, resulting in a "choroidal flush" that obscures accurate visualization.

Indocyanine green (ICG) is a soluble tricarbonate dye that was initially used to measure cardiac output. The chemical properties of ICG enable it to allow better visualization of the choroidal circulation and, therefore, it is deemed the gold standard for vascular examination of the choroid. Firstly, ICG binds to plasma proteins to a larger extent (~98%) compared to FA. This allows the majority of ICG to stay within the choroidal vasculature, instead of diffusing

Stephen H. Tsang and Peter M. J. Quinn (eds.), *Retinitis Pigmentosa*,
Methods in Molecular Biology, vol. 2560, https://doi.org/10.1007/978-1-0716-2651-1_16,

out in surrounding tissue like in FA, and delineate the vascular integrity better [1]. Secondly, ICG absorbs light at 790 nm (near-infrared) and fluoresces at 835 nm (infrared), allowing it to penetrate the retinal pigments such as melanin, xanthophyll, and pathologies such as blood, fluid, and exudates in the retinal and subretinal layers [2]. This allows better visualization of the choroid through even overlying retinal pathologies.

The use of confocal aperture with scanning laser ophthalmoscopy (CSLO) digital imaging systems further enhances the quality of ICG image produced as the set-up only allows acquisition of light from a particular focal plane (or layer of tissue), blocking out returning light from other layers or surrounding tissue. ICG angiography has now been widely implemented into clinical use and is used as an adjunct to study patients with a wide variety of diseases such as choroidal neovascularization, polypoidal choroidal vasculopathy, central serous chorioretinopathy, choroidal tumors, and uveitic inflammation of the choroid.

1.1 History of ICG Angiography

ICG itself is a water-soluble tricarbocyanine dye. The dye gained its FDA approval in 1956 and was used to study the hepatic and cardiac system [3]. ICG was known to have a high protein bonding affinity and was additionally known to display a relative lack of leakage into surrounding areas, qualities which made it an ideal candidate for angiography. Subsequent research done in Japan and the United States during the late 1980s and early 1990s introduced the developing technique of ICG angiography to the world's community of ophthalmologists. The resolution of ICGA was improved by Hayashi et al. in 1986 when the group was successfully able to develop improved filter combinations while still maintaining sufficient sensitivity for near-infrared wavelength [4]. Their findings were key in the shift from film to videotape, in their introduction of videoangiography. However, this new and improved method still had its drawbacks, as individual images could not be examined and the required light source restricted both the quality and the potential duration of the technique. In 1992, high-resolution ICG angiography images were obtained when Scheider and Schroedel used a laser ophthalmoscope in their ICG videoangiography [5]. Later that same year, Yannuzzi et al. developed an improved line resolution system accompanied by better image storage and flash synchronization, which ultimately provided the world with long-duration, high-resolution ICG angiography [6].

2 Materials

Ensure all waste disposal regulations are met when disposing of materials to prevent contamination. Test and calibrate all mechanical equipment to confirm that they are properly functioning to produce accurate, high-quality images.

1. 25-mg/5-mL ICG dye.
2. Aqueous solvent (*see* **Notes 1** and **2**).
3. 5-mL Syringe.
4. 5 mL Saline.
5. 21- to 25-gauge butterfly catheter.
6. Digital fundus camera or SLO-based systems*.
7. Excitation filter.
8. Barrier filter.
9. Digital photo processing software.
10. Armrest for injection.
11. Tourniquet.
12. Alcohol swabs.
13. Bandages.
14. Standard dilation eye drops.
15. Standard first response emergency equipment.

*Modern digital fundus camera has a field of view ranging from 35° to 200°. Some camera systems also allow for video angiography to allow real-time examination of the precise filling of the vasculature.

3 Methods

During and after the test, ensure that all waste disposal regulations are met. It is the doctors' responsibility to inform the patient of what the process will entail and any potential side effects (*see* **Notes 3** and **4**). Informing the patient of what is expected helps to alleviate any anxiety or concern. It is recommended that a clinician or trained personnel be present together with the photographer during the test so that an anaphylactic reaction to the ICG dye can be recognized and treatment can be instituted early.

3.1 Performing ICG Angiography

1. Administer dilation eye drops to the patient 30–45 min prior to the procedure. Ensure adequate dilation before proceeding (not required if done immediately after FA test) (*see* **Note 5**).
2. Ensure that the camera is fully functional and the lens is free of any dust or dirt that may obscure images (*see* **Notes 6** and **7**).

3. Position the patient's chin and forehead in line with the chinrest and headrest, respectively, to ensure the patient's head remains still throughout the test.
4. Ask the patient to blink a few times to moisten the cornea thereby producing clearer images.
5. Draw the prepared ICG dye.
6. Ensure all air is removed from the syringe to prevent a potential air embolism.
7. Locate a visible vein on the arm/hand (if no vein is clearly visible, tying rubber strips around selected areas of the arm may help increase the visibility of a vein).
8. The injecting doctor may now insert the needle into the selected vein and give verbal confirmation to the photographer manning the camera that venous access has been successful and injection will commence.
9. After venous access is achieved, the lights may be turned off. However, the injecting clinician should be able to monitor the infusion throughout the entire process in order to check if there is extravasation of dye (*see* **Note 8**).
10. The injecting clinician may now begin the bolus injection of the ICG dye.
11. A control photograph is taken at the start of the injection of ICG dye, and the timer is started to document the timings of the subsequent photographs.
12. The photographer at the camera should start taking photos immediately following the commencement of the injection of the ICG dye. For the first 45 s, focus on the macula (and/or area of interest) of the eye with pathology (or the eye which is chosen by the clinician as the study eye of choice). Images should be taken rapidly at intervals of 1 s to capture the filling of the choroid and retina.
13. After 45 s, the photographer then starts to take composite images of the periphery (unless an ultra-wide field imaging system is used). The photographer also starts to take images of the fellow eye. Additional images of both eyes are taken at 3, 5, 10, 15, and 20 min (some centers may take images up to 30 min).
14. After the procedure is complete, inform the patient to hydrate consistently to flush out any of the remaining dye through urine.
15. The doctor may also request that the patient not drive due to the dilation of pupils and potential discoloration of vision.

3.2 Interpretation of ICG Angiograms

The normal ICG angiogram can be divided into the early, middle, and late phases. The "early phase" begins when ICG dye starts appearing in the choroidal arterial circulation approximately 8–12 s after injection. The large vessels in the Haller's layer start to fill first, followed by the medium choroidal vessels in the Sattler's layer and finally the choriocapillaris. The hyperfluorescence of these vessels reaches a maximum intensity at between 1 and 2 min. Venous drainage of the choroid occurs via vortex veins systems, and they usually number from 4 to 8 in majority of people. During the middle phase (5–10 min), the outline of the choroidal vessels become less distinct, leaving a diffuse, homogenous fluorescence pattern. At this point, the fluorescence in the retinal vasculature starts to fade as well. Finally, in the late phase (15 min and beyond), there is further fading away of the fluorescence, leaving the choroidal vessels appearing as hypofluorescent channels, and the retinal vessels are not visible. The optic nerve head is dark. In the middle and late phases, lesions with abnormal hyperfluorescence stand out in stark contrast with the fading surroundings, necessitating longer examination times for ICG angiography compared to FA.

Interpretation of ICG angiograms is similar to that in fluorescein angiograms; identifying the areas of abnormal fluorescence compared to a normal ICG angiogram is key.

3.2.1 Increased ICG Fluorescence

Hyperfluorescence in ICG angiography occurs due to leakage or staining. Hyperfluorescence in the middle or late phases can be divided by its size into hot spot (less than 1 disc diameter) and plaques (1 disc diameter and more). Hyperfluorescence hot spots on ICG angiograms may represent choroidal neovascularization, polypoidal choroidal vasculopathy, or retinal angiomatous proliferation. Focal hotspots with leakage and choroidal hyperpermeability in late phase occur in central serous chorioretinopathy. Hyperfluorescence delineating internal vascular pattern is useful in the evaluation of choroidal tumors such as choroidal hemangiomas and melanomas. Lastly, hyperfluorescence due to inflammatory choroidal hyperpermeability may occur due to conditions such as Vogt-Koyanagi-Harada syndrome and other white dot syndromes [7].

3.2.2 Decreased ICG Fluorescence

Hypofluorescence on ICG angiography represents blockage (by overlying lesions such as blood), choroidal non-perfusion, or atrophy (loss). Inflammatory conditions of the choroid such as multiple evanescent white dot syndrome, multifocal choroiditis, birdshot chorioretinopathy, acute multifocal placoid pigment epitheliopathy, serpiginous choroidopathy, punctate inner choroidopathy, and acute zonal occult outer retinopathy may show hypofluorescent lesions on ICG angiography due to non-perfusion and atrophy from the inflammation [7, 8]. When evaluating inherited retinal dystrophies with ICG angiography, areas of chorioretinal atrophy are hypofluorescent. This is evident from the study by Giani et al. where they described ICGA "dark atrophy" in patients with Stargardt's disease [9].

3.3 Safety of ICG

Indocyanine green when compared to other angiographical dyes is relatively safe. The adverse reactions that may occur under the influence of ICG are only mild (nausea, vomiting, pruritus) and have only been seen in 0.15% of tests [10]. Reports of anaphylactic shock and hypotensive shock have been seen in isolated incidents but do not warrant major concern. ICG extravasation is known to be well tolerated and resolves without complications, unlike fluorescein angiography (FA). In a sterile form, ICG contains amounts of iodine and therefore carries the risk of anaphylaxis in patients with any form of iodine allergies. It is important to check for such an allergy beforehand to avoid potentially harmful effects. Additionally, the effects of ICG on an unborn fetus have not been proven, and due to the lack of research, it is advised that pregnant women should not undergo the procedure.

4 Notes

1. Indocyanine green has the ability to form polymers and bond with saline solution, so if this occurs, dilution with water is required.
2. Solvent should be obtained from the manufacturer, to ensure product integrity.
3. All allergies must be documented prior to the procedure; any renal impairment, renal dialysis, or liver dysfunction should be documented; and the dose of ICG may need to be adjusted according to drug label. The procedure is contraindicated in patients who have known allergies to the component ingredients of ICG.
4. If a patient is pregnant, ICG angiography should be avoided.
5. Both sodium fluorescein and ICG can be mixed and administered at the same time for combined examination.
6. It is vital that the camera lens be inspected and, if necessary, cleaned prior to taking photos. Any loose impurities should be blown off with an air bulb. A lens tissue should be moistened with lens cleaning fluid and then used to clean the lens surface with small circular motions beginning at the center. If needed, any remaining film with a dry lens tissue should be removed.
7. A soft cloth and water should be used to clean the body of the camera, to ensure that no water comes in direct contact with the electrical components of the camera. The headrest may be cleaned with alcohol as it comes in direct contact with patients. The camera back should be cleaned with compressed air.
8. In the event that there is extravasation of the ICG dye, immediately stop the infusion, and apply cold compression to the area. Explain to the patient that there may be temporary

discoloration of the surrounding skin. Advise patient to watch for increasing pain, redness, or swelling over the next few days and to seek appropriate medical attention if worsening of symptoms.

Conflicts of Interest

Stephen H. Tsang receives financial support from Abeona Therapeutics, Inc and Emendo. He is also the founder of Rejuvitas and is on the scientific and clinical advisory board for Nanoscope Therapeutics.

References

1. Baker KJ (1966) Binding of sulfobromophthalein (BSP) sodium and indocyanine green (ICG) by plasma alpha-1 lipoproteins. Proc Soc Exp Biol Med 122(4):957–963
2. Guex-Crosier Y, Herbort CP (1997) Prolonged retinal arterio-venous circulation time by fluorescein but not by indocyanine green angiography in birdshot chorioretinopathy. Ocul Immunol Inflamm 5(3):203–206
3. Yannuzzi LA et al (1994) Indocyanine green videoangiography: current status. Eur J Ophthalmol 4(2):69–81
4. Hayashi K, Hasegawa Y, Tokoro T (1986) Indocyanine green angiography of central serous chorioretinopathy. Int Ophthalmol 9(1):37–41
5. Scheider A, Schroedel C (1989) High resolution indocyanine green angiography with a scanning laser ophthalmoscope. Am J Ophthalmol 108(4):458–459
6. Yannuzzi LA et al (1992) Digital indocyanine green videoangiography and choroidal neovascularization. Retina 12(3):191–223
7. Borruat FX, Auer C, Piguet B (1995) Choroidopathy in multiple evanescent white dot syndrome. Arch Ophthalmol 113(12):1569–1571
8. Bernasconi O, Auer C, Herbort CP (1997) Recurrent toxoplasmic retinochoroiditis. Significance of perilesional satellite dark dots seen by indocyanine green angiography. Ocul Immunol Inflamm 5(3):207–211
9. Giani A, Pellegrini M, Carini E, Peroglio Deiro A, Bottoni F, Staurenghi G (2012 Jun 26) The dark atrophy with indocyanine green angiography in Stargardt disease. Invest Ophthalmol Vis Sci 53(7):3999–4004
10. Arevalo JF (ed) (2009) Retinal angiography and optical coherence tomography. Springer, New York

Chapter 17

Use of the Medmont Dark-Adapted Chromatic Perimeter for Assessing Rod Function in Retinitis Pigmentosa

Yan Nuzbrokh, Sara D. Ragi, and Stephen H. Tsang

Abstract

Medmont Dark-Adapted Chromatic (DAC) Perimeter enables efficient and quantifiable evaluation of rod-mediated (scotopic) vision. DAC tests rod function at multiple retinal locations, creating a topographical map of rod-mediated vision. These dynamic rod responses can be used as a functional marker to monitor disease progression and functional alterations in inherited retinal dystrophies, such as retinitis pigmentosa, Stargardt disease, cone-rod dystrophy, and choroideremia. In this chapter, we describe a protocol for the operation and analysis of the Medmont DAC in monitoring and assessing various retinal disorders.

Key words Rod vision, Two-color perimetry, Dark-adapted chromatic perimetry, Scotopic sensitivity

1 Introduction

The disease process in several inherited retinal dystrophies (IRDs), including retinitis pigmentosa, involves early changes in rod photoreceptors' function. Previously, outcomes in IRDs were measured using photopic (cone-mediated) tests, as there were few reliable methods to analyze scotopic (rod-mediated) vision. The Medmont Dark-Adapted Chromatic (DAC) Perimeter is a new, more reliable test used to assess the entire visual field of one's scotopic vision. In comparison to other scotopic microperimetry tests, the DAC has a significantly higher dynamic range [1, 2]. The DAC perimeter covers the entire range of rod-mediated vision allowing detection of subtle changes in static and dynamic rod function [1].

Objective visual function measures are critical to tracking the disease progression of IRDs. Current visual function measures include visual fields, visual acuity, and electroretinography (ERG). However, with low ERG intersessional reliability, it can be difficult to accurately measure disease progression [3]. With intra-/inter-session repeatability similar to other perimetry devices, the DAC is

Stephen H. Tsang and Peter M. J. Quinn (eds.), *Retinitis Pigmentosa*,
Methods in Molecular Biology, vol. 2560, https://doi.org/10.1007/978-1-0716-2651-1_17,

an additional objective functional measure that will be useful in both the clinic and research studies [4, 5].

Two-color perimetry can be used to identify selective impairment in rod photoreceptors. In two-color perimetry, sensitivity to a cyan (505 nm) stimulus is compared to a red (620 nm) stimulus at the same retinal location [4, 5]. Identification of rod-mediated loci can be achieved through measurement of cyan-red sensitivity differences as rods are naturally more sensitive than cones to cyan stimuli. In healthy patients, cyan stimuli elicit a 20–25 dB lower rod threshold compared to red stimuli. Contrastingly, there is a minute difference between rod and cone thresholds for the red stimulus. Thus, a relatively more significant loss of cyan sensitivity indicates an isolated loss of rod function. A cyan-red retinal sensitivity difference greater than 5 dB indicates selective rod dysfunction with normal or comparatively less diminished cone function. An equal reduction in both cyan and red sensitivity with a cyan-red difference of 0 dB indicates equally impaired cone and rod function. If the retinal loci are determined to be rod-mediated, retinal sensitivity to cyan at those locations may be compared to control values to determine rod system visual field deficits [1].

The Medmont DAC Perimeter measures a patient's response to light stimuli at various retinal locations, enabling an enhanced analysis of rod function [6]. Areas of residual functional vision in patients with IRDs can be identified through this method. Identifying these areas of remaining functional vision can be used to study the natural history of IRDs and establish benchmarks of anticipated visual loss to better target future interventions.

2 Materials

1. Medmont DAC Perimeter machine.
2. Computer with Medmont DAC Perimeter software.
3. Tropicamide 1% and phenylephrine 2.5% dilating drops.
4. Dark-adapted room.
5. Eyepatch.
6. Cylindrical and spherical trial lenses.

3 Methods

The Medmont DAC is dark bowl perimeter with 135 fixed test locations covering a field up to 72° vertically and 144° horizontally [1].

There are many preloaded test fields/grids on the computer software. These fields include binocular driving, macula, and peripheral. Test grids can be created for specific patient populations.

1. Determine subject's best-corrected visual acuity (BCVA) using a 4-m logMAR chart (*see* **Notes 1** and **2**).
2. Use the autorefractor, capture the patient's refraction for both eyes, and add +3.00 to the sphere in order to account for the distance between the patient's eye and the perimetry field prior to entering this value into patient's profile in the DAC software.
3. Using this adjusted refraction of the subject, select appropriate lenses. The lenses will be placed in the central field of the perimeter.
4. Enter the patient's refraction values into their patient profile in the computer's DAC software.
5. Dilate the preferred eye (or eyes, depending on whether the test will be administered to one or both eyes) with one drop of tropicamide 1% and one drop of phenylephrine 2.5% 5 min apart.
6. Wait 15 min following administration of dilation drops. Measure the dilation and only begin the test after dilation reaches 7 mm in diameter.
7. After dilation, walk patient over to darkened room in which perimetry testing will take place (*see* **Note 3**).
8. Position cylindrical and spherical lenses as determined by refraction with adjustment to test distance (*see* **Note 4**).
9. Place an eye patch over the eye that will undergo testing first.
10. Darken the room and instruct the patient to refrain from the use of any electronic devices.
11. Dark adapt subject for 40 min by leaving the patient comfortably in a completely darkened room.
12. Upon entering the room following dark adaptation, direct the patient to cover his or her eyes to prevent exposure to external light. After entering, instruct the patient to remove the eye patch from the eye, which will be tested first, and place on the opposite eye (*see* **Notes 5** and **6**).
13. Help position subject's head in the forehead chin rest, and align the test eye in the viewing window (*see* **Note 7**).
14. Place a handheld clicker device with clicker on side into the patient's dominant hand, and instruct the patient to click the button on this device when they see a bright flash of light.
15. Select the appropriate test grid for the participant and begin the examination. Patch contralateral eye to prevent blurry vision.

16. Testing should begin with cyan (505 nm) stimuli followed by red (605 nm) stimuli.
17. Instruct participant to focus on the red fixation light located at the center of the field. Instruct the patient to press a button whenever a flash target appears on the screen. These lights are presented to different parts of the visual field (*see* **Note 8**).
18. Monitor alignment through infrared viewing of the test eye. Reposition subject during examination when necessary with the exam paused. Quality of subject's examination can be assessed by the percentage of false-positive responses (*see* **Notes 8** and **9**).
19. After completion of first test, instruct the participant to sit back and rest until they are ready to proceed with the second perimetry exam.
20. Determine cyan-red sensitivity difference by using compare window on computer software.

4 Notes

1. Perform any necessary imaging, including spectral domain ocular coherence tomography (SD-OCT), color fundus, and near infrared reflectance (NIR) after DAC perimetry.
2. Sterilize all equipment prior to use.
3. The darkened room should be carefully crafted to facilitate minimal light. Use only red light as it is less likely to affect dark adaptation. Only use light when necessary to allow participant and examiner to function in the dark. Cover the computer screens with red light.
4. Due to difficulty of functioning in darkened room, attempt to set up most of the examination before darkening the room. Position trial lenses, align the first eye being tested, and set up computer software.
5. Position patient's head so that the forehead is placed flat against the upper rest, and then position chin on the lower rest so that the eye is properly aligned with the viewing window.
6. Contralateral eye is patched during testing to prevent blurry vision.
7. Many patients will experience flashes of light of varying color and size. Inform the patient this is normal occurrence and is part of the Medmont algorithm.
8. Encourage participant to pause as needed to prevent fatigue. Examination can be paused with the participant holding down

the testing button or the examiner pausing the test directly on the computer.

9. Instruct the participant to attempt to blink as they press the button to reduce false-negative test points.

Conflicts of Interest

Stephen H. Tsang receives financial support from Abeona Therapeutics, Inc and Emendo. He is also the founder of Rejuvitas and is on the scientific and clinical advisory board for Nanoscope Therapeutics.

References

1. Heeren TFC, Tzaridis S, Bonelli R et al (2019) Dark-adapted two-color fundus-controlled perimetry in macular telangiectasia type 2. Invest Ophthalmol Vis Sci 60(5):1760–1767. https://doi.org/10.1167/iovs.18-25360
2. Tan RS, Guymer RH, Luu CD (2018) Repeatability of retinal sensitivity measurements using a Medmont dark-adapted chromatic perimeter in healthy and age-related macular degeneration cases. Transl Vis Sci Technol 7(3):3. https://doi.org/10.1167/tvst.7.3.3
3. Seiple W, Clemens CJ, Greenstein VC et al (2004) Test–retest reliability of the multifocal electroretinogram and Humphrey visual fields in patients with retinitis pigmentosa. Doc Ophthalmol 109(3):255–272
4. Bennett LD, Klein M, Locke KG et al (2017) Dark-adapted chromatic perimetry for measuring rod visual fields in patients with retinitis pigmentosa. Transl Vis Sci Technol 6(4):15. https://doi.org/10.1167/tvst.6.4.15
5. Bennett LD, Metz G, Klein M et al (2019) Regional variations and intra-/intersession repeatability for scotopic sensitivity in normal controls and patients with inherited retinal degenerations. Invest Ophthalmol Vis Sci 60(4):1122–1131. https://doi.org/10.1167/iovs.18-25473
6. Fraser RG, Tan R, Ayton LN et al (2016) Assessment of retinotopic rod photoreceptor function using a dark-adapted chromatic perimeter in intermediate age-related macular degeneration. Invest Ophthalmol Vis Sci 57(13):5436–5442. https://doi.org/10.1167/iovs.16-19295

Chapter 18

Multi-luminance Mobility Testing Endpoint

Henry W. Zhou

Abstract

An individual's functional vision may be measured via visual assessment and performance on mobility tasks. Since traditional mobility performance tests neglect to examine the effects of illumination on performance, the multi-luminance mobility test (MLMT) was designed to quantitatively assess the effects of illumination levels on an individual's mobility performance. In this chapter, we describe how the MLMT is conducted and scored in order to properly evaluate a participant's mobility under various light conditions.

Key words Functional vision, Light perception, MLMT, Mobility performance, Mobility tasks, Multi-luminance mobility testing

1 Introduction

Functional vision is an essential component of one's ability to successfully navigate day-to-day tasks. Loss of functional vision, which may be described as the ability to independently conduct one's typical daily activities, leads to a decrease in functional ability and quality of life [1]. Evaluation of a person's functional vision requires vision assessments as well as assessment of the person's performance on mobility tasks [1, 2]. Functional vision can be considered a performance output of a person's visual function when subjected to a test involving a visually dependent activity. Several key measures of visual function can therefore influence a person's performance on mobility tasks: visual acuity, visual field, and light contrast sensitivity [3].

The total visual field plays a significant role in predicting a person's performance on mobility tasks. The smaller the total visual field, the worse the mobility performance [4]. Likewise, a person's visual acuity also plays a significant role in predicting a person's performance on mobility tasks as does their contrast sensitivity. Visual acuity is a measure of the eye's ability to perceive details from distance. Contrast sensitivity is a measure of the eye's ability to

Stephen H. Tsang and Peter M. J. Quinn (eds.), *Retinitis Pigmentosa*,
Methods in Molecular Biology, vol. 2560, https://doi.org/10.1007/978-1-0716-2651-1_18,

perceive differences in light levels. Generally, mobility appears to be more influenced by contrast sensitivity and visual field than by visual acuity [3].

Traditional assessment of mobility performance in visually impaired people typically involves calculating a percentage of preferred walking speed on a controlled mobility course [5]. However, these traditional mobility metrics fail to address the effects of illumination on mobility. Given that people typically experience a wide range of illumination levels throughout the course of a day, a person's mobility function at certain light levels must be an important factor in evaluating quality of life and overall function.

A test called the multi-luminance mobility test (MLMT) was created to meet the need for a test that quantitatively assesses the effects of illumination on speed and accuracy of navigating a controlled mobility (obstacle) course. MLMT was designed to measure changes in functional vision by using a standardized range of illumination ranging from 400 lux to 1 lux. Performance on the MLMT is dependent on the test subject's functional vision and visual function, including visual field, visual acuity, and contrast sensitivity.

In order to develop therapeutic approaches to ophthalmologic diseases, clinical study endpoints that take into account varying light conditions are essential. Therefore, the MLMT and its intentional design toward light sensitivity at varying levels of illumination serves as a useful clinical study endpoint for diseases such as inherited retinal degenerations (IRDs) that involve progressive decreases in light perception [6].

A prospective observational study conducted by Chung et al. in 2017 [3] enrolled 60 eligible subjects, with 54 completing all testing visits. The primary outcome of this study was to assess content validity and reliability of MLMT as well as assess accuracy and speed of visually impaired subjects completing the course compared to normal vision controls. The results of this study found that the MLMT consistently showed high reliability with inter-grader agreement rates of 97.9%. The MLMT showed high content validity relative to visual acuity and visual field by demonstrating cut-off effects that persisted independently of participant age [3]. The study concluded that the MLMT may be administered in outpatient settings to track functional vision. Study limitations include small sample size, "ceiling" effect at 1 lux, and variability in natural walking speed of participants.

One recent open-label, randomized, controlled phase 3 trial for gene replacement therapy in *RPE65*-mediated IRD used 1-year change in MLMT performance as the primary efficacy endpoint [7]. The study recruited 31 participants and randomized 21 to intervention and 10 to control. At 1 year, the mean change in MLMT score for the intervention group was 1.8 (standard deviation 1.1) light levels. The mean change in the control group was 0.2

(standard deviation 1.0). In total, 13 out of 21 subjects in the intervention group, as opposed to 0/10 control subjects, managed to pass the MLMT at the 1 lux luminance level. The results of this trial marked the introduction of a novel treatment for patients with *RPE65* mutations and led to the first FDA-approved gene therapy for vision loss [7].

2 Materials

1. MLMT obstacle course (Fig. 1).
2. Video recording functionality.
3. Eye patch.
4. Two independent graders.

3 Methods

The MLMT uses seven levels of illuminating ranging from 1 lux at the darkest level to 400 lux at the brightest level. These light levels can be verified by calibrated light meters at 5 different positions on the course. There are 12 different courses, each measuring 5′ × 10′. An example of one MLMT course configuration is shown in Fig. 1. For details on course standardization, *see* **Note 1**.

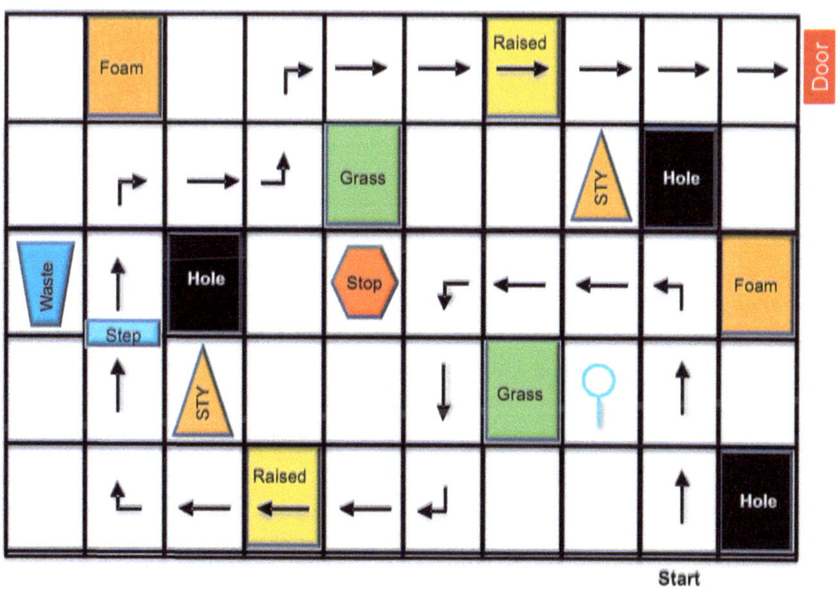

Fig. 1 Example MLMT layout. Obstacles: two raised steps with arrows (2 in. high), two grass tiles, three black tiles representing holes, two elevated foam blocks (4.5 in. high), two Styrofoam cones, one stop sign (adjustable from 40 to 72 in. high), one step-over obstacle (9 in. high), one waist-high obstacle (represented by the blue tree, 27 in. high), and one waste basket (13 in. high). (Reproduced with permission from John Wiley & Sons, 2020)

The steps for conducting the MLMT are as follows:

1. Participants are first given 40 min for dark adaptation.
2. Participants are told to follow the arrows on the course while avoiding obstacles in their path, traversing raised steps, and identifying the door at the end of the course. Each participant first completes the course with one eye patched, then complete a different configuration with the other eye patched, and finally complete yet another different configuration with no eyes patched.
3. Each participant's test runs are videotaped for both video and audio.
4. The tapes are coded, transferred to an independent reading center, and assessed by two graders. Graders mark the participant's speed and accuracy. Each course is assessed for number of obstacles hit, number of times off course, number of times re-guided, number of tiles bypassed, and time to course completion.
5. These parameters are used to calculate obstacles plus penalties, accuracy, course time, and time score. *See* **Notes 2** and **3** for details on how the time score and accuracy score are calculated.
6. The graders then assign each course completion with a "pass" or "fail" depending on a fixed time limit and a minimum number of errors at the light level being tested.
7. This process is repeated for each participant by progressing from lower to higher light levels until failing and passing levels are identified for each eye patching condition.
8. The standardized MLMT has been validated by Chung et al. as described in **Note 4**.

4 Notes

1. The traversed path is indicated with printed black arrows standardized to dimensions consistent with Snellen lettering for visual acuity of 20/200 at 2 m. In addition, each course is standardized for the number of turns and the number and type of obstacles within each course.
2. Calculating the time score involves combining the seconds needed to complete the course with the time penalties incurred (i.e., 15 s added for each instance off course, 15 s added for each tile bypassed, and 30 s added for each redirect).

3. Calculating the accuracy score involves dividing the number of accuracy penalties by the total number of obstacles in the course.
4. Chung et al. performed a validation study in 2017 that indicated the standardized MLMT showed both construct and content validity in differentiating low vision from normal vision populations and identifying a range of performance among low vision patients. Normal subjects passed time and accuracy at all light levels, while visually impaired subjects demonstrated a range of failing and passing performances. Content validity was supported by visual acuity and visual field test results.

References

1. Lepri BP (2009) Is acuity enough? Other considerations in clinical investigations of visual prostheses. J Neural Eng 6:035003. https://doi.org/10.1088/1741-2560/6/3/035003
2. Deverell L, Meyer D, Lau BT et al (2009) Optimising technology to measure functional vision, mobility and service outcomes for people with low vision or blindness: protocol for a prospective cohort study in Australia and Malaysia. BMJ Open 7:e018140. https://doi.org/10.1136/bmjopen-2017-018140
3. Chung D, McCague S, Yu Z et al (2017) Novel mobility test to assess functional vision in patients with inherited retinal dystrophies. Clin Exp Ophthalmol 46(3):247–259
4. Lovie-Kitchin JE, Soong GP, Hassan SE et al (2010) Visual field size criteria for mobility rehabilitation referral. Optom Vis Sci 87(12): E948–E957. https://doi.org/10.1097/OPX.0b013e3181ff99be
5. Soong GP, Lovie-Kitchin JE, Brown B (2001) Does mobility performance of visually impaired adults improve immediately after orientation and mobility training? Optom Vis Sci 78(9): 657–666
6. FDA Advisory Committee Meeting (2017, October 12) Spark therapeutics briefing document, pp 48–60
7. Russel S, Bennett J, Wellman JA et al (2017) Efficacy and safety of voretigene neparvovec (AAV2-hRPE65v2) in patients with RPE65-mediated inherited retinal dystrophy: a randomised, controlled, open-label, phase 3 trial. Lancet 390(10097):849–860

Chapter 19

Preclinical Models of Retinitis Pigmentosa

Mark D. Travor

Abstract

Retinitis pigmentosa (RP) is the name for a group of phenotypically-related heritable retinal degenerative disorders. Many genes have been implicated as causing variants of RP, and while the clinical phenotypes are remarkably similar, they may differ in age of onset, progression, and severity. Common inheritance patterns for specific genes connected with the development of the disorder include autosomal dominant, autosomal recessive, and X-linked. Modeling the disease in animals and other preclinical systems offers a cost-conscious, ethical, and time-efficient method for studying the disease subtypes. The history of RP models is briefly examined, and both naturally occurring and transgenic preclinical models of RP in many different organisms are discussed. Syndromic forms of RP and models thereof are reviewed as well.

Key words Retinitis pigmentosa, Preclinical models, Animal models, Retinal degeneration, Photoreceptors, Autosomal dominant, Autosomal recessive, X-linked, Transgenic, Bardet–Biedl syndrome, Usher syndrome

1 Introduction

Retinitis pigmentosa (RP) is a genetically heterogeneous disease made up of phenotypically similar retinal degenerative disorders. RP is fairly common in humans (with a prevalence around 1 in 4000 in most populations) and is typically hereditary [1]. Inheritance patterns include autosomal recessive (50–60% of cases), autosomal dominant (30–40%), and X-linked recessive (5–15%) [1]. Isolated cases may occur in patients with no family history (simplex RP), and there are also reports of mitochondrially inherited cases [2]. RP is most commonly a disease of isolated retinal involvement, but there also exist syndromic forms, including Usher and Bardet–Biedl syndromes (characterized by sensorineural deafness and obesity, respectively) [3, 4].

As a clinical entity, RP is characterized by an early loss of rods in the periphery of the retina, manifesting as night-blindness (nyctalopia) and loss of peripheral vision. Later stages of the disease involve the cones and eventually may lead to loss of central vision.

Stephen H. Tsang and Peter M. J. Quinn (eds.), *Retinitis Pigmentosa*,
Methods in Molecular Biology, vol. 2560, https://doi.org/10.1007/978-1-0716-2651-1_19,

Other hallmarks of the disease include punctate "bone spicule" pigmentation of the retina, attenuated retinal vessels, retinal pigment epithelium (RPE) or photoreceptor dysfunction (assessable by diminished electroretinogram, or ERG, response), and progressive photoreceptor death [5]. The degree and rapidity of disease progression varies by heritable subtype, causative mutation, and environmental factors [6].

While studying the disease in humans in vivo is important, it can be challenging. Modeling the disease in animals offers a cost-conscious, ethical, and less time-consuming method for studying the disease subtypes. Doing so has allowed for much better understanding of the underlying biochemical mechanisms of the disease phenotypes. Using animal models in RP is likely superior to their use in more genetically complex diseases like glaucoma, as in RP individual gene defects can be identified that produce the disease phenotype. Furthermore, working with the many identified and developed animal models has proved a fruitful method of testing novel therapeutic strategies. The main considerations in evaluating an RP model are that the genetic defect in humans corresponds to that in the model organism and that the phenotypic manifestations and progression of the disease in the animal model mirrors human RP [7].

There are naturally occurring animal models in many different organisms that have been discovered, transgenic models that have been developed using genetic engineering techniques, and even inducible models in which retinal degeneration can be initiated at the desired time [8]. Models in human induced pluripotent stem cells (hiPSCs) also exist [9].

Using preclinical models to understand human RP has its origin as early as 1924, when Dr. Keeler discovered and investigated heritable rod defects in albino mice [10]. Rodents have been a staple RP model throughout the decades since, with many naturally occurring and transgenic examples, though recently, emphasis has also been placed on larger animal models (canine, porcine, etc.) due to structural similarity with human eyes [11].

The first loci for RP were identified in the 1980s, when Bhattacharya and colleagues mapped the gene responsible for a form of X-linked RP to the X chromosome and Humphries and colleagues identified an autosomal dominant RP locus [12, 13]. The first specific mutation (*Rhodopsin* P23H) responsible for RP was identified in 1990; since then, more than 70 genes for nonsyndromic RP have been identified and another 30 or more for syndromic forms [14, 15].

The first ever transgenic animal, made via introduction of a rabbit beta-globin gene into mice zygotes, was produced in 1981, setting the precedent for myriad investigations that followed [16]. Early work in retinal transgenic models included defining the rhodopsin promoter in order to develop photoreceptor-specific promoters [17–19]. In the early 1990s, Naash and colleagues introduced a mutated opsin gene into the mouse, modeling autosomal dominant RP [20]. Now, numerous transgenic models exist where an organism bearing a mutation in a crucial pathway illustrates an RP phenotype [21].

2 Models of RP by Inheritance, Origin, and Organism

2.1 Autosomal Dominant RP

Autosomal dominant RP (adRP) is most commonly a result of mutations in the *rhodopsin* gene, though more than 25 genes have been implicated [7, 22]. Rhodopsin is a light-activated G protein-coupled receptor bound to opsin that, along with other molecules in the visual cycle, initiates the transduction cascade, leading to photoreceptor hyperpolarization and signal propagation. Often in mutants, misfolded rhodopsin protein leads to ubiquitinated aggregates, disrupting the normal architecture and physiology of affected cells [23]. There are two classes of rhodopsin mutants: Class I, where rhodopsin folding is normal but either transport or activity are compromised; and Class II, where misfolded opsin aggregates [24]. There are few naturally occurring animal models of rhodopsin mutants, but many transgenic animals will be discussed below.

Table 1 lists common preclinical models of retinitis pigmentosa, including gene, mutation, and inheritance pattern. Select models from Table 1 will be discussed in the text.

2.2 Naturally Occurring Models of adRP

2.2.1 Canine

English mastiff dogs with a naturally occurring mutation in the *Rho* gene (T4R) have been identified and represent one of the only natural models of *Rho* mutant adRP. In this model, photoreceptors develop normally, but later in life, mutants show retinal degeneration and dramatically reduced recovery of rod function after light exposure [25]. This model, being a large animal model of adRP, is useful for trials of novel therapies, especially those necessitating surgery.

2.2.2 Feline

The *Rdy* Abyssinian cat is another rare example of a naturally occurring large animal model of adRP [26]. In these cats, photoreceptor degeneration and opsin accumulation in the outer nuclear layer begin around 3 weeks of age and peak around 9 weeks [27]. The affected cats begin to go blind within the first few months of life, though more recent work has demonstrated that rods and cones may not develop normally, making this a better model for Leber's congenital amaurosis (LCA) or cone–rod dystrophy [28]. The mutated gene is the cone–rod homeobox gene (*Crx*), critical for the activation of many other genes involved in photoreceptor development [29].

Table 1
Preclinical models of nonsyndromic retinitis pigmentosa (RP)

Inheritance pattern	Gene	Model organism and trivial name	Gene product	Alteration	Reference
AD	*Chm (Rep1)*	Murine—*Chm*$^{null/WT}$ female mouse (T)	Rab escort protein-1 (REP-1)	*Chm* null/WT	[136]
AD	*Crx*	Feline—*Rdy* Abyssinian cat (N)	Cone-rod homeobox protein	Δ1 bp causing premature stop	[26–28, 188]
AD	*Prph2*	Murine—C214S *rds/rd2* mouse (T)	Peripherin/rds (retinal degeneration slow)	C214S	[36, 189]
AD	*Prph2*	Murine—P216L *rds/rd2* mouse (T)	Peripherin/rds (retinal degeneration slow)	P216L	[35]
AD	*Prph2*	Murine—*rds/rd2* mouse (N)	Peripherin/rds (retinal degeneration slow)	9 kb insertion exon 2	[30, 190]
AD	*Rd4*	Murine—*rd4* mouse (N)	Unknown	Chromosomal inversion: In (4)56Rk	[33]
AD	*Rho*	Canine—English mastiff (N)	Rhodopsin	T4R	[25]
AD	*Rho*	Murine—D190N mouse (T)	Rhodopsin	D190N	[47]
AD	*Rho*	Murine—I255/256 mouse (T)	Rhodopsin	Δ3 bp exon 4	[44, 45]
AD	*Rho*	Murine—K296E mouse (T)	Rhodopsin	K296E	[46, 191]
AD	*Rho*	Murine—P23H mouse (T)	Rhodopsin	P23H	[20, 37]
AD	*Rho*	Murine—P23H rat (T)	Rhodopsin	P23H	[39, 40]
AD	*Rho*	Murine—P347S mouse (T)	Rhodopsin	P347S	[42]
AD	*Rho*	Murine—Q344ter mouse (T)	Rhodopsin	Q344ter	[41]
AD	*Rho*	Murine—S334ter rat (T)	Rhodopsin	S334ter	[43]
AD	*Rho*	Murine—VPP mouse (T)	Rhodopsin	V20G, P23H, and P27L	[20, 38, 192]
AD	*Rho*	Piscine—Q344ter (*ovl*) zebrafish (T)	Rhodopsin	Q344ter	[53]

(continued)

Table 1 (continued)

Inheritance pattern	Gene	Model organism and trivial name	Gene product	Alteration	Reference
AD	*Rho*	Porcine—P23H Miniature pig (T)	Rhodopsin	P23H	[58]
AD	*Rho*	Porcine—P347L pig (T)	Rhodopsin	P347L	[56, 57]
AD	*Rpe65*	Murine—D477G mouse (T)	Retinoid isomerohydrolase RPE65	D477G	[193]
AD	*Timp3*	Murine—S156C knockin mouse (T)	Tissue inhibitor of metalloproteinase-3	S156C	[48]
AR	*Agtbp1*	Murine—*pcd* mouse (Purkinje cell degeneration) (N)	AGTPBP1 (ATP/GTP-Binding Protein 1)	Unknown mutation	[96, 97]
AR	*Arap1*	Murine—Arap1 KO mouse (T)	ArfGAP with RhoGAP Domain, Ankyrin repeat and PH Domain 1	Arap1 knockout	[110]
AR	*C2orf71*	Canine—Gordon setter (N)	Protein of unknown function	1 bp insertion exon 1	[73]
AR	*C2orf71*	Piscine—Zebrafish (T)	Protein of unknown function	Morpholino-induced knockdown	[115]
AR	*C8orf37*	Murine—*C8orf37* KO mouse (T)	Protein of unknown function	CRISPR/Cas9 *C8orf37* knockout	[108]
AR	*Ccdc66*	Canine—Schapendoes (N)	Coiled-coil domain-containing protein 66	1 bp insertion exon 6	[194]
AR	*Cep290*	Feline—Abyssinian retinal degeneration cat (*rdAc*) (N)	Centrosomal protein of 290 kDa	SNP in intron causing alternate splicing	[28]
AR	*Cep290*	Murine—*rd16* mouse (N)	Centrosomal protein of 290 kDa	Δ897 bp	[79]
AR	*Cerkl*	Piscine—Zebrafish (T)	CERKL (ceramide kinase-like protein)	Morpholino-induced knockdown	[116]

(continued)

Table 1
(continued)

Inheritance pattern	Gene	Model organism and trivial name	Gene product	Alteration	Reference
AR	*Cnga1*	Canine—Shetland sheepdog (N)	Cyclic nucleotide-gated cation channel alpha-1	Δ4 bp exon 9	[64]
AR	*Cngb1*	Canine—Papillon (N)	Cyclic nucleotide-gated cation channel beta-1	Δ1 bp and 6 bp insertion exon 25	[65, 195]
AR	*Cngb1*	Murine—*Cngb1-X26* mouse (T)	Cyclic nucleotide-gated cation channel beta-1	Δexon 26	[105, 106]
AR	*Crb1*	Murine—*Crb1* (*rd8)* mouse (N)	*Drosophila* Crumbs homolog 1	Δ1 bp causing premature stop at nt3481	[84, 91]
AR	*Fam161a*	Canine—Tibetan spaniel (N)	FAM161 centrosomal protein A	132 bp intronic SINE insertion near exon 5	[196]
AR	*Gc1*	Avian—*rd* (retinal degeneration) chicken (N)	Photoreceptor guanylate cyclase 1	Deletion, unknown precise location	[61, 62]
AR	*Irbp*	Murine—*IRBP* KO mouse (T)	Interphotoreceptor retinoid-binding protein	*IRBP* knockout	[109]
AR	*Mertk*	Canine—Swedish Vallhund (N)	Mertk gene (c-mer proto-oncogene tyrosine kinase)	LINE-1 insertion intron 1	[66, 67]
AR	*Mertk*	Murine—*Mer* knockdown mice (N)	Mertk gene (c-mer proto-oncogene tyrosine kinase)	Δexon	[95, 197]
AR	*Mertk*	Murine—RCS rat (N)	Mertk gene (c-mer proto-oncogene tyrosine kinase)	Δexon 2	[93, 198, 199]
AR	*Mitf*	Murine—vitiligo (*mivit*) mouse (N)	Microphthalmia-associated transcription factor	D222N	[200, 201]
AR	*Pde6a*	Canine—*rcd3* Cardigan Welsh corgi (N)	Rod PDE6 α subunit	Δ1 bp exon 15	[70, 74]
AR	*Pde6a*	Murine—*Pde6a nmf282* mouse (T-chemical mutagenesis)	Rod PDE6 α subunit	V685M	[114]

(continued)

Table 1
(continued)

Inheritance pattern	Gene	Model organism and trivial name	Gene product	Alteration	Reference
AR	*Pde6a*	Murine—*Pde6a nmf363* mouse (T-chemical mutagenesis)	Rod PDE6 α subunit	D670G	[114]
AR	*Pde6b*	Canine—*crd1* American Staffordshire terrier (N)	Rod PDE6 β subunit	Δ3 bp exon 21	[72]
AR	*Pde6b*	Canine—*rcd1* Irish setter (N)	Rod PDE6 β subunit	TGG to stop codon exon 21	[75]
AR	*Pde6b*	Canine—Sloughi dog (N)	Rod PDE6 β subunit	8 bp insertion exon 21	[71]
AR	*Pde6b*	Murine—Pde6b *H620Q* mouse (T)	Rod PDE6 β subunit	H620Q	[111]
AR	*Pde6b*	Murine—Pde6b H620Q, Pax6α::Cre mouse (T)	Rod PDE6 β subunit	H620Q, Pax6α::Cre driver	[112]
AR	*Pde6b*	Murine—Pde6b H620Q, Pde6g:: CreERT2 mouse (T)	Rod PDE6 β subunit	H620Q, Pde6g:: CreERT2 driver	[112]
AR	*Pde6b*	Murine—*rd1* mouse (*r/rd* mouse) (N)	Rod PDE6 β subunit	Y347ter and intronic insertion of Xmv-28 virus	[202–204]
AR	*Pde6b*	Murine—*rd10* mouse (N)	Rod PDE6 β subunit	R560C exon 13	[84]
AR	*Pde6g*	Murine—*Pde6g* knockout mouse (T)	Rod PDE6 ϒ subunit	*PDE6g* knockout	[113]
AR	*Prcd*	Canine—many breeds (N)	Photoreceptor disk component	G to A exon 1	[68, 205]
AR	*Prom-1*	Murine—*Prom-1* knockout mouse (T)	Prominin-1	*Prom-1 −/−*	[107]

(continued)

Table 1
(continued)

Inheritance pattern	Gene	Model organism and trivial name	Gene product	Alteration	Reference
AR	*Rd3*	Murine—*rd3* mouse (N)	RD3 (retinal degeneration 3)	R107ter	[86, 88]
AR	*Rd3* (*C1orf36*)	Canine—Collie (N)	RD3 (retinal degeneration 3)	22 bp insertion exon 4	[69]
AR	*Rpe65*	Murine—*Rpe65* (*rd12*) mouse (N)	Retinoid isomerohydrolase RPE65	R44ter	[92, 206]
AR	*Rpe65*	Murine—*Rpe65* KO mouse (T)	Retinoid isomerohydrolase RPE65	*RPE65* −/−	[98]
AR	*Sag*	Canine—Basenji (N)	S-arrestin	T to C exon 18	[207]
AR	*Slc4A3*	Canine—Golden retriever (N)	Anion exchange protein 3	1 bp insertion exon 16	[208]
AR	*Spata7*	Murine—Spata7 knockout mice (T)	Spermatogenesis-associated protein 7	*Spata7* −/−	[103, 104]
AR	*Stk38l*	Canine—Norwegian elkhound (N)	Serine/threonine-protein kinase 38-like	SINE insertion exon 4	[209]
AR	*Ttc8*	Canine—Golden retriever (N)	Tetratricopeptide repeat protein 8	Δ1 bp exon 8	[210]
Various	Many	*Drosophila* (T)	Several	Constructed with various techniques/alterations	[117]
Various	Many	human induced pluripotent stem cells (hiPSCs) (T)	Several	Reprogrammed with various techniques/alterations	[9]
XL	*Mpdz*	Avian—*rdd* chicken (retinal dysplasia and degeneration) (N)	Multiple PDZ domain protein	C to T causing premature stop	[123, 124, 126]
XL	*Rp2*	Piscine—*ZFRP2* Zebrafish (T)	Protein XRP2	Morpholino-induced knockdown	[140]

(continued)

Table 1 (continued)

Inheritance pattern	Gene	Model organism and trivial name	Gene product	Alteration	Reference
XL	*Rpgr*	Canine—XLPRA1 Siberian husky (N)	RPGR (retinitis pigmentosa GTPase regulator)	Δ5 bp ORF15	[131]
XL	*Rpgr*	Canine—XLPRA2 mongrel (N)	RPGR (retinitis pigmentosa GTPase regulator)	Δ2 bp ORF15	[131]
XL	*Rpgr*	Murine—*rd9* mouse (N)	RPGR-ORF15	Δ32 bp ORF15	[133]
XL	*Rpgr*	Murine—*RPGR* KO mouse (T)	RPGR (retinitis pigmentosa GTPase regulator)	Knockout exons 4–6	[134]
XL	*Rpgr*	Piscine—*ZFRPGR2* Zebrafish (T)	RPGR (retinitis pigmentosa GTPase regulator)	Morpholino-induced knockdown	[138]

A list of preclinical models of RP. Categorized by inheritance pattern, gene, model organism, gene product, and gene alteration. Naturally occurring or transgenic is indicated by a parenthetical "N" or "T" in model organism column. Sorted by inheritance pattern, gene, and model organism. Abbreviations: *AD* autosomal dominant, *AR* autosomal recessive, *bp* base pair, *kb* kilo base, *KO* knockout, *LINE* long interspersed nuclear element, *nt* nucleotide, *ORF* open reading frame, *SINE* short interspersed nuclear element, *SNP* single nucleotide polymorphism, *XL* X-linked, *−ter* mutation to stop codon, *Δ* deletion, −/− null mutation

2.2.3 Murine

No naturally occurring *rhodopsin* mutant models exist in mice. However, there are a few models of other implicated genes. The naturally occurring *rds/rd2* mouse, caused by a mutation in the *Prph2* (peripherin), was named "retinal degeneration slow (*rds*)" because the rate of retinal degeneration was comparatively slower versus the *rd1* mouse (discussed in Subheading 2.5.4) [30]. The genetic defect has been identified as a 9.2-kb insertion into exon 2 of the *prph2* gene, causing a frameshift and truncation of the peptide sequence [31]. *Rds/rd2* mice do not form outer segments and have no response on ERG in bright or dim light [32].

Rd4 mice carry an inversion on chromosome 4—In(4)56Rk—that is lethal in homozygotes but causes retinal degeneration in heterozygotes. In affected mice, outer nuclear layer thickness decline manifests first, followed by other typical findings in the fundus (vessel attenuation, pigment deposition, etc.) and eventual loss of ERG response [33, 34].

2.3 Transgenic Models of adRP

2.3.1 Murine

Rds mice, discussed above, have also been used to create transgenic models, with additional mutations being introduced in the peripherin gene. Two such models, C214S and P216L transgenic mice, have been produced to more closely approximate the human forms of adRP. In the P216L mice, the *rds* mutation and the P216L substitution combine to produce a phenotype that is likely a synergistic result of the two defects, approximating human *rds*-type adRP [35]. The C214S mutation, similarly, when expressed in the inner retina in *rds* mice, resulted in a loss-of-function phenotype that correlated with the human adRP patients carrying the same mutation. This suggests that a C214S mutation, in the context of an *rds* mouse, results in haploinsufficiency [36].

As opposed to naturally occurring mice, there are many transgenic *Rho* mutant mice that have been constructed. A common cause of adRP in humans, the P23H mutation, led to the early development of the P23H mouse (mentioned in Subheading 1); this Class II mutant leads to progressive loss of photoreceptors and severe visual compromise [20, 37]. More recently, the VPP mouse was created, which combines the P23H mutation with V20G and P27L mutations (all in *Rho* though these additional mutations are not thought to contribute deleteriously) [38]. These mice gradually lose photoreceptors and retinal function, despite synthesizing both mutant and wild-type rhodopsin (because they are dominant mutations). A transgenic P23H rat has also been produced, and in this model gradual loss of rods followed by cones has been illustrated and been related to increased metabolic demands [39, 40].

Q344ter mice were developed to mimic Class I mutants; in this model the last 5 amino acids of rhodopsin are truncated, leading to impaired trafficking of the mutant protein and development of abnormal aggregates [41]. A similar trafficking defect is seen in P347S mice, again causing accumulation of mutant rhodopsin protein [42]. A S334ter rat model has been produced, in which rapid photoreceptor degeneration occurs and is coupled with an increase in apoptotic mechanisms (caspase-3-like activity); in this model, intraocular injection of a caspase-3 inhibitor was shown to partially protect photoreceptors from degeneration [43].

I255/256 mice, produced by a three base pair deletion in the *Rho* gene, show rapid progression of rod cell death and absence of an ERG response early in life [44]. Studies in this model have suggested that hypoxia is capable of reversing retinal vessel attenuation and stimulating new capillary growth, which has important treatment implications [45]. K296E mice, where the mutation is in the chromophore-binding portion of the RHO protein, were hypothesized to cause photoreceptor cell death due to constitutive activation of transducin by rhodopsin. Further investigation has suggested the photoreceptor loss is due instead to persistent binding of arrestin [7, 46]. D190N mice, created by knockin of the D190N *rhodopsin* mutation mirror humans and exhibit the loss of scotopic ERG response as well as progressive rod degeneration [47]. Another feature this mouse exhibits is a hyperautofluorescence analogous to the perifoveal ring in the fundus of human patients [47].

TIMP3, the tissue inhibitor of metalloproteinase-3 gene, is expressed in the RPE and is generally mutated in patients with a form of macular degeneration called Sorsby fundus dystrophy (SFD) but has also been associated with RP [48, 49]. SFD is an adult-onset form of retinal degeneration, characterized by a rapid loss of central followed by peripheral vision, leading to eventual blindness [50]. Knockin of a causative S156C mutation in *TIMP3* leads to a more mild retinal degeneration phenotype in mice compared to analogous patients [48]. This could indicate a greater adaptive ability of the mouse retina during development, or that the full phenotype in humans is dependent on environmental or additive genetic factors [48, 51]. *TIMP3* knockout does not cause a retinal phenotype at all, suggesting that at least in mice, loss of *TIMP3* function is not causing SFD [52].

2.3.2 Piscine

Q344ter *Rho* mutant zebrafish have also been developed, analogous to the mice expressing the same mutation, and demonstrate rod apoptosis mediated by light exposure, ectopic phototransduction, and inappropriately activated adenylyl cyclase [53, 54].

2.3.3 Porcine

A known problem with murine models of RP is a smaller proportion of cones than human retinas; this issue limits the study of disease processes and potentially significant treatment possibilities related to cone preservation. Pig eyes, by contrast, have a retinal geography similar to the human retina with a cone-dominant center and a rod-dominant periphery [55]. Pig eyes are also similar in size to human eyes, allowing for improved surgical access in therapeutic interventions. Of course, pigs are less convenient to work with as model organisms due to their body size and developmental speed. Despite that limitation, a few porcine models of adRP exist. P347L pigs have been produced, demonstrating mislocalization consistent with Class I mutants, and further illustrating the loss of rods followed by cones, as one would expect in the human form of the disease [56, 57].

P23H miniature pigs have also been developed, ameliorating some of the difficulty with using full-sized pig models and giving another option for studying this most common causative mutation of human adRP. In this model, similarity to the human disease is maintained, with early loss of rod function as measured by ERG, followed by loss of cone function and outer nuclear layer degeneration [58].

2.4 Autosomal Recessive Retinitis Pigmentosa

Autosomal recessive retinitis pigmentosa (arRP), often caused by mutations affecting the rod phototransduction cascade (reactions within the cell that occur following light exposure and culminate in membrane hyperpolarization), requires two copies of a mutant allele for the disease phenotype to manifest [7]. Over 30 genes have been connected to arRP, with most being rare, causing 1% or fewer of cases [59]. One protein most frequently involved is rod phosphodiesterase (PDE), responsible for catalyzing the breakdown of cyclic GMP. PDE is a heterotetrameric complex with four subunits—one alpha, one beta, and two gamma—which are all essential for normal function. Mutations in *PDE6A* and *PDE6B* are common causes of arRP. Other genes frequently linked include subunits of the cyclic nucleotide-gated cation channel (e.g., *cnga1*, *cngb1*), *retinal pigment epithelium 65* (*rpe65*), and the *Mertk* gene (c-mer proto-oncogene tyrosine kinase).

Phenotypically, arRP, like most RP, is diverse; there are a multitude of possible mutations, different mutations in the same gene may cause different diseases, and even the same mutation can bring about different phenotypes within different related and unrelated individuals. arRP is typically considered milder than X-linked RP, which generally causes severe phenotypes in early stages of the disease. Many arRP models exist, for a wide variety of genes and in several species; notable examples will be discussed here, with others listed in Table 1.

2.5 Naturally Occurring Models of arRP

2.5.1 Avian

Chicken eyes, while more cone-dominant than human eyes, remain a viable model for RP due to their size and conservation of genetic makeup [60]. *Rd* (retinal degeneration) Rhode Island Red chickens were characterized in the 1980s and noted to be blind at birth, with many structural changes in the RPE precipitating their phenotype [61]. Further study showed that levels of cGMP are markedly reduced prior to the onset of retinal degeneration and are due to a null mutation in the photoreceptor guanylate cyclase gene (*GC1*) [62]. This chicken is most commonly used as a model of LCA, because there is a lack of ERG response even before rod and cone degeneration is detectable [63].

2.5.2 Canine

In dogs, progressive retinal atrophy (PRA) is the name for a group of hereditary retinal dystrophies and is considered the equivalent of human RP. A four base pair deletion mutation in *CNGA1*, a gene implicated in human arRP, was identified in a family of Shetland sheepdogs with PRA [64]. In a family of PRA affected Papillon dogs, a complex *CNGB1* mutation has also been identified [65]. CNGB1 is necessary for the targeting of CNGA1 to the rod outer segment, and together they form the rod cyclic nucleotide gated channel, without which rod function is lost and retinal degeneration follows [65]. The analogous mouse model is *CNGB1X-26*, discussed in Subheading 2.6.1. A novel form of PRA was identified in Swedish Vallhund dogs in 2014, and further analysis showed the involved mutation to be a large LINE-1 insertion in intron 1 of the *MERTK* gene [66, 67]. The *MERTK* gene has been implicated in arRP before, most notably in the RCS rat (discussed in Subheading 2.5.4). A subset of canine PRA, progressive rod–cone degeneration (*prcd*), is also a model for some types of human arRP. A causative gene, named *PRCD*, was identified, and mutations have been associated with human retinal degeneration as well as PRA in many different dog breeds (suggesting a founder effect) [68]. The precise functions of this protein are still being elucidated. Analogous to the *rd3* mouse, the *rd3* collie is another PRA model where the implicated gene is the canine homolog of *C1orf36/Rd3* [69]. The precise function of this gene is also poorly understood.

PDE mutants are common causes of arRP, and mutations in the alpha and beta subunits have been identified as causing progressive retinal atrophy in dog breeds [70–73]. Alpha subunit mutations have been identified in Cardigan Welsh corgis and in American Staffordshire terriers as well; both are characterized by small intraexon deletions [70, 72]. In the corgi, a frameshift occurs leading to a loss of catalytic activity in the PDE protein. Similar to *PDE6B* mutant Irish setters, the corgi photoreceptor development halts at an early age, and degeneration begins after 3 weeks old [74]. American Staffordshire terriers exhibit early photoreceptor morphology defects and are in an advanced state of degeneration by 2 years of age, exhibiting a phenotype similar to *rd10* mice [72]. In Irish setters, a premature stop codon in *PDE6B* (beta subunit) leads to a nonfunctional PDE. Similar to *rd1* mice, cGMP accumulates and leads to sustained depolarization of rods. In these dogs, retinal development occurs normally until 13 days after birth, then photoreceptor development ceases, and degeneration begins within a month. Rod loss occurs over 5 months, and cone loss occurs within 1 year [7, 75]. Sloughi dogs also have a mutation affecting exon 21 of *PDE6B* leading to a similar phenotype [71].

2.5.3 Feline

Abyssinian retinal degeneration cats (*rdAc*) were first described in 1982 and have since become an important model of arRP, as well as Senior–Løken syndrome (discussed in Subheading 2.19) [28, 76, 77]. At birth, cats have normal vision but exhibit retinal degeneration beginning around 1.5–2 years of age. The disease progresses with initial rod degeneration followed by cone disruption, and end-stage disease/blindness occurs by 3–5 years of age [78]. The mutation responsible is an SNP in the *CEP290* gene causing a new splice site, a 4 base pair insertion, a frame shift, and a premature stop codon [28]. The truncated centrosomal protein, involved in the ciliary trafficking system, is unable to maintain photoreceptor integrity. Similar mutants in *rd16* mice have also been identified [79].

2.5.4 Murine

Retinal degenerations have long been observed in naturally occurring mice and were named based on the order in which they were discovered (*rd1* through *rd16*) [11, 80]. As mentioned, Keeler first discovered the *rd1* mouse (also called *rodless*, *rd*, and *r*), wherein the defect is a nonsense *PDE6B* mutation [10]. The *rd1* mice first lose rods at developmental stage P10 and start losing cones around P35 [81]. As such, the *rd1* mouse is a model for a severe, early onset, rapid retinal degeneration. The inability to breakdown cGMP from the nonfunctional PDE causes accumulated cGMP and possibly contributes to apoptotic cell death [82]. There do exist criticisms of the *rd1* mouse, as the disease overlaps with normal development; normal development does not finish before degeneration begins, making it less appropriate as a model of late-onset human arRP [83]. *Rd10* mice, by contrast, carry a missense (R560C) *PDE6B* mutation and are characterized by a slower onset of retinal degeneration with detectable PDE6B protein levels in early development followed by a more gradual loss of rods [84, 85].

The *rd3* mouse, initially discovered in 1993, was one of the first mouse models of arRP where photoreceptors were initially normal and then degenerate [86]. The identified gene, named *Rd3*, produces a protein of yet unknown function, but premature truncation in mutants causes retinal degeneration beginning at 2–3 weeks of life and completed by 8–16 weeks [87, 88]. *Rd5*, or *tubby* mutant mice, are used as a model for some of the retinitis pigmentosa syndromes due to the presence of obesity and hearing loss as well as retinal degeneration in mutants [84]. *Rd6* mice show a phenotype with white retinal flecks, and this mouse has been more commonly used as a model for Stargardt disease or retinitis punctata albescens [89].

Frameshift mutations in the *CRB1* gene have been shown to cause both RP and Leber's congenital amaurosis (LCA), which is the defect identified in *rd8* mice [90, 91]. Similar to *Drosophila crumbs* mutants, the adherens junction is disrupted in affected cells, and photoreceptor degeneration occurs as well [91].

Rd12 mice have mutations in *RPE65*, which result in the absence of this protein crucial for phototransduction. This mouse model is used to study both LCA and arRP, as there is a lack of RPE65 protein at birth, though overt degeneration doesn't occur until 6 weeks of age [92]. *Rd16* mice carry a deletion in the centrosomal protein CEP290 and exhibit a similar phenotype to the Abyssinian cat model discussed in Subheading 2.5.3. In mutants, there is an altered interaction between the CEP290 protein and RPGR, another important ciliary protein [79].

The RPE cell layer is crucial for the functioning of photoreceptors, playing important structural and physiologic roles. Perturbations of the RPE have been associated with human RP. Two important models of arRP that involve RPE disruption are the Royal College of Surgeon's (RCS) rat and the *mer* knockout mouse. The RCS rat has a deletion affecting the *mertk* gene, where *mertk* normally codes for a protein that binds photoreceptors and has a tyrosine kinase domain [93]. This impairs the RPE's ability to phagocytose photoreceptor outer segments, leading to accumulation and retinal degeneration [94]. The *mer* knockout mouse displays a similar phenotype, again with accumulation of photoreceptor debris and retinal degeneration [95].

The Purkinje cell degeneration mouse (*pcd*) is a model of retinitis pigmentosa that exhibits syndromic qualities (there is early ataxia due to Purkinje cell degeneration, as well as olfactory cell death) in addition to photoreceptor cell degeneration [96]. The precise mutation is unknown but may occur in the regulatory region of the *Agtpbp1* (*Nna1*) gene, which encodes a nuclear protein identified to be involved in neuronal regeneration, raising interesting links between regeneration and degeneration [97].

2.6 Transgenic Models of arRP

2.6.1 Murine

Many transgenic mouse models of arRP exist; some will be highlighted here, with others listed in Table 1. RPE65 knockout mice, created in 1998, lack 11-cis-retinal and accumulate retinyl esters in the RPE [98]. This mouse exhibits normal rod photoreceptor development, but rods degenerate after about 6 months of age; cone degeneration occurs much more quickly [99–102]. This mouse is most commonly used to model LCA. Spata7 (spermatogenesis associated protein 7) mutations have been implicated in forms of LCA and juvenile RP [103]. The protein localizes to the connecting cilium of photoreceptors and directly interacts with the RPGR-interacting protein (often mutated in LCA) [104]. *Spata7* knockout mice display mislocalization of rhodopsin followed by apoptosis of photoreceptors suggesting Spata7 plays an important role (along with the RPGR-interacting protein) in protein trafficking across the photoreceptor connecting cilium [104].

The *Cngb1-X26* mouse model, made by excision of exon 26 in the *Cngb1* gene, has a genetic basis and phenotype similar to the Papillon *Cngb1* model (Subheading 2.5.1) [65, 105]. The *Cngb1-X26* mouse expresses no CNGB1 protein, and in the absence of CNGB1, CNGA1 is also absent from rod outer segments; slowly progressive rod apoptosis ensues [106].

Prominin-1 (Prom-1) is a cholesterol-binding protein whose function has been suggested to involve stabilization or formation of new photoreceptive disks but is not fully understood [107]. Mice with *Prom-1* knockout exhibit progressive loss of function and degeneration of both rods and cones, as well as impaired disk morphogenesis in the outer segments [107]. *C8orf37*, a gene of unknown function, is associated with arRP, Bardet–Biedl, and cone–rod dystrophy and is possibly involved in the secretory pathway of membrane proteins [108]. Knockout of this gene in mice produced a retinal phenotype analogous to that seen in affected humans, with disorganization of the outer segment disks and progressive degeneration of rods and cones [108].

IRBP, or interphotoreceptor retinoid-binding protein, is a protein necessary for the exchange of retinoids between the RPE and photoreceptor cells. In mice with the *IRBP* gene knocked out, a loss of photoreceptor nuclei and disruption of outer segments was observed, followed by decreased ERG photic response [109]. *Arapl*, a gene whose mechanism of action is unknown, causes photoreceptor degeneration when knocked out. These mice undergo normal development but show photoreceptor degeneration at 4 weeks of age and a fundus phenotype similar to human RP [110]. *Arapl* is expressed in Müller glial cells, not photoreceptors themselves, indicating these cells play a significant role in the development of some forms of RP [110].

Phosphodiesterase (PDE) is important for the regulation of phototransduction as discussed previously. The *rd1* mouse has criticisms mentioned above (Subheading 2.5.1), so transgenic mice with mutations in the *PDE6B* gene have been created to better represent human disease. An H620Q mutation was introduced in the *PDE6B* gene, leading to normal photoreceptor development (not present in *rd1* mice) followed by later degeneration and loss of rod function that was rescuable, making it a better model for study of human RP and future treatments [111]. A PDE6B-based model was created to investigate whether the presence of dying photoreceptor cells impacts nearby cells that have been transfected with gene therapeutic techniques, as these techniques are often scattershot and do not uniformly treat areas of retina [112]. To assess this hypothesis, mosaic mice with either rescued or untreated *Pde6B-H620Q* were developed and drivers were used to express the mutants and induce rescue under specific conditions [112]. The results of this study showed that dying rods did not cause cell death of surrounding rescued photoreceptors; however, structural abnormalities in the outer segment of rescued photoreceptors persisted [112]. In a separate experiment, the inhibitory gamma subunit of PDE6 (*PDE6G/PDE6Y*), when disrupted in mice, resulted in a paradoxical decrease in PDE activity and caused rapid photoreceptor degeneration, suggesting an essential role for the gamma subunit in maintaining the activity of PDE and the integrity of photoreceptors [113].

While not strictly speaking transgenic, mice with mutations in the *Pde6a* gene have been produced using a chemical mutagenesis method [114]. In these two mouse models of *Pde6a* disease ($Pde6a^{nmf282}$ and $Pde6a^{nmf363}$), highly conserved amino acids are altered, causing RP phenotypes [114]. In both mice, PDE activity was decreased, though to different degrees, and this was demonstrated to be due to the allelic differences between the mice. The $Pde6a^{nmf282}$ mouse has a V685M amino acid change and apparently causes a nonfunctional PDE6A protein. The $Pde6a^{nmf363}$ mouse (D670G) had a less severe phenotype and had a partially active PDE6A; dark rearing these mice also slowed degeneration possibly by either reducing oxidative stress or increasing the cGMP levels [114]. These mice exhibit the first small animal models of PDE6A disease, where previously only the Welsh corgi model was an option.

2.6.2 Piscine

C2orf71, a protein of unknown function but which localizes to photoreceptor outer segments/cilia, has been identified as a cause of arRP in a naturally occurring Gordon setter line and was suppressed in a zebrafish model through the use of morpholino-induced knockdown [73, 115]. Another zebrafish model was used to investigate the role of the *ceramide kinase-like* (*cerkl*) gene, leading to the discovery that it is involved in protecting against oxidative stress and that knockdown can lead to increased apoptosis and photoreceptor degeneration [116].

2.6.3 Other

Drosophila models of human RP exist, with six models of either arRP or adRP being produced to study human disease [117]. In these models, mutations in the *Drosophila* ortholog of the implicated human gene cause retinal degeneration in the fly as well. These models mimic both autosomal dominant and autosomal recessive forms of human RP but will be grouped and discussed here. These transgenic models include mutations in genes such as *Rho*, *Crb1*, *Cerkl*, and *Prom-1*, which we have discussed previously [117]. The highly advanced genetic tools available in the fruit fly, as well as the similarity of the genetic profile, make for a valuable model organism in which to study human retinal disease.

Human induced pluripotent stem cells (hiPSCs) have been used to model human RP, with precision genome-editing allowing for highly specific therapeutic design and studies of disease mechanism. 2D and 3D cell models have been developed, allowing for the maintenance of organ structure. Similar to *Drosophila*, many models that have been produced are in genes commonly mutated in existing models, e.g., *Prph2*, *Rho*, *Mfrp*, *Mertk*, *Cep290*, and *Rpgr* [9]. Patient hiPSCs, coupled with gene-editing techniques, open the exciting possibility of autologous treatment approaches.

2.7 X-Linked Retinitis Pigmentosa

X-linked retinitis pigmentosa (XLRP) is typically considered the most severe form of hereditary RP, due to its early age of onset and rapidly progressive phenotype. Affected individuals have severe visual impairment by the third or fourth decade of life. A vast majority (>70%) of XLRP in humans is caused by mutations in the retinitis pigmentosa GTPase regulator (*RPGR*) gene, with another significant percentage being caused by variants in the *RP2* gene [118]. The *RPGR* transcript undergoes alternative splicing leading to the expression of both the constitutive (exon 1–19) and open-reading frame 15 (ORF15) variants. The *RPGR* gene is commonly mutated in ORF15, which seems to be a mutational hotspot, and all disease-causing mutations are present in this region of the gene [119, 120]. The function of RPGR is still being elucidated, but it has been shown to localize to the cilia of the photoreceptor through binding to an RPGR-interacting protein (RPGRIP) and likely plays a role in transporting phototransduction elements across said connecting cilium [121, 122]. Models are listed in Table 1.

2.8 Naturally Occurring Models of XLRP

2.8.1 Avian

Rdd (retinal dysplasia and degeneration) chickens were first identified in 1979 and shown to have a sex-linked form of retinal disease very similar to X-linked human RP [123]. *Rdd* chickens are sighted at birth, but vision deteriorates rapidly; holes in the RPE form first, followed by progressive thinning of all retinal layers and degeneration of the photoreceptors [123–125]. Initially, it was suspected that the responsible mutated gene was the *PDE6A* gene, based on linkage mapping and phenotype [125]. However, more recent work has identified a premature stop mutation in the *mpdz* gene as the culprit [126]. MPDZ (multiple PDZ domain protein), whose function is still being elucidated but is known to interact with many other proteins, localizes to the outer limiting membrane (OLM) in the retina and has been shown to interact with CRB1 there [126, 127]. This model is therefore useful for study of OLM disruptive retinal disease as well as future treatment modalities that may take advantage of this OLM disruption for cell transplantation therapies [128, 129].

2.8.2 Canine

In dogs, X-linked progressive retinal atrophy (XLPRA) is the naturally occurring mimic of XLRP. The Siberian husky and Samoyed dogs, with known mutations in the *RPGR* gene causing XLPRA1, have a very similar phenotype to human XLRP. The affected dogs have rod outer segment dysfunction beginning around 6 months of age, eventually leading to complete rod loss, followed by cone degeneration [130]. The XLPRA1-causing mutation is a small deletion causing a frameshift and premature stop codon in *RPGR*-ORF15 [131]. A similar mutant, XLPRA2, is also due to a small deletion in ORF15 leading to many additional basic amino acids and then a premature stop codon further downstream [131]. The XLPRA2 mutant phenotype is more severe, with a faster degeneration and more impaired development. In these dogs, abnormal photoreceptors were seen prior to 4 weeks of age and followed by increased cell death and inner retinal remodeling [132]. This more severe progression is presumably due to a toxic gain of function of the mutant RPGR-ORF15 protein, which aggregates in the endoplasmic reticulum [131]. The phenotype of XLPRA2 was noted to be similar to that of the *Rdy* cat model of adRP (Subheading 2.2.2 [132].

2.8.3 Murine

The *Rd9* mouse, another XLRP model, is caused by a 32 base pair deletion in the *RPGR* gene's ORF15 leading to a frameshift [133]. The truncated protein is unstable and does not localize normally. The phenotype of *Rd9* is relatively mild compared to the human forms of the disease caused by similar mutations but leads to mislocalization of opsin and early reduction of ERG function followed by progressive ERG amplitude loss with age [133]. This model is similar in phenotype and progression to the *Rpgr*-KO mouse discussed in Subheading 2.9.1, which is understandable given that neither mouse expresses RPGR-ORF15.

2.9 Transgenic Models of XLRP

2.9.1 Murine

An *RPGR* knockout mouse was produced in 2000, which undergoes development normally, but begins mislocalizing opsin and degenerating around 2 months of age [134]. ERG responses were substantially reduced, and there was disorganization of the newly formed disks in the outer segment [134]. Interestingly, the cilium appears structurally intact in these mice despite the lack of this important protein in that location [7].

Choroideremia is a rare, X-linked degeneration of the choroid, typically caused by mutations in the Rab escort protein-1 manifesting as progressive nyctalopia and in some cases eventual blindness [135]. *CHM* is the name of the gene that codes for the Rab escort protein-1 (REP-1). Choroideremia has been mistaken for XLRP in patients [135]. Full knockout of the *CHM* gene in mice was embryonically lethal in males, so conditional knockout models were produced (leading to viable $CHM^{null/WT}$ heterozygous female mice) [136]. In these conditional knockout models, the disease progression is similar to that seen in human patients, with fundal hypopigmentation, decreased ERG response, and degeneration of both photoreceptors and the RPE [136]. The same study also mentions that RPE and photoreceptor degeneration are independent processes. Of note, while the phenotype in this heterozygote female model approximates that seen in human males with the disease, there is a clear difference as human males with *CHM* null mutations do not die in embryologic development [137].

2.9.2 Piscine

Zebrafish models of *RPGR* defects have been produced as well. Due to a genome duplication that occurred in their evolutionary history, the zebrafish has two *RPGR* genes (*ZFRPGR1* and *ZFRPGR2*) [138]. Using morpholino-induced knockdown of *ZFRPGR2*, model zebrafish exhibited systemic developmental abnormalities similar to those seen in other ciliopathies, affecting gastrulation and head and tail morphology [138]. This is in contrast to the human *RPGR* mutation, which is largely an isolated retinal phenotype, suggesting that in humans the *RPGR* activity related to systemic polarity in early development is redundant [139].

RP2, mutated in approximately 20% of human XLRP, has also been modeled in zebrafish, using a morpholino-induced knockdown approach [140]. The RP2 protein has been identified as likely being important in maintaining photoreceptor intracellular transport around the centriole [141]. The zebrafish form of the analogous gene (*ZFRP2*), when knocked down, led to decreased eye size and abnormal photoreceptors lacking outer segments with increased levels of apoptotic retinal neurons [140]. The *ZFRP2* gene has also been implicated in ciliopathies, with zebrafish mutants exhibiting renal abnormalities and left–right patterning abnormalities through an interaction with the polycystin (PKD2) protein, though in human *RP2*-mediated disease these other features are absent [140, 142]. This model will help further elucidate ciliopathies and *RP2* mutations.

2.10 Syndromic RP

There are a large number of syndromes associated with RP, wherein there are extraocular manifestations in addition to a retinal phenotype. The most common will be discussed here, and some preclinical models will also be discussed. Bardet–Biedl and Usher syndromes are the most prevalent: Usher syndrome affects about 1 in 23,000 in the USA [143]. Bardet–Biedl has a prevalence that varies widely among populations, affecting about 1 in 150,000 in North American populations and closer to 1 in 15,000 in other populations [4]. Other, far less common conditions that will be discussed include Joubert syndrome, Bietti syndrome, and Alström syndrome. Leber congenital amaurosis will be treated as a distinct condition, and not as a subset of RP, and therefore not discussed in detail, though some models that are used to study LCA have been briefly mentioned in the preceding subheadings. Select models of syndromic RP are listed in Table 2.

2.11 Alström Syndrome

Alström syndrome is a ciliopathy (phenotypically similar to Bardet–Biedl syndrome) characterized by retinal degeneration, hearing loss, obesity, cardiomegaly, endocrine abnormalities, and pulmonary and hepatic dysfunction [144]. *Alms1*, a gene encoding a protein of unknown function, is mutated in Alström syndrome, and a few mouse models with *Alms1* alterations have been produced which display the retinal phenotype [144]. *Alms1* mutant mice, homozygous for an L1231X mutation, have been developed and show altered transport of rhodopsin [145]. *Alms1* knockout mice similarly exhibit rhodopsin mislocalization as well as accumulation of vesicles in photoreceptor inner segments [146]. A similar retinal phenotype to *Alms1* knockout is seen in *BBS4* null mice as well as in tubby (*rd5*) mice (Subheading 2.5.4) [147, 148].

2.12 Bardet–Biedl Syndrome

Bardet–Biedl syndrome (BBS) is an autosomal recessive ciliopathy characterized by the presence of retinal dystrophy in addition to renal dysfunction, polydactyly, obesity, hypogonadism, and cognitive defects [149]. The degree to which each affected individual manifests these traits is variable. Early clinical signs of retinal disease are typical of RP, with early rod loss followed by cone degeneration, though in BBS the macula is involved early [150]. At least 16 causative BBS genes have been identified, with most mutations occurring in *BBS1* and *BBS10* [149]. Several of the other ciliopathies, some of which will be discussed, have some overlapping features with BBS, suggesting that these diseases are on a spectrum.

Mouse models of the retinal degeneration in BBS have been produced. *BBS2* knockout causes retinal degeneration as well as other features of the syndrome in mice [151]. *BBS3* null mice demonstrate degeneration of photoreceptors and ONL loss, similar

Table 2
Models of syndromic retinitis pigmentosa

Disease	Gene	Model organism and trivial name	Gene product	Alteration	Reference
Alström	*Alms1*	Murine—*Alms1* L1231X mutant mouse (T)	Centrosome and basal body associated protein (unknown function)	L1231X	[145]
Alström	*Alms1*	Murine—*Alms1* null mouse (T)	Centrosome and basal body associated protein (unknown function)	*Alms1* −/−	[146]
Bardet–Biedl	*Bbs1*	Murine—*Bbs1* M390R knockin mouse (T)	Bardet–Biedl syndrome 1	M390R	[155]
Bardet–Biedl	*Bbs2*	Murine—*Bbs2* null mouse (T)	Bardet–Biedl syndrome 2	*Bbs2* −/−	[151]
Bardet–Biedl	*Bbs3*	Murine—*Bbs3* null mouse (T)	Bardet–Biedl syndrome 3	*Bbs3* −/−	[152]
Bardet–Biedl	*Bbs4*	Murine—*Bb4* null mouse (T)	Bardet–Biedl syndrome 4	*Bbs4* −/−	[147]
Bardet–Biedl	*Bbs6* (*Mkks*)	Murine—*Bbs6* (*Mkks*) null mouse (T)	Bardet–Biedl syndrome 6 (McKusick–Kaufman syndrome)	*Bbs6* −/−	[211]
Bietti	*Cyp4v2* (*Cyp4v3* in mice)	Murine—*Cyp4v3* knockout mouse (T)	Cytochrome P450 4 V2	*Cyp4v3* KO	[156]
Cockayne	*Csb*	Murine—Csb mutant mouse (T)	Cockayne syndrome B protein (ERCC excision repair 6)	Premature stop	[162, 163]
GACR	*Oat*	Murine—*Oat* null mouse (T)	Ornithine aminotransferase	*Oat* −/−	[165]
GACR	*Oat*	Murine—*rhg* (retarded hair growth) mouse (N)	Ornithine aminotransferase	G to C exon 9 *Oat* gene	[167]
Joubert	*Ahi1*	Murine—*Ahi1* knockout mouse (T)	Abelson helper integration site 1	*Ahi1* KO	[171]

(continued)

Table 2 (continued)

Disease	Gene	Model organism and trivial name	Gene product	Alteration	Reference
Joubert	*Cep290*	Murine—*Cep290* knockout mouse (T)	Centrosomal protein of 290 kDa	*Cep290* KO	[173]
NARP	*ATP6*	Murine—*ATP6* mRNA disruption mouse (T)	Mitochondrial ATP synthase membrane subunit 6	AAV-vectored ribozyme introduced for mRNA disruption	[174]
Senior–Løken	*Cep290*	Feline—Abyssinian retinal degeneration cat (*rdAc*) (N)	Centrosomal protein of 290 kDa	SNP in intron causing alternate splicing	[28]
Senior–Løken	*Cep290*	Murine—*rd16* mouse (N)	Centrosomal protein of 290 kDa	Δ897 bp	[79]
Senior–Løken	*Nphp1*	Murine—*Nphp1 del20* mouse (T)	Nephrocystin 1	Deletion exon 20	[179]
Senior–Løken	*Nphp11/ Tmem67*	Murine—*bpck* mouse (N)	Meckelin protein	Deletion 6 genes chromosome 4	[181]
Senior–Løken	*Nphp11/ Tmem67*	Murine—*wpk* rat (N)	Meckelin protein	P394L	[212]
Senior–Løken	*Nphp4*	Murine—*nmf192* mouse (T)	Nephrocystin 4	Nonsense mutation exon 4	[180]
Usher	*Tub*	Murine—tubby (*rd5*) mouse (N)	Tubby bipartite transcription factor	G to T eliminating splice site chromosome 7	[148, 187, 213]
Usher	*Ush1c*	Murine—*Ush1c c.216G > A* knockin mouse (T)	USH1 harmonin protein	*Ush1c* c.216G > A knockin	[185]
Usher	*Ush2a*	Murine—*Ush2a* KO mouse (T)	Usherin protein	*Ush2a* KO	[186]

A list of preclinical models of syndromic retinitis pigmentosa. Categorized by disease, gene, model organism, gene product, and gene alteration. Naturally occurring or transgenic is indicated by a parenthetical "N" or "T" in model organism column. Sorted by disease, gene, and model organism. Abbreviations: *AAV* adeno-associated virus, *bp* base pair, *KO* knockout, *nt* nucleotide, *SNP* single nucleotide polymorphism, *−ter* mutation to stop codon, *Δ* deletion, −/− null mutation to the others mentioned here [152]. *BBS4* null mice undergo apoptotic death of ciliated photoreceptor cells [147, 153]. *BBS6* (*MKKS*) knockout mice have been shown to further exhibit progressive retinal degeneration, specifically in the outer segment, similar to *BBS4* knockout mice [154]. A *BBS1* knockin mouse model expressing a homozygous M390R mutation (a common mutation affecting humans with BBS1-mediated disease) was produced and also shows gradual retinal degeneration [155].

2.13 Bietti Syndrome

Bietti crystalline dystrophy (BCD) is a disease characterized by crystalline corneal deposits and RP-type features [156]. The most common gene mutated is the cytochrome P450 4V2 enzyme (*CYP4V2*), resulting in systemic dyslipidemia [156].

A model of the disease with a knockout of the mouse ortholog of human *CYP4V2*, *CYP4V3*, was produced and exhibited some of the features of the human disease: corneal and retinal crystalline deposits and systemic dyslipidemia [156]. However, there are a few crucial differences making this *CYP4V3* mouse a poor model for BCD. First, the systemic lipid abnormalities seen in human patients and in this model differ substantially: levels of the lipid C18:0 are decreased in *CYP4V3* mice compared with wild-type mice, whereas in human BCD patients the levels of C18:0 are increased compared to healthy controls [156, 157]. Not only does this fail to mimic the human disease, the trend is in the opposite direction and indicates that the biochemical abnormalities differ in the mouse and BCD patient. C18:1, C18:2, and C18:3 levels in the mouse model also do not mimic those lipid levels seen in human patients [156, 157]. Furthermore, while these mice do exhibit crystal deposition, it does not lead to vision loss or RPE atrophy. This is not sufficient as a phenotype, as crystal deposits are only one of the manifestations of BCD, and crystal deposition in the retina is not specific to BCD [158–160]. Therefore, this model fails to mimic BCD in multiple crucial aspects (both phenotypic and molecular) including character and mechanism of systemic dyslipidemia, presence of retinal degeneration and visual loss, and nature and result of crystal deposition.

2.14 Cockayne Syndrome

Cockayne syndrome is an autosomal recessive disorder characterized by cachectic dwarfism, neurologic dysfunction, RP, deafness, and other developmental issues leading to death in early adolescence [161]. Defects in DNA repair have been hypothesized as the underlying mechanism for the disease [161]. Mice generated with a mutation in the *CSB* gene, which encodes part of the nucleotide excision repair pathway, showed spontaneous loss of photoreceptors with age and a loss of a majority of rods by age 18 months, as well as increased apoptosis when exposed to radiation [162, 163].

2.15 Gyrate Atrophy of the Choroid and Retina (GACR)

Another rare disease with retinal degeneration (initially described as a form of atypical RP) is gyrate atrophy of the choroid and retina (GACR) [164]. GACR is an autosomal recessive blinding disorder of chorioretinal degeneration caused by a deficiency of the ornithine aminotransferase enzyme (OAT) and characterized by progressive narrowing of the visual fields and accumulation of ornithine [165]. In addition, myopia, early cataracts, and cystoid macular edema are hallmarks of the disease, and circular areas of chorioretinal atrophy occur in the peripheral retina on fundoscopy [166]. Naturally occurring *rhg* (*Oat* missense) mice have been presented as a model for GACR and display retinal degeneration, hyperornithinemia, and cataract formation [167]. This is a milder phenotype than the *Oat* null mouse (transgenic) which causes retinal degeneration and hyperornithinemia but also causes all homozygotes to die within a few days of birth unless given arginine supplementation [165].

There are key differences between these mice and humans, however, making them less than ideal models. The *rhg* mouse is not explicitly noted to have visual loss or reduced ERG response; and while retinal degeneration is present, it is not the same as that seen in humans, where humans exhibit outer retinal tubulation structures and hyperreflective deposits in addition to the common feature of RPE disruption [166, 167]. Both *rhg* mouse and human demonstrate hyperornithinemia of a similar magnitude as adults, but the flow of the OAT catalyzed reaction is different in mouse neonates leading to a different time course of mouse versus human disease progression [167, 168]. Cataracts are present in the *rhg* mouse, but it is not specified what type. In humans they are typically posterior sutural cataracts present by the second decade, while in the mice they present at least as early as 2 months of age but the type is unknown [166, 169]. Macular edema is not noted in the rhg mouse [167].

OAT null mice have been shown to have a rapid course of retinal degeneration compared to humans, assessed by ERG response [165]. Another key distinction, besides the early lethality of the null mice mentioned already, is the distribution of retinal degeneration: in humans the retinal degeneration begins in the periphery, while in this mouse model it involves more of the central retina [165, 170]. Again, no macular edema is noted, and cataract formation is also not mentioned in this model [165].

2.16 Joubert Syndrome

Joubert syndrome is another ciliopathy, characterized by disease of the retina, kidney, and cerebellar vermis [171]. Symptoms can include hypotonia, ataxia, breathing abnormalities, abnormal facial features, nephronophthisis, and retinal degeneration [172]. *Ahi1* is a gene that has been implicated in a form of Joubert syndrome highly penetrant for retinal degeneration. An *Ahi1* knockout mouse model fails to form outer segments and also exhibits opsin mislocalization, followed by photoreceptor cell death [171]. Another gene implicated in the development of Joubert syndrome is the *cep290* gene, discussed in Subheadings 2.5.3 and 2.5.4 [173]. This gene is known to cause some forms of BBS as well. The *rd16* mouse involves the *cep290* gene, but the phenotype is isolated to the retina, whereas in this mouse model of *cep290* knockout visual loss occurs as expected (no outer segment formation and no connecting cilium) in addition to hydrocephalus and kidney pathology [173].

2.17 Neuropathy, Ataxia, and RP (NARP) Syndrome

An adeno-associated virus (AAV) method was used to disrupt the mRNA of the mitochondrial ATP synthase 6 gene (*ATP6*), in order to create a mouse model of the NARP syndrome [174]. The syndrome is mitochondrially inherited and is characterized by sensory neuropathy, ataxia, dementia, RP, and in some cases cardiac or other neurologic dysfunction [175].

2.18 Refsum Disease

Refsum disease causes RP in most cases, as well as limb deformities, anosmia, ataxia, hearing loss, and other defects in human patients [176]. The disease is a peroxisomal disorder that involves defects in phytanic acid metabolism. To date however, no animal model of Refsum disease exists that has the ocular manifestations seen in human patients [177].

2.19 Senior–Løken Syndrome

Senior–Løken syndrome (SLS) is an autosomal recessive disease involving RP-like retinal dystrophy and nephronophthisis (a cystic kidney disease) [178]. The *nephrocystin* gene family, encoding proteins that are found in photoreceptor connecting cilia and in kidney cell primary cilia, has been identified as causing SLS [178]. While many genes have been identified and modeled, not all of the models display retinal phenotypes, and of those that do, most do not display renal phenotypes and thus are not true models of the human disease.

Nphp1 mice with deletion of exon 20 display retinal degeneration due to a defect in intraflagellar transport [179]. *Nphp4* mutant mice exhibit severe photoreceptor degeneration by 9 weeks of age, dysfunction of outer segments, and mislocalization of proteins within photoreceptors [180]. *Cep290* (*Nphp6*) mutants are also used to model SLS, such as the rd16 mouse and the *rdAc* Abyssinian cat, both of which were discussed previously (Subheadings 2.5.3, 2.5.4, and 2.16) [76, 79].

Meckelin/Nphp11/Tmem67 is a gene implicated in SLS and other forms of syndromic RP, and in the *bpck* mouse model, it is absent, resulting in early photoreceptor degeneration as well as absence of the photoreceptor outer segment [181]. A similar phenotype is seen in the *wpk* rat, caused by a P394L mutation in the same gene [182].

2.20 Usher Syndrome

Usher syndrome is a disorder characterized by hearing loss in addition to visual loss and is the most common cause of deaf-blindness [7]. It is classified into three subtypes based upon severity and progression of hearing and visual loss [183]. Many models exist for the hearing loss and vestibular dysfunction aspects of the syndrome, such as the Jackson shaker, waltzer, and deaf circler mice [183]. However, these mice do not display profound retinal degeneration despite some mild dysfunction on ERG, making them less appropriate as models for retinal disease [184].

The mouse models for Usher syndrome that do exhibit retinal dysfunction include a mutant knockin model of *Ush1c*, a *Ush2a* knockout mouse, and *Rd5* [144]. The *Ush1c* knockin mouse has an abnormal ERG by 1 month, and loses photoreceptors between 6 and 12 months of age [185]. The *Ush2a* (encoding the Usherin protein) knockout mouse exhibits slowly progressive photoreceptor degeneration, consistent with the human RP phenotype [186]. Rd5, or *tubby* mutant mice, mentioned in Subheading 2.5.4, are also used as a model for Usher syndrome and other ciliopathies, exhibiting early vessel changes followed by pigmentary deposits and loss of ERG response [187].

3 Future Directions

The use of preclinical models for RP has a history encompassing nearly a century. The future of RP modeling will likely involve identifying the common molecular pathways and proteins implicated in the diverse mechanisms of photoreceptor cell degeneration and RP phenotypes, allowing for treatments to be specifically tailored [2]. Similarly, application of insights gleaned from hiPSC models will allow patients to have their specific mutations corrected using their own cells. Gene therapy methods used in existing animal models of RP have had promising results thus far. The CRISPR/Cas9 revolution will also continue to make gene therapy more viable and versatile. As new treatment modalities are developed, the wide variety of available models will be indispensable for assessing efficacy and safety before moving to human trials. Doubtless, new models will continue to be discovered and developed and will be instrumental in the pursuit of effective treatments or even a cure for these devastating diseases.

References

1. Hartong DT, Berson EL, Dryja TP (2006) Retinitis pigmentosa. Lancet 368:1795–1809
2. Zhang Q (2016) Retinitis pigmentosa: progress and perspective. Asia Pac J Ophthalmol (Phila) 5:265–271
3. Usher syndrome. https://ghr.nlm.nih.gov/condition/usher-syndrome
4. Bardet-Biedl syndrome. https://ghr.nlm.nih.gov/condition/bardet-biedl-syndrome

5. Petrs-Silva H, Linden R (2013) Advances in gene therapy technologies to treat retinitis pigmentosa. Clin Ophthalmol 8:127–136
6. Berger W, Kloeckener-Gruissem B, Neidhardt J (2010) The molecular basis of human retinal and vitreoretinal diseases. Prog Retin Eye Res 29:335–375
7. Fletcher EL, Jobling AI, Vessey KA et al (2011) Animal models of retinal disease. In: Progress in molecular biology and translational science. Elsevier, pp 211–286
8. Hafezi F, Grimm C, Simmen BC et al (2000) Molecular ophthalmology: an update on animal models for retinal degenerations and dystrophies. Br J Ophthalmol 84:922–927
9. Artero Castro A, Lukovic D, Jendelova P et al (2018) Concise review: human induced pluripotent stem cell models of retinitis pigmentosa. Stem Cells 36:474–481
10. Keeler CE (1924) The inheritance of a retinal abnormality in white mice. Proc Natl Acad Sci 10:329–333
11. Baehr W, Frederick JM (2009) Naturally occurring animal models with outer retina phenotypes. Vis Res 49:2636–2652
12. Bhattacharya SS, Wright AF, Clayton JF et al (1984) Close genetic linkage between X-linked retinitis pigmentosa and a restriction fragment length polymorphism identified by recombinant DNA probe L1.28. Nature 309: 253
13. Farrar GJ, McWilliam P, Sharp EM et al (1989) Autosomal dominant retinitis pigmentosa: exclusion of a gene from extensive regions of chromosomes 6, 13, 20, and 21. Genomics 5:612–618
14. Dryja TP, McGee TL, Reichel E et al (1990) A point mutation of the rhodopsin gene in one form of retinitis pigmentosa. Nature 343: 364–366
15. RetNet: Summaries. https://sph.uth.edu/retnet/sum-dis.htm
16. Wagner TE, Hoppe PC, Jollick JD et al (1981) Microinjection of a rabbit beta-globin gene into zygotes and its subsequent expression in adult mice and their offspring. PNAS 78:6376–6380
17. Flannery JG (1999) Transgenic animal models for the study of inherited retinal dystrophies. ILAR J 40:51–58
18. Zack DJ, Bennett J, Wang Y et al (1991) Unusual topography of bovine rhodopsin promoter-lacZ fusion gene expression in transgenic mouse retinas. Neuron 6:187–199
19. Lem J, Applebury ML, Falk JD et al (1991) Tissue-specific and developmental regulation of rod opsin chimeric genes in transgenic mice. Neuron 6:201–210
20. Naash MI, Hollyfield JG, Ubaidi MR et al (1993) Simulation of human autosomal dominant retinitis pigmentosa in transgenic mice expressing a mutated murine opsin gene. PNAS 90:5499–5503
21. Chader GJ (2002) Animal models in research on retinal degenerations: past progress and future hope. Vis Res 42:393–399
22. Daiger SP, Bowne SJ, Sullivan LS (2015) Genes and mutations causing autosomal dominant retinitis pigmentosa. Cold Spring Harb Perspect Med 5:a017129
23. Saliba RS, Munro PMG, Luthert PJ et al (2002) The cellular fate of mutant rhodopsin: quality control, degradation and aggresome formation. J Cell Sci 115:2907–2918
24. Rossmiller B, Mao H, Lewin AS (2012) Gene therapy in animal models of autosomal dominant retinitis pigmentosa. Mol Vis 18: 2479–2496
25. Kijas JW, Cideciyan AV, Aleman TS et al (2002) Naturally occurring rhodopsin mutation in the dog causes retinal dysfunction and degeneration mimicking human dominant retinitis pigmentosa. PNAS 99:6328–6333
26. Barnett KC, Curtis R (1985) Autosomal dominant progressive retinal atrophy in Abyssinian cats. J Hered 76:168–170
27. Chong NHV, Alexander RA, Barnett KC et al (1999) An immunohistochemical study of an autosomal dominant feline rod/cone dysplasia (Rdy Cats). Exp Eye Res 68:51–57
28. Narfström K, Holland Deckman K, Menotti-Raymond M (2011) The domestic cat as a large animal model for characterization of disease and therapeutic intervention in hereditary retinal blindness. J Ophthalmol 2011: 906943
29. Hennig AK, Peng G-H, Chen S (2008) Regulation of photoreceptor gene expression by Crx-associated transcription factor network. Brain Res 1192:114–133
30. van Nie R, Iványi D, Démant P (1978) A new H-2-linked mutation, rds, causing retinal degeneration in the mouse. Tissue Antigens 12:106–108
31. Travis GH, Brennan MB, Danielson PE et al (1989) Identification of a photoreceptor-specific mRNA encoded by the gene responsible for retinal degeneration slow (rds). Nature 338:70–73
32. Sanyal S, Jansen HG (1981) Absence of receptor outer segments in the retina of rds mutant mice. Neurosci Lett 21:23–26

33. Roderick TH, Chang B, Hawes NL et al (1997) A new dominant retinal degeneration (Rd4) associated with a chromosomal inversion in the mouse. Genomics 42:393–396
34. Kitamura E, Danciger M, Yamashita C et al (2006) Disruption of the gene encoding the β1-subunit of transducin in the Rd4/+ mouse. Invest Ophthalmol Vis Sci 47: 1293–1301
35. Kedzierski W, Lloyd M, Birch DG et al (1997) Generation and analysis of transgenic mice expressing P216L-substituted rds/peripherin in rod photoreceptors. Invest Ophthalmol Vis Sci 38:498–509
36. Stricker HM, Ding X-Q, Quiambao A et al (2005) The Cys214-->Ser mutation in peripherin/rds causes a loss-of-function phenotype in transgenic mice. Biochem J 388: 605–613
37. Olsson JE, Gordon JW, Pawlyk BS et al (1992) Transgenic mice with a rhodopsin mutation (Pro23His): a mouse model of autosomal dominant retinitis pigmentosa. Neuron 9:815–830
38. Liu X, Wu T-H, Stowe S et al (1997) Defective phototransductive disk membrane morphogenesis in transgenic mice expressing opsin with a mutated N-terminal domain. J Cell Sci 110:2589–2597
39. Machida S, Kondo M, Jamison JA et al (2000) P23H rhodopsin transgenic rat: correlation of retinal function with histopathology. Invest Ophthalmol Vis Sci 41:3200–3209
40. Acosta ML, Shin Y-S, Ready S et al (2010) Retinal metabolic state of the proline-23-histidine rat model of retinitis pigmentosa. Am J Physiol Cell Physiol 298:C764–C774
41. Sung CH, Makino C, Baylor D et al (1994) A rhodopsin gene mutation responsible for autosomal dominant retinitis pigmentosa results in a protein that is defective in localization to the photoreceptor outer segment. J Neurosci 14:5818–5833
42. Li T, Snyder WK, Olsson JE et al (1996) Transgenic mice carrying the dominant rhodopsin mutation P347S: evidence for defective vectorial transport of rhodopsin to the outer segments. Proc Natl Acad Sci U S A 93:14176–14181
43. Liu C, Li Y, Peng M et al (1999) Activation of caspase-3 in the retina of transgenic rats with the rhodopsin mutation s334ter during photoreceptor degeneration. J Neurosci 19: 4778–4785
44. Gryczan CW, Kuszak JR, Novak L et al (1995) A transgenic mouse model for autosomal dominant retinitis pigmentosa caused by a three base pair deletion in codon 255/256 of the opsin gene. Invest Ophthalmol Vis Sci 36: S423
45. Penn JS, Li S, Naash MI (2000) Ambient hypoxia reverses retinal vascular attenuation in a transgenic mouse model of autosomal dominant retinitis pigmentosa. Invest Ophthalmol Vis Sci 41:4007–4013
46. Chen J, Shi G, Concepcion FA et al (2006) Stable rhodopsin/arrestin complex leads to retinal degeneration in a transgenic mouse model of autosomal dominant retinitis pigmentosa. J Neurosci 26:11929–11937
47. Sancho-Pelluz J, Tosi J, Hsu C-W et al (2012) Mice with a D190N mutation in the gene encoding rhodopsin: a model for human autosomal-dominant retinitis pigmentosa. Mol Med 18:549–555
48. Weber BHF, Lin B, White K et al (2002) A mouse model for Sorsby fundus dystrophy. Invest Ophthalmol Vis Sci 43:2732–2740
49. Jones SE, Jomary C, Neal MJ (1994) Expression of TIMP3 mRNA is elevated in retinas affected by simplex retinitis pigmentosa. FEBS Lett 352:171–174
50. Sorsby A, Mason MEJ, Gardener N (1949) A fundus dystrophy with unusual features (late onset and dominant inheritance of a central retinal lesion showing oedema, haemorrhage and exudates developing into generalised choroidal atrophy with massive pigment proliferation). Br J Ophthalmol 33:67–97
51. Marmorstein AD, Marmorstein LY (2007) The challenge of modeling macular degeneration in mice. Trends Genet 23:225–231
52. Leco KJ, Waterhouse P, Sanchez OH et al (2001) Spontaneous air space enlargement in the lungs of mice lacking tissue inhibitor of metalloproteinases-3 (TIMP-3). J Clin Invest 108:817–829
53. Nakao T, Tsujikawa M, Notomi S et al (2012) The role of mislocalized phototransduction in photoreceptor cell death of retinitis pigmentosa. PLoS One 7:e32472
54. Link BA, Collery RF (2015) Zebrafish models of retinal disease. Annu Rev Vis Sci 1: 125–153
55. Hendrickson A, Hicks D (2002) Distribution and density of medium- and short-wavelength selective cones in the domestic pig retina. Exp Eye Res 74:435–444
56. Petters RM, Alexander CA, Wells KD et al (1997) Genetically engineered large animal model for studying cone photoreceptor survival and degeneration in retinitis pigmentosa. Nat Biotechnol 15:965–970

57. Li ZY, Wong F, Chang JH et al (1998) Rhodopsin transgenic pigs as a model for human retinitis pigmentosa. Invest Ophthalmol Vis Sci 39:808–819
58. Ross JW, de Castro JPF, Zhao J et al (2012) Generation of an inbred miniature pig model of retinitis pigmentosa. Invest Ophthalmol Vis Sci 53:501–507
59. Ferrari S, Di Iorio E, Barbaro V et al (2011) Retinitis pigmentosa: genes and disease mechanisms. Curr Genomics 12:238–249
60. Burt DW, Bruley C, Dunn IC et al (1999) The dynamics of chromosome evolution in birds and mammals. Nature 402:411–413
61. Ulshafer RJ, Allen CB (1985) Ultrastructural changes in the retinal pigment epithelium of congenitally blind chickens. Curr Eye Res 4: 1009–1021
62. Semple-Rowland SL, Lee NR, Hooser JPV et al (1998) A null mutation in the photoreceptor guanylate cyclase gene causes the retinal degeneration chicken phenotype. PNAS 95:1271–1276
63. Ulshafer RJ, Allen C, Dawson WW et al (1984) Hereditary retinal degeneration in the Rhode Island Red chicken. I. Histology and ERG. Exp Eye Res 39:125–135
64. Wiik AC, Ropstad EO, Ekesten B et al (2015) Progressive retinal atrophy in Shetland sheepdog is associated with a mutation in the CNGA1 gene. Anim Genet 46:515–521
65. Winkler PA, Ekenstedt KJ, Occelli LM et al (2013) A large animal model for CNGB1 autosomal recessive retinitis pigmentosa. PLoS One 8:e72229
66. Cooper AE, Ahonen S, Rowlan JS et al (2014) A novel form of progressive retinal atrophy in Swedish Vallhund dogs. PLoS One 9: e106610
67. Everson R, Pettitt L, Forman OP et al (2017) An intronic LINE-1 insertion in MERTK is strongly associated with retinopathy in Swedish Vallhund dogs. PLoS One 12:e0183021
68. Zangerl B, Goldstein O, Philp AR et al (2006) Identical mutation in a novel retinal gene causes progressive rod-cone degeneration in dogs and retinitis pigmentosa in humans. Genomics 88:551–563
69. Kukekova AV, Goldstein O, Johnson JL et al (2009) Canine RD3 mutation establishes rod-cone dysplasia type 2 (rcd2) as ortholog of human and murine rd3. Mamm Genome 20:109–123
70. Petersen–Jones SM, Entz DD, Sargan DR (1999) cGMP phosphodiesterase-α mutation causes progressive retinal atrophy in the Cardigan Welsh Corgi dog. Invest Ophthalmol Vis Sci 40:1637–1644
71. Dekomien G, Runte M, Gödde R et al (2000) Generalized progressive retinal atrophy of Sloughi dogs is due to an 8-bp insertion in exon 21 of the PDE6B gene. Cytogenet Cell Genet 90:261–267
72. Goldstein O, Mezey JG, Schweitzer PA et al (2013) IQCB1 and PDE6B mutations cause similar early onset retinal degenerations in two closely related terrier dog breeds. Invest Ophthalmol Vis Sci 54:7005–7019
73. Downs LM, Bell JS, Freeman J et al (2013) Late-onset progressive retinal atrophy in the Gordon and Irish Setter breeds is associated with a frameshift mutation in C2orf71. Anim Genet 44:169–177
74. Tuntivanich N, Pittler SJ, Fischer AJ et al (2009) Characterization of a canine model of autosomal recessive retinitis pigmentosa due to a PDE6A mutation. Invest Ophthalmol Vis Sci 50:801–813
75. Suber ML, Pittler SJ, Qin N et al (1993) Irish setter dogs affected with rod/cone dysplasia contain a nonsense mutation in the rod cGMP phosphodiesterase beta-subunit gene. PNAS 90:3968–3972
76. Narfström K, Nilsson SE (1985) Hereditary retinal degeneration in the Abyssinian cat: correlation of ophthalmoscopic and electroretinographic findings. Doc Ophthalmol 60: 183–187
77. Jacobson SG, Kemp CM, Narfström K et al (1989) Rhodopsin levels and rod-mediated function in Abyssinian cats with hereditary retinal degeneration. Exp Eye Res 49: 843–852
78. Narfström K, Nilsson SE (1986) Progressive retinal atrophy in the Abyssinian cat. Electron microscopy. Invest Ophthalmol Vis Sci 27: 1569–1576
79. Chang B, Khanna H, Hawes N et al (2006) In-frame deletion in a novel centrosomal/ciliary protein CEP290/NPHP6 perturbs its interaction with RPGR and results in early-onset retinal degeneration in the rd16 mouse. Hum Mol Genet 15:1847–1857
80. Han J, Dinculescu A, Dai X et al (2013) Review: the history and role of naturally occurring mouse models with Pde6b mutations. Mol Vis 19:2579–2589
81. Farber DB, Flannery JG, Bowes-Rickman C (1994) The rd mouse story: seventy years of research on an animal model of inherited retinal degeneration. Prog Retin Eye Res 13: 31–64

82. Acosta ML, Fletcher EL, Azizoglu S et al (2005) Early markers of retinal degeneration in rd/rd mice. Mol Vis 11:717–728
83. Blanks JC, Adinolfi AM, Lolley RN (1974) Photoreceptor degeneration and synaptogenesis in retinal-degenerative (rd) mice. J Comp Neurol 156:95–106
84. Chang B, Hawes NL, Hurd RE et al (2002) Retinal degeneration mutants in the mouse. Vis Res 42:517–525
85. Chang B, Hawes NL, Pardue MT et al (2007) Two mouse retinal degenerations caused by missense mutations in the beta-subunit of rod cGMP phosphodiesterase gene. Vis Res 47: 624–633
86. Chang B, Heckenlively JR, Hawes NL et al (1993) New mouse primary retinal degeneration (rd-3). Genomics 16:45–49
87. Heckenlively JR, Chang B, Peng C et al (1993) Variable expressivity of rd-3 retinal degeneration dependent on background strain. In: Hollyfield JG, Anderson RE, LaVail MM (eds) Retinal degeneration: clinical and laboratory applications. Springer US, Boston, pp 273–280
88. Friedman JS, Chang B, Kannabiran C et al (2006) Premature truncation of a novel protein, RD3, exhibiting subnuclear localization is associated with retinal degeneration. Am J Hum Genet 79:1059–1070
89. Kameya S, Hawes NL, Chang B et al (2002) Mfrp, a gene encoding a frizzled related protein, is mutated in the mouse retinal degeneration 6. Hum Mol Genet 11:1879–1886
90. den Hollander AI, ten Brink JB, de Kok YJ et al (1999) Mutations in a human homologue of Drosophila crumbs cause retinitis pigmentosa (RP12). Nat Genet 23:217–221
91. Mehalow AK, Kameya S, Smith RS et al (2003) CRB1 is essential for external limiting membrane integrity and photoreceptor morphogenesis in the mammalian retina. Hum Mol Genet 12:2179–2189
92. Pang J-J, Chang B, Hawes NL et al (2005) Retinal degeneration 12 (rd12): a new, spontaneously arising mouse model for human Leber congenital amaurosis (LCA). Mol Vis 11:152–162
93. D'Cruz PM, Yasumura D, Weir J et al (2000) Mutation of the receptor tyrosine kinase gene Mertk in the retinal dystrophic RCS rat. Hum Mol Genet 9:645–651
94. Dowling JE, Sidman RL (1962) Inherited retinal dystrophy in the rat. J Cell Biol 14: 73–109
95. Duncan JL, LaVail MM, Yasumura D et al (2003) An RCS-like retinal dystrophy phenotype in mer knockout mice. Invest Ophthalmol Vis Sci 44:826–838
96. Mullen RJ, Eicher EM, Sidman RL (1976) Purkinje cell degeneration, a new neurological mutation in the mouse. PNAS 73:208–212
97. Fernandez-Gonzalez A, La Spada AR, Treadaway J et al (2002) Purkinje cell degeneration (pcd) phenotypes caused by mutations in the axotomy-induced gene, Nna1. Science 295: 1904–1906
98. Redmond TM, Yu S, Lee E et al (1998) Rpe65 is necessary for production of 11-cis--vitamin A in the retinal visual cycle. Nat Genet 20:344–351
99. Van Hooser JP, Aleman TS, He YG et al (2000) Rapid restoration of visual pigment and function with oral retinoid in a mouse model of childhood blindness. Proc Natl Acad Sci U S A 97:8623–8628
100. Lai C-M, Yu MJ, Brankov M et al (2004) Recombinant adeno-associated virus type 2-mediated gene delivery into the Rpe65−/− knockout mouse eye results in limited rescue. Genet Vaccines Ther 2:3
101. Rohrer B, Lohr HR, Humphries P et al (2005) Cone opsin mislocalization in Rpe65−/− mice: a defect that can be corrected by 11-cis retinal. Invest Ophthalmol Vis Sci 46:3876–3882
102. Znoiko SL, Rohrer B, Lu K et al (2005) Downregulation of cone-specific gene expression and degeneration of cone photoreceptors in the Rpe65−/− mouse at early ages. Invest Ophthalmol Vis Sci 46:1473–1479
103. Wang H, den Hollander AI, Moayedi Y et al (2009) Mutations in SPATA7 cause Leber congenital amaurosis and juvenile retinitis pigmentosa. Am J Hum Genet 84:380–387
104. Eblimit A, Nguyen T-MT, Chen Y et al (2015) Spata7 is a retinal ciliopathy gene critical for correct RPGRIP1 localization and protein trafficking in the retina. Hum Mol Genet 24:1584–1601
105. Petersen-Jones SM, Occelli LM, Winkler PA et al (2018) Patients and animal models of CNGβ1-deficient retinitis pigmentosa support gene augmentation approach. J Clin Invest 128:190–206
106. Hüttl S, Michalakis S, Seeliger M et al (2005) Impaired channel targeting and retinal degeneration in mice lacking the cyclic nucleotide-gated channel subunit CNGB1. J Neurosci 25:130–138
107. Zacchigna S, Oh H, Wilsch-Bräuninger M et al (2009) Loss of the cholesterol-binding protein prominin-1/CD133 causes disk

dysmorphogenesis and photoreceptor degeneration. J Neurosci 29:2297–2308
108. Sharif AS, Yu D, Loertscher S et al (2018) C8ORF37 is required for photoreceptor outer segment disc morphogenesis by maintaining outer segment membrane protein homeostasis. J Neurosci 38:3160–3176
109. Liou GI, Fei Y, Peachey NS et al (1998) Early onset photoreceptor abnormalities induced by targeted disruption of the interphotoreceptor retinoid-binding protein gene. J Neurosci 18:4511–4520
110. Moshiri A, Humpal D, Leonard BC et al (2017) Arap1 deficiency causes photoreceptor degeneration in mice. Invest Ophthalmol Vis Sci 58:1709–1718
111. Davis RJ, Tosi J, Janisch KM et al (2008) Functional rescue of degenerating photoreceptors in mice homozygous for a hypomorphic cGMP phosphodiesterase 6 b allele (Pde6b H620Q). Invest Ophthalmol Vis Sci 49:5067–5076
112. Koch SF, Duong JK, Hsu C-W et al (2017) Genetic rescue models refute nonautonomous rod cell death in retinitis pigmentosa. PNAS 114:5259–5264
113. Tsang SH, Gouras P, Yamashita CK et al (1996) Retinal degeneration in mice lacking the γ subunit of the rod cGMP phosphodiesterase. Science 272:1026–1029
114. Sakamoto K, McCluskey M, Wensel TG et al (2009) New mouse models for recessive retinitis pigmentosa caused by mutations in the Pde6a gene. Hum Mol Genet 18:178–192
115. Nishimura DY, Baye LM, Perveen R et al (2010) Discovery and functional analysis of a retinitis pigmentosa gene, C2ORF71. Am J Hum Genet 86:686–695
116. Li C, Wang L, Zhang J et al (2014) CERKL interacts with mitochondrial TRX2 and protects retinal cells from oxidative stress-induced apoptosis. Biochim Biophys Acta 1842:1121–1129
117. Lehmann M, Knust E, Hebbar S (2019) Drosophila melanogaster: a valuable genetic model organism to elucidate the biology of retinitis pigmentosa. In: Weber BHF, Langmann T (eds) Retinal degeneration: methods and protocols. Springer New York, New York, pp 221–249
118. Pelletier V, Jambou M, Delphin N et al (2007) Comprehensive survey of mutations in RP2 and RPGR in patients affected with distinct retinal dystrophies: genotype-phenotype correlations and impact on genetic counseling. Hum Mutat 28:81–91
119. Vervoort R, Lennon A, Bird AC et al (2000) Mutational hot spot within a new RPGR exon in X-linked retinitis pigmentosa. Nat Genet 25:462–466
120. Tee JJL, Smith AJ, Hardcastle AJ et al (2016) RPGR-associated retinopathy: clinical features, molecular genetics, animal models and therapeutic options. Br J Ophthalmol 100: 1022–1027
121. Khanna H, Hurd TW, Lillo C et al (2005) RPGR-ORF15, which is mutated in retinitis pigmentosa, associates with SMC1, SMC3, and microtubule transport proteins. J Biol Chem 280:33580–33587
122. Khanna H, Davis EE, Murga-Zamalloa CA et al (2009) A common allele in RPGRIP1L is a modifier of retinal degeneration in ciliopathies. Nat Genet 41:739–745
123. Randall CJ, McLachlan I (1979) Retinopathy in commercial layers. Vet Rec 105:41–42
124. Randall CJ, Wilson MA, Pollock BJ et al (1983) Partial retinal dysplasia and subsequent degeneration in a mutant strain of domestic fowl (rdd). Exp Eye Res 37: 337–347
125. Burt DW, Morrice DR, Lester DH et al (2003) Analysis of the rdd locus in chicken: a model for human retinitis pigmentosa. Mol Vis 9:164–170
126. Ali M, Hocking PM, McKibbin M et al (2011) Mpdz null allele in an avian model of retinal degeneration and mutations in human Leber congenital amaurosis and retinitis pigmentosa. Invest Ophthalmol Vis Sci 52: 7432–7440
127. van de Pavert SA, Kantardzhieva A, Malysheva A et al (2004) Crumbs homologue 1 is required for maintenance of photoreceptor cell polarization and adhesion during light exposure. J Cell Sci 117:4169–4177
128. West EL, Pearson RA, Tschernutter M et al (2008) Pharmacological disruption of the outer limiting membrane leads to increased retinal integration of transplanted photoreceptor precursors. Exp Eye Res 86:601–611
129. Pearson RA, Barber AC, West EL et al (2010) Targeted disruption of outer limiting membrane junctional proteins (Crb1 and ZO-1) increases integration of transplanted photoreceptor precursors into the adult wild-type and degenerating retina. Cell Transplant 19: 487–503
130. Zeiss CJ, Acland GM, Aguirre GD (1999) Retinal pathology of canine X-linked progressive retinal atrophy, the locus homologue of RP3. Invest Ophthalmol Vis Sci 40: 3292–3304

131. Zhang Q, Acland GM, Wu WX et al (2002) Different RPGR exon ORF15 mutations in Canids provide insights into photoreceptor cell degeneration. Hum Mol Genet 11: 993–1003
132. Beltran WA, Hammond P, Acland GM et al (2006) A frameshift mutation in RPGR exon ORF15 causes photoreceptor degeneration and inner retina remodeling in a model of X-linked retinitis pigmentosa. Invest Ophthalmol Vis Sci 47:1669–1681
133. Thompson DA, Khan NW, Othman MI et al (2012) Rd9 is a naturally occurring mouse model of a common form of retinitis pigmentosa caused by mutations in RPGR-ORF15. PLoS One 7:e35865
134. Hong D-H, Pawlyk BS, Shang J et al (2000) A retinitis pigmentosa GTPase regulator (RPGR)- deficient mouse model for X-linked retinitis pigmentosa (RP3). PNAS 97: 3649–3654
135. Guo H, Li J, Gao F et al (2015) Whole-exome sequencing reveals a novel CHM gene mutation in a family with choroideremia initially diagnosed as retinitis pigmentosa. BMC Ophthalmol 15:1–7
136. Tolmachova T, Anders R, Abrink M et al (2006) Independent degeneration of photoreceptors and retinal pigment epithelium in conditional knockout mouse models of choroideremia. J Clin Invest 116:386–394
137. Simunovic MP, Jolly JK, Xue K et al (2016) The spectrum of CHM gene mutations in choroideremia and their relationship to clinical phenotype. Invest Ophthalmol Vis Sci 57: 6033–6039
138. Shu X, Zeng Z, Gautier P et al (2010) Zebrafish Rpgr is required for normal retinal development and plays a role in dynein-based retrograde transport processes. Hum Mol Genet 19:657–670
139. Raghupathy RK, McCulloch DL, Akhtar S et al (2014) Pathogenesis of X-linked RP3: insights from animal models. Adv Exp Med Biol 801:477–485
140. Shu X, Zeng Z, Gautier P et al (2011) Knockdown of the zebrafish ortholog of the retinitis pigmentosa 2 (RP2) gene results in retinal degeneration. Invest Ophthalmol Vis Sci 52: 2960–2966
141. Evans RJ, Schwarz N, Nagel-Wolfrum K et al (2010) The retinitis pigmentosa protein RP2 links pericentriolar vesicle transport between the Golgi and the primary cilium. Hum Mol Genet 19:1358–1367
142. Hurd T, Zhou W, Jenkins P et al (2010) The retinitis pigmentosa protein RP2 interacts with polycystin 2 and regulates cilia-mediated vertebrate development. Hum Mol Genet 19: 4330–4344
143. Boughman JA, Vernon M, Shaver KA (1983) Usher syndrome: definition and estimate of prevalence from two high-risk populations. J Chronic Dis 36:595–603
144. Norris DP, Grimes DT (2012) Mouse models of ciliopathies: the state of the art. Dis Model Mech 5:299–312
145. Li G, Vega R, Nelms K et al (2007) A role for Alström syndrome protein, Alms1, in kidney ciliogenesis and cellular quiescence. PLoS Genet 3:e8
146. Collin GB, Cyr E, Bronson R et al (2005) Alms1-disrupted mice recapitulate human Alström syndrome. Hum Mol Genet 14: 2323–2333
147. Mykytyn K, Mullins RF, Andrews M et al (2004) Bardet–Biedl syndrome type 4 (BBS4)-null mice implicate Bbs4 in flagella formation but not global cilia assembly. PNAS 101:8664–8669
148. Stubdal H, Lynch CA, Moriarty A et al (2000) Targeted deletion of the tub mouse obesity gene reveals that tubby is a loss-of-function mutation. Mol Cell Biol 20: 878–882
149. Forsythe E, Beales PL (2013) Bardet–Biedl syndrome. Eur J Hum Genet 21:8–13
150. Hamel CP (2007) Cone rod dystrophies. Orphanet J Rare Dis 2:7
151. Nishimura DY, Fath M, Mullins RF et al (2004) Bbs2-null mice have neurosensory deficits, a defect in social dominance, and retinopathy associated with mislocalization of rhodopsin. PNAS 101:16588–16593
152. Zhang Q, Nishimura D, Seo S et al (2011) Bardet-Biedl syndrome 3 (Bbs3) knockout mouse model reveals common BBS-associated phenotypes and Bbs3 unique phenotypes. PNAS 108:20678–20683
153. Abd-El-Barr MM, Sykoudis K, Andrabi S et al (2007) Impaired photoreceptor protein transport and synaptic transmission in a mouse model of Bardet–Biedl syndrome. Vis Res 47:3394–3407
154. Ross AJ, May-Simera H, Eichers ER et al (2005) Disruption of Bardet-Biedl syndrome ciliary proteins perturbs planar cell polarity in vertebrates. Nat Genet 37:1135–1140
155. Davis RE, Swiderski RE, Rahmouni K et al (2007) A knockin mouse model of the Bardet–Biedl syndrome 1 M390R mutation has cilia defects, ventriculomegaly, retinopathy, and obesity. PNAS 104:19422–19427

156. Lockhart CM, Nakano M, Rettie AE et al (2014) Generation and characterization of a murine model of Bietti crystalline dystrophy. Invest Ophthalmol Vis Sci 55:5572–5581
157. Lai TYY, Chu K-O, Chan K-P et al (2010) Alterations in serum fatty acid concentrations and desaturase activities in Bietti crystalline dystrophy unaffected by CYP4V2 genotypes. Invest Ophthalmol Vis Sci 51:1092–1097
158. Audo I, Vanakker OM, Smith A et al (2007) Pseudoxanthoma elasticum with generalized retinal dysfunction, a common finding? Invest Ophthalmol Vis Sci 48:4250–4256
159. Roth BM, Yuan A, Ehlers JP (2012) Retinal and choroidal findings in oxalate retinopathy using EDI-OCT. Ophthalmic Surg Lasers Imaging 43:S142–S144
160. Choi RY, Chortkoff SC, Gorusupudi A et al (2016) Crystalline maculopathy associated with high-dose lutein supplementation. JAMA Ophthalmol 134:1445–1448
161. Karikkineth AC, Scheibye-Knudsen M, Fivenson E et al (2017) Cockayne syndrome: clinical features, model systems and pathways. Ageing Res Rev 33:3–17
162. van der Horst GTJ, van Steeg H, Berg RJW et al (1997) Defective transcription-coupled repair in Cockayne syndrome B mice is associated with skin cancer predisposition. Cell 89:425–435
163. Gorgels TGMF, van der Pluijm I, Brandt RMC et al (2007) Retinal degeneration and ionizing radiation hypersensitivity in a mouse model for Cockayne syndrome. Mol Cell Biol 27:1433–1441
164. Jacobsohn E (1888) Ein Fall von Retinitis pigmentosa atypica. Klin Monatsbl Augenheilkd 26:202–206
165. Wang T, Milam AH, Steel G et al (1996) A mouse model of gyrate atrophy of the choroid and retina. Early retinal pigment epithelium damage and progressive retinal degeneration. J Clin Invest 97:2753–2762
166. Sergouniotis PI, Davidson AE, Lenassi E et al (2012) Retinal structure, function, and molecular pathologic features in gyrate atrophy. Ophthalmology 119:596–605
167. Bisaillon JJ, Radden LA, Szabo ET et al (2014) The retarded hair growth (rhg) mutation in mice is an allele of ornithine aminotransferase (Oat). Mol Genet Metab Rep 1: 378–390
168. Wang T, Lawler AM, Steel G et al (1995) Mice lacking ornithine–δ–amino–transferase have paradoxical neonatal hypoornithinaemia and retinal degeneration. Nat Genet 11: 185–190
169. Curtain M, Donahue LR, Ward-Bailey PF (2009) Cataracts and retarded hair growth in rhg. MGI Direct Data Submission:7
170. Kaiser-Kupfer MI, Ludwig IH, de Monasterio FM et al (1985) Gyrate atrophy of the choroid and retina: early findings. Ophthalmology 92:394–401
171. Louie CM, Caridi G, Lopes VS et al (2010) AHI1 is required for photoreceptor outer segment development and is a modifier for retinal degeneration in nephronophthisis. Nat Genet 42:175–180
172. Joubert syndrome. https://ghr.nlm.nih.gov/condition/joubert-syndrome
173. Rachel RA, Yamamoto EA, Dewanjee MK et al (2015) CEP290 alleles in mice disrupt tissue-specific cilia biogenesis and recapitulate features of syndromic ciliopathies. Hum Mol Genet 24:3775–3791
174. Bongorno J, Guy J, Lewin AS (2004) 437. Developing a mouse model of the mitochondrial NARP syndrome using AAV-ribozymes for ATP6. Mol Ther 9:S167
175. NARP. https://ghr.nlm.nih.gov/condition/neuropathy-ataxia-and-retinitis-pigmentosa
176. Refsum disease. https://ghr.nlm.nih.gov/condition/refsum-disease
177. Wierzbicki AS, Lloyd MD, Schofield CJ et al (2002) Refsum's disease: a peroxisomal disorder affecting phytanic acid α-oxidation. J Neurochem 80:727–735
178. Ronquillo CC, Bernstein PS, Baehr W (2012) Senior–Løken syndrome: a syndromic form of retinal dystrophy associated with nephronophthisis. Vis Res 75:88–97
179. Jiang S-T, Chiou Y-Y, Wang E et al (2009) Essential role of nephrocystin in photoreceptor intraflagellar transport in mouse. Hum Mol Genet 18:1566–1577
180. Won J, de Evsikova CM, Smith RS et al (2011) NPHP4 is necessary for normal photoreceptor ribbon synapse maintenance and outer segment formation, and for sperm development. Hum Mol Genet 20:482–496
181. Collin GB, Won J, Hicks WL et al (2012) Meckelin is necessary for photoreceptor intraciliary transport and outer segment morphogenesis. Invest Ophthalmol Vis Sci 53: 967–974
182. Tammachote R, Hommerding CJ, Sinders RM et al (2009) Ciliary and centrosomal defects associated with mutation and depletion of the Meckel syndrome genes MKS1 and MKS3. Hum Mol Genet 18:3311–3323
183. Williams DS (2008) Usher syndrome: animal models, retinal function of Usher proteins,

and prospects for gene therapy. Vis Res 48: 433–441

184. Johnson KR, Gagnon LH, Webb LS et al (2003) Mouse models of USH1C and DFNB18: phenotypic and molecular analyses of two new spontaneous mutations of the Ush1c gene. Hum Mol Genet 12:3075–3086
185. Lentz JJ, Gordon WC, Farris HE et al (2010) Deafness and retinal degeneration in a novel USH1C knock-in mouse model. Dev Neurobiol 70:253–267
186. Liu X, Bulgakov OV, Darrow KN et al (2007) Usherin is required for maintenance of retinal photoreceptors and normal development of cochlear hair cells. PNAS 104:4413–4418
187. Noben-Trauth K, Naggert JK, North MA et al (1996) A candidate gene for the mouse mutation tubby. Nature 380:534–538
188. Menotti-Raymond M, Deckman KH, David V et al (2010) Mutation discovered in a feline model of human congenital retinal blinding disease. Invest Ophthalmol Vis Sci 51: 2852–2859
189. Nour M, Fliesler SJ, Naash MI (2008) Genetic supplementation of RDS alleviates a loss-of-function phenotype in C214S model of retinitis pigmentosa. Adv Exp Med Biol 613:129–138
190. Cai X, Conley SM, Naash MI (2010) Gene therapy in the retinal degeneration slow model of retinitis pigmentosa. In: Anderson RE, Hollyfield JG, LaVail MM (eds) Retinal degenerative diseases. Springer New York, New York, pp 611–619
191. Li T, Franson WK, Gordon JW et al (1995) Constitutive activation of phototransduction by K296E opsin is not a cause of photoreceptor degeneration. PNAS 92:3551–3555
192. Peachey NS, Wang M, Naash MI (1997) The Vpp Mouse. In: LaVail MM, Hollyfield JG, Anderson RE (eds) Degenerative retinal diseases. Springer US, Boston, pp 89–97
193. Choi EH, Suh S, Sander CL et al (2018) Insights into the pathogenesis of dominant retinitis pigmentosa associated with a D477G mutation in RPE65. Hum Mol Genet 27:2225–2243
194. Dekomien G, Vollrath C, Petrasch-Parwez E et al (2010) Progressive retinal atrophy in Schapendoes dogs: mutation of the newly identified CCDC66 gene. Neurogenetics 11: 163–174
195. Ahonen SJ, Arumilli M, Lohi H (2013) A CNGB1 frameshift mutation in Papillon and Phalène dogs with progressive retinal atrophy. PLoS One 8:e72122
196. Downs LM, Mellersh CS (2014) An intronic SINE insertion in FAM161A that causes exon-skipping is associated with progressive retinal atrophy in Tibetan Spaniels and Tibetan Terriers. PLoS One 9:e93990
197. Scott RS, McMahon EJ, Pop SM et al (2001) Phagocytosis and clearance of apoptotic cells is mediated by MER. Nature 411:207
198. McHenry CL, Liu Y, Feng W et al (2004) MERTK arginine-844-cysteine in a patient with severe rod-cone dystrophy: loss of mutant protein function in transfected cells. Invest Ophthalmol Vis Sci 45:1456–1463
199. Gal A, Li Y, Thompson DA et al (2000) Mutations in MERTK, the human orthologue of the RCS rat retinal dystrophy gene, cause retinitis pigmentosa. Nat Genet 26: 270–271
200. Smith SB (1992) C57BL/6J-vit/vit mouse model of retinal degeneration: light microscopic analysis and evaluation of rhodopsin levels. Exp Eye Res 55:903–910
201. Tang M, Pawlyk BS, Kosaras B et al (1997) ERG abnormalities in relation to histopathologic findings in vitiligo mutant mice. Exp Eye Res 65:215–222
202. Pittler SJ, Keeler CE, Sidman RL et al (1993) PCR analysis of DNA from 70-year-old sections of rodless retina demonstrates identity with the mouse rd defect. PNAS 90: 9616–9619
203. Farber DB (1995) From mice to men: the cyclic GMP phosphodiesterase gene in vision and disease. The Proctor lecture. Invest Ophthalmol Vis Sci 36:263–275
204. Wu W-H, Tsai Y-T, Justus S et al (2016) CRISPR repair reveals causative mutation in a preclinical model of retinitis pigmentosa. Mol Ther 24:1388–1394
205. Bunel M, Chaudieu G, Hamel C et al (2019) Natural models for retinitis pigmentosa: progressive retinal atrophy in dog breeds. Hum Genet 138:441–453
206. Cai X, Conley SM, Naash MI (2009) RPE65: role in the visual cycle, human retinal disease, and gene therapy. Ophthalmic Genet 30:57
207. Goldstein O, Jordan JA, Aguirre GD et al (2013) A non-stop S-antigen gene mutation is associated with late onset hereditary retinal degeneration in dogs. Mol Vis 19:1871–1884
208. Downs LM, Wallin-Håkansson B, Boursnell M et al (2011) A frameshift mutation in golden retriever dogs with progressive retinal atrophy endorses SLC4A3 as a candidate gene for human retinal degenerations. PLoS One 6:e21452
209. Goldstein O, Kukekova AV, Aguirre GD et al (2010) Exonic SINE insertion in STK38L causes canine early retinal degeneration (erd). Genomics 96:362–368

210. Downs LM, Wallin-Håkansson B, Bergström T et al (2014) A novel mutation in TTC8 is associated with progressive retinal atrophy in the golden retriever. Canine Genet Epidemiol 1:4
211. Fath MA, Mullins RF, Searby C et al (2005) Mkks-null mice have a phenotype resembling Bardet–Biedl syndrome. Hum Mol Genet 14: 1109–1118
212. Smith UM, Consugar M, Tee LJ et al (2006) The transmembrane protein Meckelin (MKS3) is mutated in Meckel-Gruber syndrome and the wpk rat. Nat Genet 38: 191–196
213. Ohlemiller KK, Hughes RM, Lett JM et al (1997) Progression of cochlear and retinal degeneration in the tubby (rd5) mouse. Audiol Neurootol 2:175–185

Chapter 20

Electroretinogram (ERG) to Evaluate the Retina Using Mouse Models

Pei-Kang Liu, Wan-Chun Huang, and Nan-Kai Wang

Abstract

Electroretinogram (ERG) is a sensitive and useful tool for the measurement of the retina's electrical response to flash stimuli. It provides a functional evaluation of the photoreceptors and downstream associated retinal cells. Similar to those conducted on humans, mouse ERGs include the amplitudes of a- and b-waves as well as the implicit time from those ERGs. Applications of ERGs include identification of retinal phenotypes, measurement of retinal function (at one and various time points), and evaluation of treatment efficacy. However, there are some differences between the manifestation of disease in patients as compared to mouse models that should be taken into consideration when implementing mouse ERGs. Herein, this chapter will introduce how to perform and obtain mouse ERGs.

Key words Electroretinogram (ERG), Mouse model, Full-field ERG, Serial intensity ERG

1 Introduction

Basic research on human inherited retinal degeneration relies on the well-established animal models, which allow researchers to study the mechanism underlying human eye diseases or to investigate the efficacy of potential therapeutic strategies. The electroretinogram (ERG) serves as an objective, sensitive, noninvasive, and useful tool for assessing retinal function in the process, and it permits the animal to breed after being tested. First, it reveals characterizing functional changes of the retina that result from the interruption of visual signals of the retina in a mouse model with genetic modification [1, 2]. When an animal model is generated, researchers can use ERG testing to determine whether the phenotype of the model corresponds to the phenotype of human disease. Second, ERG can be used to test the therapeutic effects or to evaluate drug toxicity in mouse models. As the disease progresses, ERGs can be used to evaluate the retinal function or the severity of retinal degeneration at different time points [3–6].

Stephen H. Tsang and Peter M. J. Quinn (eds.), *Retinitis Pigmentosa*,
Methods in Molecular Biology, vol. 2560, https://doi.org/10.1007/978-1-0716-2651-1_20,

Given that cones account for only 3–5% of photoreceptors in mice and humans, the protocols of mouse ERGs are similar to human ERG recording settings [7]. However, there are some differences between human and mouse ERGs. Anesthesia is required to obtain ERG recordings from animal models [8]. More proper preparation and procedures before mouse ERG recordings is required. Additionally, the ERG settings may vary in different laboratories as well as based on different experimental designs. According to the experiment designs of our laboratory, our mouse models are assessed with the full-field ERG testing (similar to human full-field ERG to assess rod responses, maximal responses, and cone responses) and serial intensity ERGs. In the following paragraphs, we describe the methods for performing ERGs in mice, including the materials we used, the details of the examination procedure, and the analysis of ERG testing in this chapter.

2 Materials

2.1 Equipment

1. An advanced real-time acquisition system with integrated power isolation, a direct pattern generator, isolated auxiliary line outlets to meet medical leakage current standards, and a machined aluminum case with all-digital filtering.
2. A ColorDome with a flash luminance range between 10^{-9} and 3000 cd·s/m^2 and full color control of stimulus.
3. A heating pad for maintaining normal body temperature of the anesthetized mouse during ERG recordings.
4. A small stage on which the anesthetized mouse lies.
5. Electrode preparation.
   (a) Assembling the electrode ball, which is a magnetic ball used for finely adjusting the position of rodent corneal electrodes.
   (b) Recording electrodes. Metal (platinum, gold, silver, and copper) wire-loop electrodes or Bayer–Mittag contact lens electrodes could be applied for active electrodes, which connect to the positive input for recording full-field ERGs [9]. In our settings, we use two gold wire-loop electrodes as active electrodes.
   (c) Two platinum needle electrodes: One platinum needle electrode is used for a reference and the other one for a ground electrode.
      (i) Reference electrodes: The needle is inserted under the skin at the cheek.
      (ii) Ground electrode: The needle is inserted under the skin at the back.

2.2 Other Materials

1. Mydriatic agents (e.g., tropicamide or phenylephrine).
2. Lubricant agents (e.g., methylcellulose drops).
3. Anesthetic agents (e.g., ketamine and xylazine).
4. One syringe (1 mL) for intraperitoneal injection.
5. Balance scale.
6. Headlamp with dim red light.
7. Microisolator cage and cage lid.
8. Large container wrapped with aluminum foil, and a black light proof cloth for covering whole the large container.
9. Black light proof curtains for blocking out the light for dark adaptation before examination.
10. ERG rooms decorated with black light proof curtains to avoid any undesired light.

2.3 Mice

1. A control group is mandatory in each set of ERG recordings given that several factors are involved in ERG recordings (*see* **Note 1**).
2. C57BL/6 J mice can be used as a control group, but the most appropriate control for testing is the wild-type littermate inbred strain. In that case, the genetic background and the age of experimental and control groups would be the same.

3 Methods

3.1 One Day Before Examination

1. Confirm the mice strain, gender, or marks/numbers to be compatible with what are listed in the mouse data sheets before dark adaptation. Keeping all the mice that will be measured in the same dark adaptation condition is better.
2. Placing the cages for an overnight dark adaptation without any light leakage (*see* **Note 2**).

3.2 Preparation of ERG Recordings

1. Preparing fresh mouse anesthetic agents (dosage: 1 mL of ketamine and 0.1 mL of xylazine in 8.9 mL of PBS) (*see* **Note 3**).
2. Turn off the room light and eliminate undesired light leakage. All procedures must be done under a dim red light until the end of the ERG recording.
3. Place the mouse cages into a large container under a dim red light and use black light proof cloth to cover the whole container (*see* **Note 4**).
4. Transport the large container back to the ERG room, and make sure no undesired light enters the door gap before testing.

5. Open the container and dilate pupils with mydriatic agents. Making an extra mark on the tail enables the examiner to identify the dilated mice.
6. Input the basic information for each mouse (e.g., mice code, the group name in any given experiment, date of birth, gender).
7. Check the pupils and make sure that maximal dilation is reached. Then, select a mouse to test.
8. Document any cataract or corneal opacification in both eyes (*see* **Note 5**).
9. Measure the body weight of each mouse and calculate the appropriate amount of anesthetic dose for each mouse. For example, 0.2 mL of Mouse Anesthetic Mix is appropriate for a mouse with 20 g (*see* **Note 6**).
10. Intraperitoneal injection of the mixture into the mouse with a 1-mL syringe.
11. Put the mouse back to the cage and wait until fully anesthetized.
12. Evaluate adequate anesthesia regularly by monitoring for at least one indicator of deep pain recognition (e.g., pedal reflex, pinna reflex).
13. Apply mydriatic eye drops to both eyes again and wait until pupils are fully dilated.
14. Place the anesthetized mouse on the heating pad on the stage. Stabilizing the body temperature of the mouse during examination is important.
15. The mouse head should be positioned at the center of Ganzfeld bowl on a transparent plate so that the eyes are stimulated uniformly from all directions.
16. Insert the reference electrode subcutaneously at the middle of the forehead or at the middle of the cheek; apply the ground electrode at the middle of the back near the tail (*see* **Note 7**).
17. Apply lubricant to both eyes to moisten active electrodes and to keep the corneal surface moist.
18. Wait until the lubricant is evenly distributed and cover the ColorDome down carefully (*see* **Note 8**).
19. Check all impedances before ERG recordings or replace electrodes if the signals show an aberrant drifting or fluctuations (*see* **Note 9**).

3.3 ERG Recording Protocols

3.3.1 Full-Field ERG

1. Similar to the human full-field ERG, the mouse full-field ERG helps to differentiate rod or cone system dysfunction and generalized outer or inner retinal dysfunction.
2. Stimulation: The dark-adapted (DA, scotopic) and light-adapted (LA, photopic) ERGs are performed to assess the generalized retinal activities. The ERG recordings start from dim light after dark adaption. The first step of ERG recordings is to measure rod response, followed by maximum response (combined rod–cone response) and cone response, since the rod photoreceptors are very photosensitive. It takes approximately 0.5 hour to finish the recordings. Trigger the stimulus and record data simultaneously, as described below.
3. Scotopic (DA) ERGs:
   (a) Rod responses: DA ERGs provide the function of rod photoreceptors and downstream retinal cells. The b-wave can be recorded after a pulse intensity of 0.001 cd·s/m^2 (white-6500 K pulse color). At this stage, the a-wave is nearly not captured due to very weak response of rod photoreceptors. The waves of ten repeated stimuli are averaged, and the minimum interval between each flash is 5 seconds (*see* Fig. 1a).
   (b) Maximum response: Using a brighter pulse intensity of 3.0 cd·s/m^2 with the same color, ERGs have input from both rod and cone photoreceptors, and a- and b-waves are recorded. The waves of five repeated stimuli were averaged, and the minimum interval between each flash is 15 seconds (*see* Fig.1b).
4. Photopic (LA) ERGs:
   (a) Cone response: The standard period of light adaptation with a constant background luminance of 30 cd/m^2 (white-6500 K pulse color) in the Ganzfeld is 10 minutes. LA ERGs provide measures of generalized cone photoreceptors function, which are obtained using a flash strength of 30 cd·s/m^2. The waves of twenty repeated stimuli are averaged, and the minimum interval between each flash is 1 second. The single flash LA ERGs are composed of a- and b-waves. The b-waves are prominent, but the a-waves are relatively not obvious (*see* Fig.1c).

3.3.2 Serial Intensity ERGs

1. Serial intensity ERGs provide more sensitive and detailed measures of retinal functions in retinal degeneration mouse models. By using different intensity stimuli that impact the rod and cone photoreceptors, researchers can collect more precise data of retinal functions. Scotopic serial intensity ERGs provide information on the function of the rod photoreceptors, whereas photopic serial intensity ERGs reveal the cone

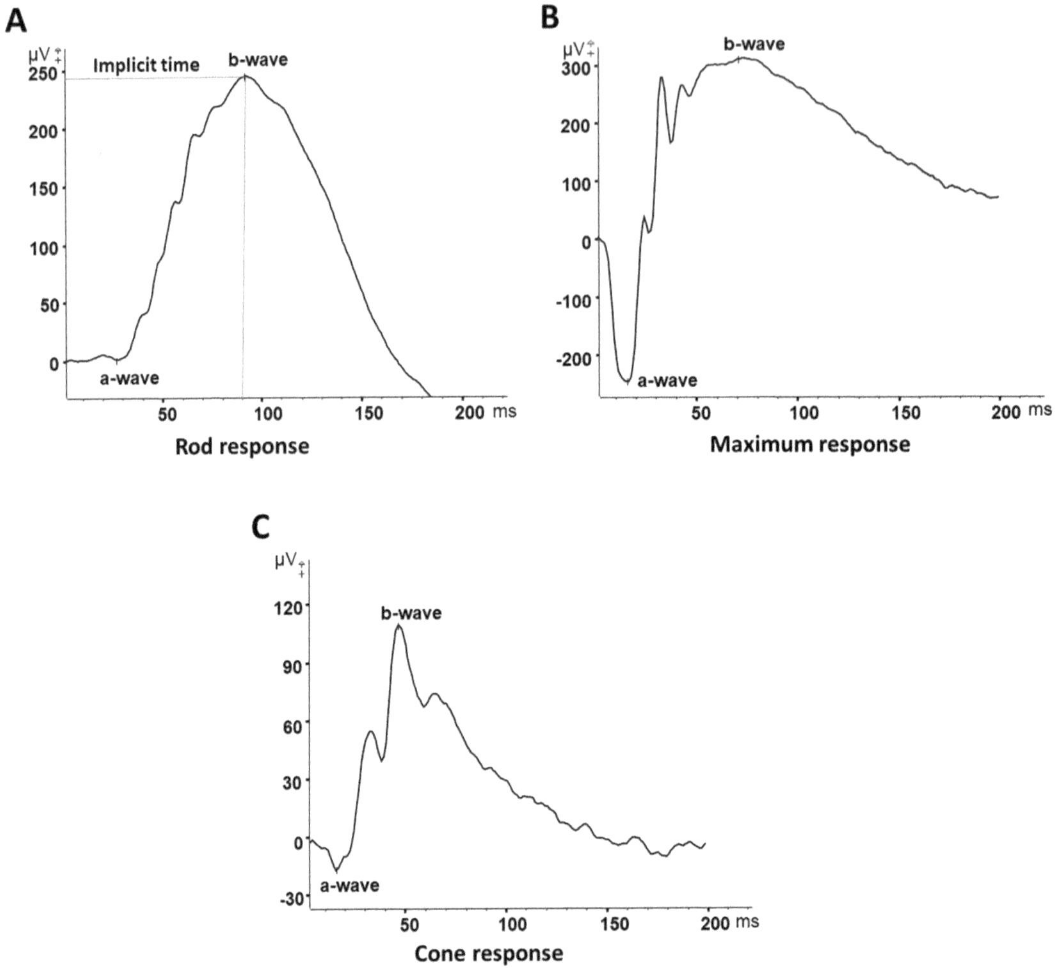

Fig. 1 Representative full-field electroretinograms (ERGs) of wild-type mice (C57BL/6 J, 6 months old). (**a**) Scotopic rod response (dark adapted, 0.001 cd·s/m^2). (**b**) Scotopic maximum response (dark adapted, 3 cd·s/m^2) ERGs. (**c**) Photopic cone response (light adapted, 30 cd.s/m^2)

photoreceptors integrity. In our lab, both scotopic and photopic serial ERGs have eight steps, respectively. The stimuli intensities will increase gradually (Table 1), and the whole measurement takes around 30 minutes.

2. Scotopic serial intensity ERGs: The light intensities of stimuli for scotopic serial intensity ERGs are −6.0, −5.0, −4.0, −3.0, −2.0, −1.0, 0.0, and 1.0 log cd·s/m^2 in sequence. The intervals between each stimulus are from 2 to 30 seconds, and the numbers of repeats are from 3 to 20 times. For the total recovery of the photoreceptors after stimuli, the intervals between each stimulus increase, but the numbers of repeats decrease with the strengthening of the stimuli (*see* Table 1). Normally, the intensity of the first stimulus (−6.0 log cd·s/m^2)

Table 1
Protocols for serial intensity electroretinograms (ERGs)

Steps	Stimulus intensity (log cd·s/m^2)	Interstimulus interval (s)	Number of repeats
Scotopic serial intensity[a]			
1	−6.0	2	20
2	−5.0	2	20
3	−4.0	5	15
4	−3.0	5	10
5	−2.0	5	10
6	−1	10	10
7	0	10	5
8	1.0	30	3
Photopic serial intensity[b]			
1	−1	1	10
2	0	1	10
3	0.3	2	10
4	0.6	2	10
5	1	5	10
6	1.48	5	5
7	2.0	10	5
8	2.3	10	3

[a]Overnight dark adaption
[b]Photopic background illuminance: 30 cd/m^2; light adaptation duration: 10 minutes

is very weak so that the a- and b-waves are not obvious. As the light intensities increase, the b-wave will become more and more obvious. The a-wave will become more prominent when the pulse intensity increases to −2.0 log cd·s/m^2. Both a- and b-waves become very prominent when the intensities are above −2.0 log cd·s/m^2 (*see* Fig. 2a).

3. Photopic serial intensity ERGs: The light intensities of stimuli for photopic serial intensity ERGs are −1.0, 0.0, 0.3, 0.6, 1.0, 1.48, 2.0, and 2.3 log cd·s/m^2 in sequence. The intervals between each stimulus are from 1 to 10 seconds, and the numbers of repeats are from 3 to 10 times (*see* Table 1). The a-waves are not prominent in photopic serial intensity ERGs. The b-waves enlarge with increasing light intensities. The b-waves dominate the photopic serial intensity ERGs assessment (*see* Fig. 2b).

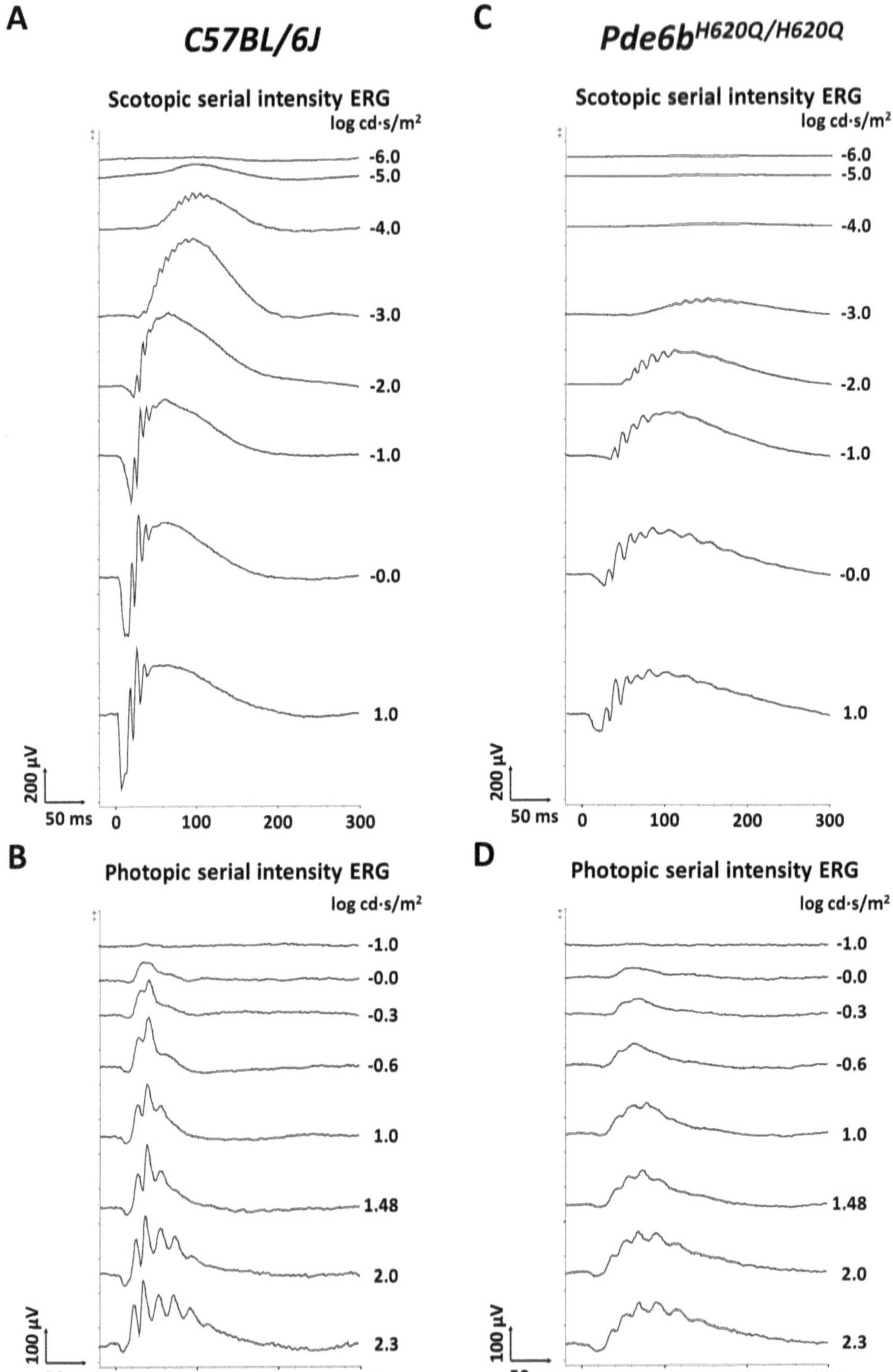

Fig. 2 Serial intensity electroretinograms (ERGs). (**a** and **b**) Scotopic (**a**) and photopic (**b**) serial intensity ERGs of a wild-type mouse (C57BL/6 J, 6 months old). The a-wave is recordable when the pulse intensity increases to −2.0 log cd·s/m^2. With increasing pulse intensity, both a- and b-waves become more and more prominent.

3.4 ERG Response Analysis

Similar to human ERGs, the interpretation of amplitudes and implicit time (peak time) of the a- and b-wave in mouse ERGs are important. The a-wave is the initial negative deflection, which represents the response of the photoreceptors to the flash. The b-wave is the first positive deflection derived from the inner layer of retina (predominantly bipolar cells), which reflects the response of downstream retinal neurons to the activated photoreceptors. The amplitude of the a-wave is from the baseline to the lowest point of the a-wave. The b-wave amplitude is generally measured from the bottom of the a-wave to the top of the tallest curve. The implicit time is the interval from the onset of the stimulus to the peak of the b-wave (*see* Fig. 1a).

A decreased amplitude correlates to the extent of retinal dysfunctions and numbers of photoreceptors. The delay in the implicit time represents diffuse photoreceptors dysfunction of whole retina. Here, we use the ERGs of $Pde6b^{H620Q/H620Q}$ mice as an example. $Pde6b^{H620Q/H620Q}$ mice represent a severe form of RP where retinal degeneration begins within 2 weeks and reach a nearly complete loss of photoreceptors by 8 weeks after birth [10]. Compared to the normal data of wild-type mice, scotopic and photopic serial intensity ERGs in these $Pde6b^{H620Q/H620Q}$ mice reveal a decrease in both a- and b-wave amplitudes. The implicit times are delayed as well, compatible with diffuse retinal degeneration. Performing serial intensity ERGs in animal models provides more detailed information to be gathered, allowing researchers to observe trends and differences (*see* Figs. 2a–d and 3a–c).

4 Notes

1. The importance of control groups: The ERG recordings may be affected by the techniques of operators and the equipment (please refer to the chapter regarding human ERG). Many factors may influence the results in series testing, such as the time of dark adaption, the depth of anesthesia, the position of the electrodes, the stability of the machine, and the room temperature of ERG room, even if the same machine is operated by the same examiners. Lower room temperature may be associated with lower ERG recording responses. For a new examiner, the comparison between the control groups and the nomograms of the lab help to solve the technical problems.

Fig. 2 (continued) (**c** and **d**) Scotopic (**c**) and photopic (**d**) serial intensity ERGs of a $Pde6b^{H620Q/H620Q}$ mouse (3 weeks old) demonstrate decreases of the amplitudes and delays of implicit times, which correspond to the degeneration of rod and cone photoreceptors in the retina

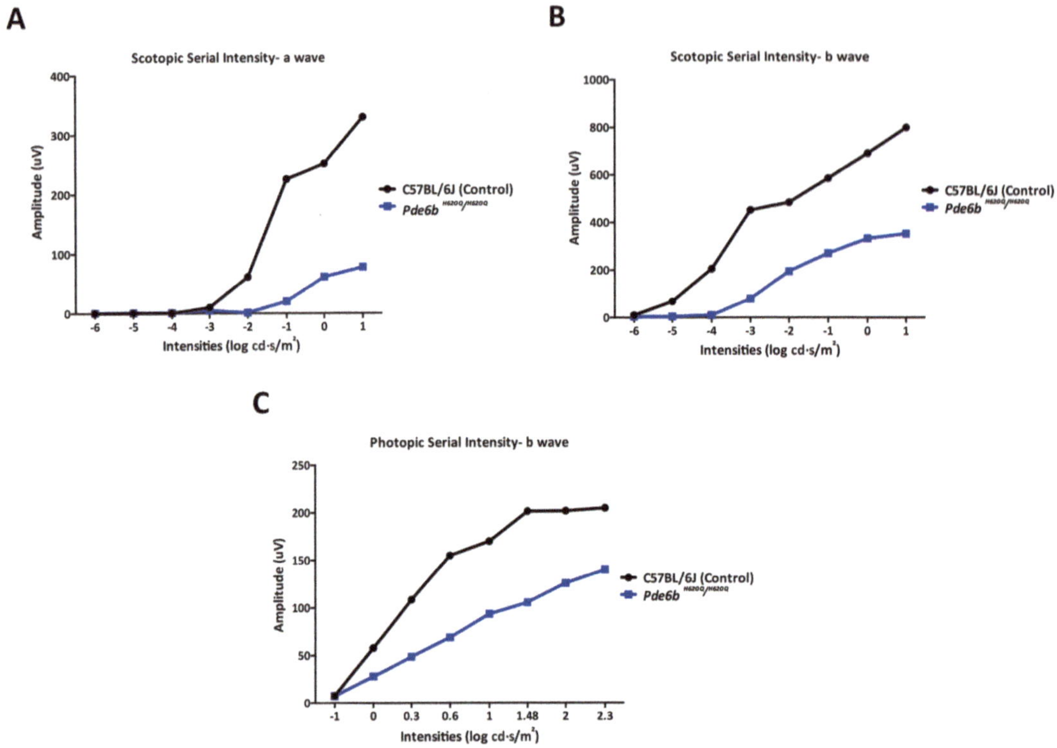

Fig. 3 (**a** and **b**) The a- and b-wave amplitudes of scotopic serial intensity ERGs of a *Pde6b*$^{H620Q/H620Q}$ mouse (3 weeks old) are lower than a wild-type mouse. (**c**) The b-wave amplitudes of photopic serial intensity ERGs of a *Pde6b*$^{H620Q/H620Q}$ mouse (3 weeks old) is lower than a wild type mouse. The results are compatible with diffuse rod and cone photoreceptors degeneration in a 3-week-old *Pde6b*$^{H620Q/H620Q}$ mouse

2. The length of dark adaption: We suggest overnight dark adaption and consistency. Remarks regarding the dark adaption length to the results are necessary.
3. Validity period of the anesthetic agents: The best timing to prepare the anesthetic agent is just before the tests. The anesthetic effects will be best. Generally, the mice would be anesthetized within 1 minute after injection. Longer storage time of anesthetic agents corresponds with worse anesthetic effects.
4. As with humans, all the tests should be performed under dim red light. Bright red light may affect the recordings.
5. Any visual axis opacity (e.g., cataract, corneal opacity) may preclude the light from entering the retina. The ERG recordings may be less reliable.
6. Adjusting the dose of anesthetic agents: The amount of anesthetic solution may be adjusted according to different conditions. After injecting a normal amount of drug, the mice will be anesthetized for about 1 hour. If the duration of testing is longer than 1 hour, the amount may be increased. If the mice

have lower body weight (<10 g), the dose of anesthetic agents should be decreased to prevent death after anesthesia. Mice with lower body weight are more sensitive to the anesthetic agents. In contrast, pregnant mice or mice tested immediately or shortly after delivery have poor response to the anesthetic drugs, and they may need a larger dose.

7. The position of the reference electrode: We recommend placing the reference electrode at the middle of the forehead or cheek. An alternative position is at the tongue, but electrode displacement may occur.
8. If the lubricant flows through the ocular surface of the mice, the ERG recordings will be unstable. Start recording the waves after even distribution of the lubricant.
9. We recommend checking the impedances regularly. If the signals remain unstable even after correcting all the above factors, correction of the ERG recording machine may be considered.

References

1. Peachey NS, Ball SL (2003) Electrophysiological analysis of visual function in mutant mice. Doc Ophthalmol 107(1):13–36
2. Tanimoto N, Muehlfriedel RL, Fischer MD et al (2009) Vision tests in the mouse: functional phenotyping with electroretinography. Front Biosci (Landmark Ed) 14:2730–2737
3. Perlman I (2009) Testing retinal toxicity of drugs in animal models using electrophysiological and morphological techniques. Doc Ophthalmol 118(1):3–28. https://doi.org/10.1007/s10633-008-9153-6
4. Weber BH, Schrewe H, Molday LL et al (2002) Inactivation of the murine X-linked juvenile retinoschisis gene, Rs1h, suggests a role of retinoschisin in retinal cell layer organization and synaptic structure. Proc Natl Acad Sci U S A 99(9):6222–6227. https://doi.org/10.1073/pnas.092528599
5. Biel M, Seeliger M, Pfeifer A et al (1999) Selective loss of cone function in mice lacking the cyclic nucleotide-gated channel CNG3. Proc Natl Acad Sci U S A 96(13):7553–7557. https://doi.org/10.1073/pnas.96.13.7553
6. Duncan JL, LaVail MM, Yasumura D et al (2003) An RCS-like retinal dystrophy phenotype in mer knockout mice. Invest Ophthalmol Vis Sci 44(2):826–838. https://doi.org/10.1167/iovs.02-0438
7. Carter-Dawson LD, LaVail MM (1979) Rods and cones in the mouse retina. I. Structural analysis using light and electron microscopy. J Comp Neurol 188(2):245–262. https://doi.org/10.1002/cne.901880204
8. Frishman LJ, Wang MH (2011) Electroretinogram of human, monkey and mouse. In: Levin LA, SFE N, Hoeve JV, Wu S, Kaufman PL, Alm A (eds) Adler's physiology of the eye, 11th edn. Elsevier Health Sciences, pp 480–501
9. Bayer AU, Cook P, Brodie SE et al (2001) Evaluation of different recording parameters to establish a standard for flash electroretinography in rodents. Vis Res 41(17):2173–2185. https://doi.org/10.1016/s0042-6989(01)00103-1
10. Davis RJ, Tosi J, Janisch KM et al (2008) Functional rescue of degenerating photoreceptors in mice homozygous for a hypomorphic cGMP phosphodiesterase 6 b allele (Pde6bH620Q). Invest Ophthalmol Vis Sci 49(11):5067–5076. https://doi.org/10.1167/iovs.07-1422

Chapter 21

Autofluorescence Imaging to Evaluate Retinal Disease Progression in Rodent

Chia-Hua Cheng, Xuan Cui, and Stephen H. Tsang

Abstract

Fundus autofluorescence (FAF) imaging is a noninvasive retinal imaging methodology that allows mapping of lipofuscin distribution in the retinal pigment epithelium cell (RPE). Excessive accumulation of lipofuscin granules in the lysosomal compartment of RPE cells represents a common downstream pathogenetic pathway in various hereditary and complex retinal diseases, including age-related macular degeneration. The clinical applications of FAF coupled with its ease of use, and the noninvasive nature of characterizing retinal diseases, are increasingly valuable to the field of ophthalmology and in assessing the progression of retinitis pigmentosa (RP). Quantitative AF (qAF) enhances the understanding of retinal disease processes, serves as a diagnostic aid, and allows for the monitoring of the effects of therapeutic interventions. This chapter introduces basic principles of FAF and general protocols of FAF evaluating retinal disease progression in rodents.

Key words Bisretinoid compounds, FAF imaging, Fundus autofluorescence imaging, Lipofuscin, Retinal pigment epithelium

1 Introduction

Fundus autofluorescence (FAF) imaging is a noninvasive imaging method that can provide a distribution map of the predominant retinal fluorophore, lipofuscin, in the retinal pigment epithelium (RPE). Specifically, FAF provides information about lipofuscin distribution and RPE health, and consequently an increased accumulation of lipofuscin has been correlated with aging and development of certain retinal conditions [1].

RPE lipofuscin is mainly composed of bisretinoid compounds that are produced in photoreceptor cells. The fluorescence emission of all these bisretinoid chromophores is broad, peaking at approximately 610 nm; however, these pigments exhibit various excitation maxima in the visible spectrum, including 430 nm (all-trans-retinal dimer), 439 nm (A2E), 426 nm (iso-A2E), 490 nm (A2-dihydro-pyridine-phosphatifylethanolamine, A2-DHP-PE), and 510 nm

Stephen H. Tsang and Peter M. J. Quinn (eds.), *Retinitis Pigmentosa*,
Methods in Molecular Biology, vol. 2560, https://doi.org/10.1007/978-1-0716-2651-1_21,

(all-transretinal dimer-phosphatidylethanolamine and all-trans-retinal dimer-ethanolamine) [2]. This range of excitation wavelengths could affect FAF imaging. Depending on whether one is imaging with a cSLO and 488-nm excitation or with a modified fundus camera and longer wavelengths (535–580-nm excitation), contributions to the images from different subgroups of the lipofuscin fluorophores may vary [2, 3].

There are several instruments with different hardware configurations and settings capable of acquiring FAF images. Each of the methods provides different results according to the purposes [4]. For example, a series of single FAF images are usually recorded for enhancing the signal-to-noise ratio of fundus images. With the eye-tracking function, we are able to align single images to correct for eye movements during acquisition. Normalized and averaged FAF images get better visualization; however, the mean or normalized images only provide the autofluorescence distribution and could not be used for quantification [3].

Quantitative measurement of autofluorescence is independent of detector gain and laser power over clinically relevant ranges [5]. A2E measurement by high-performance liquid chromatography (HPLC) also indicated the quantitative AF (qAF) is feasible in mice. The qAF method enables measurement of in vivo lipofuscin and the detection of genotype and age-associated differences [6].

2 Methods

2.1 Anesthesia of Mice

1. Pupils were dilated using topical 2.5% phenylephrine hydrochloride and 1% tropicamide (Akorn Inc., Lakeforest, IL) 5–10 min before anesthesia (*see* **Note 1**).
2. Weigh the mouse and give anesthesia solution intraperitoneally with 1-cc syringe with a final concentration at 10 mg/100 g body weight (BW) for ketamine and 1 mg/100 g BW for xylazine.
3. Repeat dilating the pupils as described in **step 1**.
4. Apply one drop of Gonioscopic Prism solution to both eyes of the mouse to keep the cornea moisture (*see* **Note 1**). And mouse was placed on heating pad to keep body temperature.
5. Wait until the,mouse was fully anesthetized, mouse was placed on the specific platform, and ready to take images.

2.2 FAF Imaging

1. Autofluorescence images were obtained with the Spectralis optical coherence tomography scanning laser confocal ophthalmoscope (OCT-SLO Spectralis; Heidelberg Engineering, Heidelberg, Germany) (*see* **Note 2**).

2. During the procedure, body temperature was maintained at 40 °C by a heating pad. Clean the Gonioscopic gel from right eye by balanced saltwater, apply proper Gonioscopic Prism solution again on left eye to keep it in moisture. Place the mouse on the platform and adjust its right eye toward the camera for imaging.
3. Adjust the lens and move the camera to focus on the cornea of the mouse clearly in IR (820 nm) mode. Then move the camera forward to focus on the superficial vessels as well as center the optic nerve. Move forward until the light was fully and evenly light the whole fundus in the camera.
4. Take an image at a resolution of 768 × 768 pixels using the 55° wide-field lens mounted on a Heidelberg Spectralis device in IR mode. It was critical to centrally align the camera to avoid obstruction by the iris.
5. The laser was switched to the blue (488 nm) excitation mode, and move the camera to keep the image refocused until the whole field reached its maximum intensity.
6. Moisture the cornea with few drops of balanced saltwater.
7. Take an image at a resolution of 768 × 768 pixels using the 55° wide-field lens mounted on a Heidelberg Spectralis device in AF mode. And choose the qAF (mean of 9 images) mode for further quantification.
8. Apply Gonioscopic Prism solution on the right eye to keep it in moisture after imaging. Clean the left eye by balanced saltwater and repeat the imaging steps.

2.3 Recovery

1. Place the rodent on an adjustable temperature-controlled heating pad and place in a recovery cage with a non-particulate absorbent surface and observe until it is able to right itself and ambulate; it is then returned to a clean cage.
2. The mouse awakes after about 30 min and appears groggy for 1–2 h but suffers no obvious pain.
3. Animals will be monitored daily for 3 days for any sign of distress or illness such as ruffled fur, lethargy, decreased appetite, or others. Once any postoperative animal is found ill, it will be euthanized as soon as possible.

3 Notes

1. Be sure to keep the eyes of mouse in moisture to avoid temporary cataract forming and blocking the excitation light from the fundus. The excitation light was significantly blocked by the

dry cornea. Keep drop the balanced saltwater on the cornea when collecting images.

2. The system of Spectralis HRA + OCT is a cSLO technique based on confocal principle. It uses a point source that projects a low-power beam on the retina and a point detector, which has a common focal point so that scattered light does not fall on the detector, improving the signal/background ratio.

Conflicts of Interest

Stephen H. Tsang receives financial support from Abeona Therapeutics, Inc and Emendo. He is also the founder of Rejuvitas and is on the scientific and clinical advisory board for Nanoscope Therapeutics.

References

1. Pichi F, Abboud EB, Ghazi NG et al (2018) Fundus autofluorescence imaging in hereditary retinal diseases. Acta Ophthalmol 96: e549–e561. https://doi.org/10.1111/aos.13602
2. Sparrow JR, Wu Y, Nagasaki T et al (2010) Fundus autofluorescence and the bisretinoids of retina. Photochem Photobiol Sci 9: 1480–1489. https://doi.org/10.1039/c0pp00207k
3. Schmitz-Valckenberg S, Holz FG, Bird AC et al (2008) Fundus autofluorescence imaging: review and perspectives. Retina 28:385–409. https://doi.org/10.1097/IAE.0b013e318164a907
4. Zhang L, Cui X, Jauregui R et al (2018) Genetic rescue reverses microglial activation in preclinical models of retinitis pigmentosa. Mol Ther 26: 1953–1964. https://doi.org/10.1016/j.ymthe.2018.06.014
5. Delori F, Greenberg JP, Woods RL et al (2011) Quantitative measurements of autofluorescence with the scanning laser ophthalmoscope. Invest Ophthalmol Vis Sci 52:9379–9390. https://doi.org/10.1167/iovs.11-8319
6. Sparrow JR, Blonska A, Flynn E et al (2013) Quantitative fundus autofluorescence in mice: correlation with HPLC quantitation of RPE lipofuscin and measurement of retina outer nuclear layer thickness. Invest Ophthalmol Vis Sci 54:2812–2820. https://doi.org/10.1167/iovs.12-11490

Chapter 22

Large Animal Models of Retinitis Pigmentosa in Therapy Development and Preclinical Testing

Laurence M. Occelli and Simon M. Petersen-Jones

Abstract

Large animal models are valuable for developing and testing translational therapies for inherited retinal dystrophies such as retinitis pigmentosa (RP). Gene augmentation therapy has been developed utilizing such models. Adeno-associated viral (AAV) vectors have been frequently utilized and delivered by intravitreal or subretinal injection. In vivo longitudinal assessments of therapeutic outcomes are essential. These include regular ophthalmic examinations as well as detailed fundus assessments including confocal scanning laser ophthalmoscopy (cSLO) and high-resolution cross-sectional imaging of the retina by spectral domain-optical coherence tomography (SD-OCT). Retinal function assessment includes vision testing and electroretinography (ERG).

Key words Large animal model, Retinitis pigmentosa, Therapy, In vivo assessment techniques

1 Introduction

Large animal models of retinal dystrophies, including retinitis pigmentosa, are being used for development and testing of translational therapeutic approaches such as gene therapy (*see* Table 1). Successful gene augmentation therapy for recessively inherited loss-of-function mutations has been achieved by subretinal delivery of adeno-associated virus (AAV) vectors delivering a normal copy of the mutant gene often driven by a cell-specific promoter. Dominant diseases where the mutant allele is expressed and has a deleterious effect typically require a more complex strategy including a "knock-down" of the mutant allele.

The in vivo assessment of therapeutic outcomes in large animal models includes:

1. Ophthalmoscopic examination for detection of inflammation or other adverse effects as well as for evaluation of fundus appearance for assessment of retinal preservation. Techniques include anterior segment slit lamp examination and fundus

Stephen H. Tsang and Peter M. J. Quinn (eds.), *Retinitis Pigmentosa*,
Methods in Molecular Biology, vol. 2560, https://doi.org/10.1007/978-1-0716-2651-1_22,

Table 1
Spontaneous retinal dystrophy dog models reported in gene therapy studies. Listed by gene

Phototransduction	Cilia/transport	Other
CNGB1 [1] (ARRP)	NPHP5 [2] (LCA)	BEST1 [3] (bestrophinopathy)
CNGB3 [4] (achromatopsia)	RPGR [5] (XLRP)	RPE65 [6] (LCA)
PDE6A [7] (ARRP)	RPGRIP1 [8] (ARRP)	
PDE6B [9] (ARRP)		
Rhodopsin [10] (ADRP)		

Key: *ARRP* autosomal recessive retinitis pigmentosa, *ADRP* autosomal dominant retinitis pigmentosa, *LCA* Leber congenital amaurosis, *XLRP* X-linked retinitis pigmentosa

examination with indirect ophthalmoscopy and retinal imaging by a video ophthalmoscope (fundus imaging) and confocal scanning laser ophthalmoscope (cSLO).

2. Electroretinography (ERG).
3. Evaluation of functional vision–vision testing.
4. In vivo cross-sectional retinal imaging to assess and measure retinal morphology and layer thicknesses using spectral domain-optical coherence tomography (SD-OCT).

Animals require general anesthesia to perform detailed electroretinography (ERG) and spectral domain-optical coherence tomography (SD-OCT) and confocal scanning laser ophthalmoscopy (cSLO). Ophthalmic examination can be performed in conscious animals. Fundus imaging can be performed without the need for anesthesia in most instances (if a contact camera is used, topical anesthesia will be needed). If the animal is being anesthetized for other parts of the study, fundus images can also be taken then. Prior to anesthesia, the animals will require a general physical examination. They must be fasted and a premedication given prior to anesthesia induction.

2 Materials

All the experiments should comply with the appropriate animal use regulations, including prior approval from the Institutional Animal Care and Use Committee, and be in compliance with the ARVO Statement for the Use of Animals in Ophthalmic and Visual Research.

2.1 Animals

1. Access to the appropriate animal model and control animals is required.

2.2 Anesthesia

Protocols may vary and should be developed in conjunction with trained anesthesia personnel.

1. Appropriate anesthetic machine for delivery of inhaled isoflurane in oxygen.
2. Variety of syringes, needles, catheter, catheter caps, heparinized saline (2 units/mL), Ringer lactate solution and fluid lines, hair clippers, 70% ethanol and chlorhexidine solution, medical tape.
3. Premedication: acepromazine 2 mg/mL and buprenorphine 0.3 mg/mL or butorphanol 10 mg/mL.
4. Induction: propofol 10 mg/mL and various size of endotracheal tubes and light or laryngoscope.
5. Maintenance: isoflurane mixed with oxygen +/− mechanical (anesthetic ventilator) or manual ventilation through a Bain breathing system for animals less than 10 kg and through a rebreathing circle system for animals 10 kg or more.
6. Monitoring: stethoscope, monitor displaying heart rate (HR), respiratory rate (RR), blood pressure (BP), oxygen saturation (SpO2) and end-tidal carbon dioxide (EtCO2), ECG, temperature (T) monitoring or esophageal stethoscope and temperature probe, digital thermometer.
7. A method for maintaining body temperature during anesthesia is required such as towels/blankets circulating water heating mat or Bair Hugger.

2.3 Intravitreal Injection

AAV vectors are being developed that have improved retinal penetration from the vitreous.

1. Equipment for a standard intravitreal injection includes a lid speculum, forceps to grasp the conjunctiva for stabilization (e.g., Bishop–Harmon forceps), and the syringe and fine gauge needle—27 G.
2. If the protocol requires injection close to the retinal surface, the equipment needed is similar to that for a subretinal injection (see below).

2.4 Subretinal Injection

1. This is a specialist procedure and should be performed by the appropriately qualified and trained personnel. In large animal models, a subretinal injection can be achieved without the need to perform a vitrectomy.

1. Adjustable surgical table, vacuum pack beads pillow (Olympic Vac-Pac, Natus Medical Inc.).
2. Surgical microscope and sterile knobs.

3. Surgical drapes, surgical gowns and gloves, Betadine and 2% diluted Betadine, sterile q-tip and gauzes.
4. Surgical supplies and surgical instrument box including, for example: different size Barraquer eyelid speculums, tenotomy scissors, Bishop–Harmon forceps, mosquito forceps ×2, Castroviejo 0.12 tying forceps, Castroviejo calipers, Castroviejo needle holder, curved Westcott tenotomy scissors, small suture scissors, tying forceps ×2, 27 G cannula, Balanced Salt Solution (BSS), small cups, small gauzes, and cellulose eye sponge spears.
5. Other surgical devices and instruments possibly needed depending on exact approach used such as microvitreoretinal (MVR) blades, scleral ports (23 or 25 G), light pipe for posterior segment illumination, and a wet-field cautery.
6. Braided non-absorbable silk 6-0 or 4-0 stay sutures for positioning the eye, conjunctival sutures 6-0 polyglactin 910 absorbable sutures.
7. Syringe to deliver vector such as Hamilton gas tight luer lock syringes (50–500 μL) (e.g., Hamilton Company), regular 30 G hypodermic needles. Subretinal injector, e.g., DORC subretinal injector with an extendable 41 G cannula or other subretinal injection cannula (DORC). The RetinaJect [1] (which has a 25 G needle and advanceable 39 G cannula) (SurModics) is unfortunately no longer manufactured.
8. System for visualizing the posterior segment of the eye through the operating microscope, e.g., a contact vitrectomy lens (Volk) which is coupled with sterile lubricating gel or an irrigating vitrectomy lens (e.g., Machemer Magnifying Vitrectomy Lens (Ocular Instruments)). It is even possible to use a 10- to 14-mm microscope coverslip in conjunction with sterile ocular lubricating gel. Alternatively, a non-contact system such as the oculus BIOM (Oculus Surgical, Inc.) with the associated ocular inverter can be used.

2.5 Vision Testing

1. Four exit choice device as described by Gearhart et al. [2].
2. Maze device as described by Garcia et al. [3].
3. Variable light intensities adjustable by a rheostat to allow vision testing at scotopic, mesopic, and photopic lighting levels. A photometer to help select the needed light intensities.
4. Corneal opaque corneal contact lens, topical anesthesia proparacaine 0.5%, coupling corneal gel (e.g., hypromellose 2.5%, e.g., Gonak (Akorn) or Optixcare ophthalmic gel (CLC Medical)).
5. Video recorder system.

2.6 Electro-retinography

1. Electroretinogram machine, e.g., Espion system (Diagnosys LLC), or the systems manufactured by LKC system or Roland.
2. A room that can be darkened completely with minimal electrical interference (Faraday cage like).
3. Recording electrode: monopolar (e.g., ERG-Jet lens (e.g., Fabrinal SA)) or bipolar (Burian Allen (Hansen Ophthalmic Development Lab)).
4. Platinum subdermal ground and reference electrodes (e.g., Genuine Grass).
5. Coupling gel such as hypromellose 2.5%, Optixcare plus, eyewash.
6. Stay sutures, e.g., silk 6-0 or 4-0 sutures.
7. Plastic eyelid speculum: to fit size of animal.
8. Dilating drops tropicamide 1%, phenylephrine 2.5%, atropine 1%.
9. A darkroom safelight or LED headlamp with a dim red light.
10. Each laboratory should be standardizing their protocol with normal controls for their ERG machine and for each one of the recording lenses.

2.7 Spectral Domain-Optical Coherence Tomography

1. SD-OCT imaging system such as the Spectralis OCT+ HRA (Heidelberg) with measuring software (HEYEX) with 30° and 55° lens and infrared imaging (820 nm laser).
2. Stay sutures, e.g., silk 6-0 or 4-0 sutures.
3. Barraquer eyelid speculum: to fit size of animal.
4. Eyewash solution (sodium chloride or regular eye wash), 20 G plastic catheter tip or cannula mounted on a 10- or 20-mL syringe filled with eye wash to keep the cornea constantly moist.

2.8 Fundus Imaging or Ophthalmic Examination

1. Slit lamp. Handheld are easiest to use in large animals, e.g., SL17 (Kowa), PSL (Keeler).
2. Indirect ophthalmoscope and indirect condensing lenses, e.g., 20 D, 30 D or 2.2 pan retinal (Volk).
3. Tonometer to evaluate intraocular pressure: rebound, e.g., TonoVet (iCare) or applanation tonometer, e.g., Tono-Pen Vet (Metronic) or Tono-Pen Avia (Reichert).
4. Fundus imaging system: Handheld cameras are easier to use than table-mounted imaging systems. Examples include Retcam II or Retcam shuttle (Clarity Medical Systems) or Micron X (Phoenix technology group) or Kowa Genesis fundus camera. There are now several options that mount on to smart phones. When contact systems are used in awake animals,

a topical corneal anesthetic such as proparacaine is needed and a coupling gel between the camera and cornea—e.g., artificial tear gel or preservative free ultrasound coupling gel.

5. Confocal scanning laser ophthalmoscope (cSLO) which is often combined with a spectral domain-optical coherence tomography system (e.g., Spectralis OCT+HRA, Heidelberg) with 30° and 55° lens and infrared imaging (820-nm laser) and fluorescent imaging (488-nm laser).
6. Fluorescein injectable 10% if fluorescein angiography assessment is desired.

3 Methods

3.1 Animals

Access to the appropriate animal model and control animals is required.

3.2 Anesthesia

A veterinary anesthesiologist or a veterinarian or licensed veterinary technician trained in anesthesia should oversee all anesthesia to ensure safety of the animals and personnel and adequate levels of anesthesia and analgesia. The following are example of suitable protocols.

General anesthesia is required for subretinal or intravitreal injection, ERG, SD-OCT, and cSLO. Fundus imaging can also be performed under general anesthesia after ERG or SD-OCT/cSLO or in most awake large animal models.

1. Perform a general physical examination including chest auscultation (using a stethoscope), record heart rate (HR), respiratory rate (RR), temperature (T), mucous membrane color, and capillary refill time.
2. Premedicate the dog with acepromazine 0.01–0.03 mg/kg (ERG) and buprenorphine 0.02–0.04 mg/kg or butorphanol 0.2–0.3 mg/kg (for SD-OCT/cSLO) intramuscularly or subcutaneously 30 min before induction of anesthesia depending on how easy the animal is to handle.
3. Apply one drop of tropicamide 1% +/− phenylephrine 2.5% to ocular surface twice, 10 min apart. Atropine 1% can be used but has a slower onset.
4. After clipping a 3 × 5 cm hair area in the regions of one of the cephalic veins, scrub with 70% ethanol then chlorhexidine scrub for 5 min contact then dry, a cephalic catheter is placed with an injection cap and secured with medical tape and flushed with heparinized saline.

5. General anesthesia is induced using 4–6 mg/kg intravenous propofol to effect. Intubation is performed with an appropriate size of endotracheal tube. An examination light or laryngoscope is used to help visualization of the larynx. The endotracheal tube is then connected to the anesthesia system.
6. The animal is placed sternally for ERG/SD-OCT/cSLO/fundus imaging and dorsally for subretinal/intravitreal injection on a heated water blanket covered by towels. For subretinal and intravitreal surgery, a vacuum pack positioning pillow is placed under the patient as well to help position the head so the corneal surface will be horizontal when the eye is rotated into the primary gaze position. Some blankets or thermal wraps are also placed on top of the animal to maintain body temperature during the procedure.
7. General anesthesia is maintained with isoflurane (1–3%) mixed with oxygen +/− mechanical or manual ventilation through a Bain breathing system for animals less than 10 kg (oxygen rate: 300–600 mL/kg/min) or through a rebreathing system for animals 10 kg or more (oxygen rate: 100 mL/kg/min). The catheter is flushed with heparinized saline and intravenous Ringer lactate supplied at 2–5 mL/kg/h.
8. The animal is attached to a patient monitor during anesthesia for monitoring of vital parameters including ECG, heart rate (HR), respiratory rate (RR), blood pressure (BP), oxygen saturation (SpO2), and end-tidal carbon dioxide (EtCO2). The temperature is monitored either manually using a digital thermometer or via an esophageal temperature probe.

3.3 Intravitreal Injection

1. Following induction of anesthesia, the ocular surface, conjunctival sac, and lids are cleaned with 2% povidone-iodine.
2. A lid speculum is placed.
3. An injection is made using a suitable sized needle, e.g., 27–30 G. The needle is passed through the sclera in the region of the pars plana (about 6 mm posterior to the limbus for adult dogs) directed toward the posterior of the eye to avoid the lens. The injection can be made into the central vitreous.
4. Following injection (a volume of 100 μL is acceptable), the needle is usually held in place for 30–120 s to avoid reflux of fluid.
5. If the protocol calls for a more accurate positioning of the injection (such as adjacent to the retinal surface), the procedure can be done under direct visualization as described below for subretinal injections. The shadow of the needle can be used to help assess its distance from the retinal surface to avoid contact.
6. Possible complications are indicated in **Notes 1** and **2**.

3.4 Subretinal Injection

A vitrectomy is not necessary prior to a subretinal injection in large animals. If desired, it can be performed and generally does make it a little easier to start the detachment. The description here is for the procedure without a vitrectomy.

1. After anesthesia is induced, and the anesthesia monitoring leads attached, the animal is placed in dorsal recumbency with the neck flexed such that the corneal surface is horizontal. A vacuum-positioning pillow is useful for positioning the head.
2. The eye is prepared for aseptic surgery using 2% Betadine solution as described above for the intravitreal injection. The operating microscope is positioned, and the surgeons prepare for aseptic surgery (surgical mask and head covering, perform routine scrub, and then gown and glove).
3. The sterile surgical instruments tray is opened in a sterile fashion and placed on an instrument stand which is covered by a sterile drape.
4. Sterile positioning knobs are placed on the surgical microscope and the animal draped in a routine fashion for ocular surgery.
5. An eyelid speculum is placed to hold the lids open. If the exposure is limited, a lateral canthotomy is performed using tenotomy scissors.
6. Two stay sutures are placed through the perilimbal conjunctiva at 4 and 8 o'clock using 6-0 Silk in smaller animals and 4-0 Silk in larger animals. These sutures are clamped with mosquito artery forceps to manipulate the eye position and keep it in central gaze.
7. The next stage depends on the subretinal injector to be used. Most injectors and cannulas require a separate sclerotomy. The RetinaJect has a sharp outer 25 G needle that can be used to penetrate the sclera, but this system is no longer manufactured. Initially the conjunctiva is reflected over the sclerotomy site which is measured and marked with Castroviejo calipers. The sclerotomy is made at the 10–11 o'clock position avoiding the major scleral blood vessels. It is performed 2.5–4 mm from the limbus in puppies and 5–7 mm in adult dogs. An MVR blade of the desired width can be used (prior wet-field cautery can be used to reduce scleral bleeding and an effort is made to avoid scleral vessels). The lens must be avoided during sclerotomy and introduction of instruments. They should be directed at an angle toward the optic nerve to avoid contacting the lens. An aqueocentesis is then performed with a short 30 G needle at the limbus removing ~0.1–0.2 mL of aqueous humor to "make space" for the fluid to be injected.

8. An injection cannula and attached Hamilton syringe is prefilled with the viral vector diluted to the desired titer (RetinaJect, Hamilton needle, or other injectors). The cannula tip can be cut to give a slight bevel to ensure a tight seal with the retinal surface and help penetration to the subretinal space. The injector is introduced through the sclerotomy and a posterior segment viewing system used. This can be an irrigating vitrectomy lens, or a non-irrigating system used with coupling gel. A second port with a light pipe is generally not required in the dog. The room lights are switched off to help visualization. If a light pipe is used, the microscope light is also switched off. The microscope is focused on the retina and zoomed in to give excellent visualization of the cannula tip and retinal surface.
9. Subretinal injection is performed by gently pressing the cannula tip on to the retinal surface at the desired location. Once the cannula tip touches the retina, an assistant gives a slight quick push on the syringe plunger to start the retinal detachment (*see* Fig. 1). Once the detachment starts, the pressure should be reduced so the retinal detachment slowly increases until the desired size is achieved. An infusion pump from a vitrectomy machine can also be used for the subretinal injection.
10. The sclerotomy is closed (6-0 to 7-0 polyglactin suture) if needed (25 G sclerotomy may not require suturing) and the conjunctival incision (peritomy) can be closed using the same suture.
11. Fundus imaging is performed to record the immediate post-injection size of the subretinal blebs.
12. If performed, the lateral canthotomy is also closed with 6-0 polyglactin suture performed a single buried suture, a figure of 8 skin suture to reform the lateral canthus and single interrupted sutures to close the rest of the wound.
13. Subconjunctival injection of steroid and antibiotic is used as desired.
14. The patient is recovered from anesthesia and postoperative analgesics provided.
15. Possible complications are indicated in **Notes 1** and **2**.

3.5 Vision Testing

At regular time points, as defined by the study protocol, the animal will undergo vision testing to assess rescue of functional vision. This is often performed under a range of different light levels (scotopic, mesopic, and photopic).

1. *Four-exit choice vision testing device* as described by Gearhart et al. [2]. This consists of a central box with four exit tunnels that can be closed at the far end. Only one of the four tunnels is open at the far end for each "run," and if the animal can see

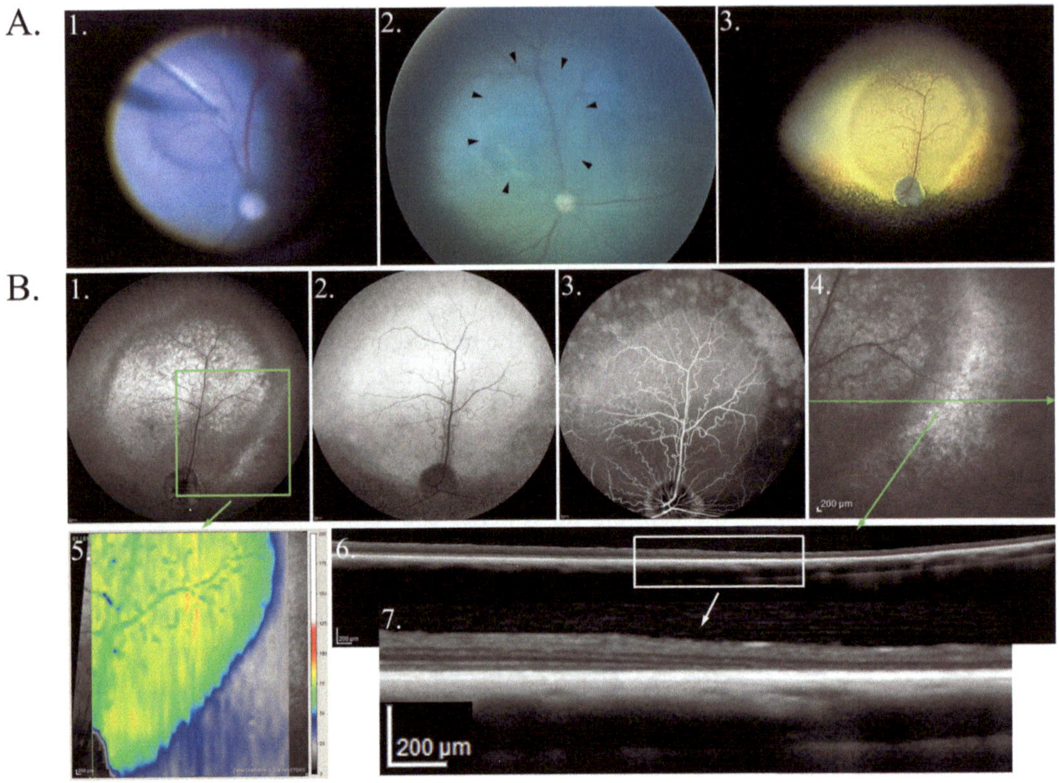

Fig. 1 (**a**) Fundus images. (1). Intraoperative image showing a subretinal injection using a Retinoject subretinal injector (video grab). (2). Fundus image immediately after subretinal injection in a 27-day-old *Pde6a−/−* dog (RetCam II). The black arrowheads demark the edge of the retinal detachment from the subretinal injection. (3). Fundus image 1-year post subretinal injection of an AAV-PDE6A construct. The retina is preserved in the treated region and degenerated in the surrounding untreated region (RetCam II image of same eye as in A.2). (**b**) cSLO and SD-OCT images of the same eye as in A.2 (Spectralis, Heidelberg Engineering). (1). Infrared cSLO fundus image 1-year post-injection. (2). Autofluorescent cSLO image 1-year post-injection. (3). cSLO fluorescein angiography 2 years post-injection showing vascular preservation in the treated region. (4). cSLO showing the location of the SD-OCT high-resolution retinal cross section shown in 6 and 7. (5). Color heat map (location indicated in 4) at 1-year post-injection representing the bleb area REC+. Showing the preservation in the treated area. (6). High-resolution SD-OCT retinal cross section across the injected–non-injected area 1-year post-injection. Note the retinal preservation in the treated area and degeneration in the untreated area. (7). Magnified view of area in 6 demarcated by the white box

open tunnel end, it will choose and exit through this tunnel. A range of light intensities ranging from very dim light to test rods to mesopic light (testing both rods and cones) to bright light testing cones only is used. A photometer is used to adjust the light levels as required. Eyes can be tested separately by placing an opaque corneal contact lens over the eye that is not being tested (topical anesthesia such as proparacaine is administered and the opaque contact lens fitted). The animal is placed in the central box. The first exit entered (correct or incorrect) is noted and time to exit recorded. 7–14 runs are performed for each light intensity with at least 5-min light adaption between different light intensities when progressing from the dimmer light to the brightest light. Light intensities can be chosen randomly but a period of dark adaptation of 20 min between light intensities is needed when progressing from a brighter to dimmer light.

2. *Maze/obstacle course vision testing* as described by Garcia et al. [3]. This consists of a walkway which has a series of panels that can be moved to obstruct part of the pathway. Animals with normal vision would go from one end of the course to the other weaving between the barriers and not bumping into them. The session is video recorded, and the time taken to traverse the course and the number of barriers/walls that are bumped into recorded. Light levels can be adjusted for testing scotopic to photopic vision. An opaque contact lens can be placed to allow vision of each eye to be tested separately as described above. Possible complications are indicated in **Note 3**.

3.6 Electroretinography [4]

1. Prior to ERG, the animal is dark-adapted for a minimum of 1 h. It is then premedicated, pupil dilated with tropicamide +/− phenylephrine or atropine and anesthesia induced as described above. This is performed with aid of a dim-red light so the animal remains dark-adapted.
2. Anesthesia is induced, the animal intubated and attached to the anesthetic and monitoring machines.
3. The animal is placed in sternal recumbency with the head on a raised block. The head can be stabilized with medical tape. The eyelids are held open with a plastic eyelid speculum and the globes positioned in primary gaze using conjunctival sutures placed immediately adjacent to the limbus at the 6 and 12 o'clock position (e.g., 4-0–6-0 Silk). The positioning sutures are attached to mosquito forceps and secured on the muzzle and head using medical tape.
4. The ground electrode is placed subcutaneously at the back of the neck.
5. The contact lens electrode (e.g., ERG-Jet lens) is placed onto the cornea using some coupling gel (e.g., hypromellose 2.5%), and the reference electrode (e.g., Grass platinum needle subdermal electrode) is placed subcutaneously near the lateral canthus. The distance the reference electrode is positioned from the lateral canthus must be consistent for the ERG recordings to be comparable.

6. The Ganzfeld stimulator is positioned to evenly illuminate the eye(s) and the baseline and impedance checked. The dark-adapted (scotopic) ERGs are recorded first followed by the light-adapted (photopic) ERG. Our typical protocol is to perform a dark-adapted luminance-response series (−4 to 1.4 log cd.s/m^2) to include a rod 5-Hz flicker at 0.025 cd.s/m^2, followed by light adaptation (10 min of a 30 cd/m^2 white light), and a light-adapted series (−2.4 to 1.4 log cd.s/m^2) and a cone flicker response (we use 33 Hz at 3 cd.s/m^2 to avoid averaging in any 60-Hz interference which is a potential issue if exactly 30-Hz flicker is used). The number of sweeps averaged will depend on the signal-to-noise ratio. For very low-amplitude signal, much more averaging may be necessary than for large-amplitude signal.
7. Once the recording is completed, the electrodes and stay sutures are removed. The corneas are flushed with eyewash and some lubricant is placed on the eye (e.g., Optixcare). The patient is then recovered from anesthesia and monitored until fully recovered.
8. ERG recordings are saved and ERG a- and b-wave amplitudes and implicit times are measured in a standard fashion.
9. Possible complications are indicated in **Notes 3** and **4**.

3.7 Spectral Domain-Optical Coherence Tomography (SD-OCT) and Confocal Scanning Laser Ophthalmoscopy (cSLO) (e.g., Spectralis, Heidelberg Engineering) [5, 6]

1. Prior to SD-OCT and cSLO, the animal is premedicated, pupils dilated with tropicamide +/− phenylephrine or atropine, and anesthesia is induced as described above.
2. After general anesthesia induction, the animal is attached to the anesthetic machine and monitoring devices.
3. The animal is placed in sternal position and the head stabilized with medical tape. The eyelids are kept open using a Barraquer eyelid speculum. To adjust position of the globe, 4-0 Silk sutures are placed in the ventro-nasal conjunctiva close to the limbus and attached to mosquito forceps.
4. The head is moved toward the SD-OCT/cSLO machine and positioned so the cornea is perpendicular to the machine lens. During the entirety of the procedure, the corneal surface is irrigated every 15–20 s with eyewash or saline using a 10- or 20-mL syringe attached to a plastic cannula or 20 G catheter. This will help to keep the cornea moist, prevent ulceration, and keep a clear transparent media for the imaging.
5. SD-OCT/cSLO images are then captured. The order of the imaging does not matter (SD-OCT or cSLO first) as long as it is consistent in the study.

6. A specific protocol is developed for each study depending on the procedure performed and goals. The following is a typical protocol: SD-OCT high-resolution retinal cross-sectional images are captured using combination of single scan lines and volume scan images using the 820-nm wavelength laser. Images are captured from the central retina to include the *area centralis* and from the four retinal quadrants as well as the optic nerve. Effort is made to focus on the injected/treated fundus region to include capturing images of the region of the sub-retinal injection but also the junction between treated–untreated regions. Prior to capturing images, caution must be made to focus onto the retinal region of interest (follow the instrument manual to achieve this). The 30° lens is more commonly used for SD-OCT image acquisition while the 55° lens more commonly used to capture cSLO images. Single scan lines can be captured using the 30° or 55° lens averaging 50–100 images by Automatic Real Time (ART). SD-OCT images are acquired in conjunction with the infrared (IR; 820 nm) or autofluorescent (AF; 488 nm) cSLO images. Volume scan can be performed up to 30° × 30° with the 30° lens and up to 55° × 45° with the 55° lens. For volume scan, the ART is usually set between 9 and 16 images. When using the 30° lens, 120 μm is a commonly used distance between line scan. Distance can be adjusted depending on the detail required. Once images are captured, they need to be saved and archived for later analysis. Measurement of different retinal layers can be performed using the manufacturer's software (e.g., Heidelberg Eye Explorer (HEYEX) software, Heidelberg) or custom-made software. Some software allows creation of 3D images from the volume scan as well as "heat maps" to show regional variation in layer thicknesses (*see* Fig. 1).
7. cSLO images are acquired from the *area centralis* and the four quadrants and depending on the study and the treated retinal regions. Both infrared imaging (IR) (820-nm laser) and autofluorescent imaging (AF) (488-nm laser) can be performed. The ART is usually set from 25 to 100 images. The sensitivity is adjusted for the best quality image. To compare autofluorescence between animals, the normalize setting needs to be turned off and a standardized sensitivity setting used (*see* Fig. 1).
8. For fluorescein angiography, a 20 or 22 G catheter is placed in one of the cephalic veins and fitted with an injection cap. The animal is positioned as described above. The cSLO live image using a 55° is focused on the region of interest using first the IR then the AF settings. Once the desired position is obtained, the AF sensitivity is adjusted to 35 (for the Spectralis Heidelberg machine; pretesting should be done in each lab to define the

best start sensitivity). 20 mg/kg of 10% fluorescein for injection is injected in the cephalic vein as a bolus and the timer started at the end of injection, and a video captured typically for 60 s. After this, images are captured every minute for a further 5 min, then if needed at 10- and 20-min post-injection. For these single images, each quadrant can be imaged to allow assessment of the entire retina (*see* Fig. 1).

9. Once the SD-OCT, cSLO, or fluorescein angiography imaging is completed, stay sutures are gently removed as well as the tape securing the head in place. The corneas are flushed with eyewash and some lubricant is placed on the eye (e.g., Optixcare). The patient is then recovered from anesthesia and monitored until fully recovered.
10. Possible complications are indicated in **Notes 3** and **4**.

3.8 Fundus Imaging and/or Ophthalmic Examination

1. Fundus imaging and/or ophthalmic examination can be performed in awake animals. If being performed before or after SD-OCT/cSLO, it can be done under anesthesia. If a contact video fundus camera is used (e.g., RetCam), coupling gel is needed so this should be performed after the SD-OCT/cSLO session is completed.
2. A standard ophthalmic examination can be performed. Prior to pupil dilation, the pupillary light reflex should be assessed. Intraocular pressure is typically measured (rebound, e.g., TonoVet, or applanation tonometer, e.g., Tono-Pen Vet or Tono-Pen Avia). A standard protocol is used for the examination; this typically starts with an assessment of the eyelids and adnexa then the cornea, anterior chamber, and lens, initially with a focal light source and then with a slit lamp. The fundus is then assessed using an indirect ophthalmoscope with a 20 D or 30 D or 2.2 pan retinal indirect lens (Volk). Any findings should be recorded—a standard examination form is useful for this purpose.
3. Fundus imaging system is performed using a fundus camera such as a Retcam II or other fundus camera (portable fundus cameras are a lot easier to use for imaging large animals than table-mounted fundus cameras). The RetCam II is a contact system and therefore requires coupling gel (non-preservative ultrasound gel). If the imaging is done awake it can be performed after topical anesthesia such as proparacaine is applied twice at 2-min intervals prior to imaging, alternatively, imaging can be performed under general anesthesia. Wide-field images are captured in the different fundus quadrants and with different light intensities. They are then recorded and saved (*see* Fig. 1). After imaging, the corneas were rinsed with eyewash and some corneal lubricant applied (e.g., Optixcare).
4. Possible complication is indicated in **Note 4**.

4 Notes

1. Complications can occur during or post-intravitreal or subretinal injections detailed, respectively, in Subheadings 3.3 and 3.4. In both procedures, intraocular bleeding from scleral vessels can occur. Careful positioning and avoidance of vessels can reduce the risk. Typically, mild intraocular bleeding resolves quickly. If the lens is touched during the procedures, the capsule may be damaged. This can lead to increased intraocular inflammation and cataract formation. During subretinal injection if the retinal vessels are damaged, some retinal bleeding may occur. This usually resorbs in the post-surgery period, but close monitoring is also recommended. In some instances, when attempting a subretinal injection, the retina does not detach as planned; in some cases, the retinal detachment does not start and the fluid to be injected leaks into the vitreous. If the cannula is advanced too far, it can penetrate the RPE and an intrachoroidal injection may result.
2. Post-therapy delivery (*see* Subheadings 3.3 and 3.4), animals are monitored for therapeutic outcome. Regular eye examinations (*see* Subheading 3.7) are also essential to evaluate any adverse effect such as uveitis. If uveitis develops, additional medical treatment (such as topical or oral anti-inflammatory medications) may be necessary depending on its severity. Suture dehiscence of the lateral canthotomy can occur, usually those can be left to heal by second intention (antibiotic ophthalmic medication can be used if needed).
3. Mild conjunctivitis and/or some focal conjunctival bleeding from suture placement (*see* Subheadings 3.5 and 3.7) can occur. They usually resolve within 24–48 h but should be monitored. Corneal ulceration is extremely rare post-therapy assessment techniques but could result from contact lens abrasion during vision testing or the recording electrode during ERG or the lack of proper hydration of the cornea during SD-OCT. The use of ocular lubricants after each testing session reduces the risk of corneal lesions. Regular ophthalmic examinations should be performed and ophthalmic antibiotic medication applied if needed.
4. Difficulty in performing surgery (*see* Subheadings 3.3 and 3.4) or post-therapy assessment (e.g., ERG (*see* Subheading 3.6), SD-OCT (*see* Subheading 3.7), and fundus examination (*see* Subheading 3.8)) can occur if the animal pupils are not well dilated, as visualization of the fundus will be compromised.

References

1. Petersen-Jones SM et al (2018) Patients and animal models of CNGbeta1-deficient retinitis pigmentosa support gene augmentation approach. J Clin Invest 128(1):190–206
2. Gearhart PM et al (2008) A novel method for objective vision testing in canine models of inherited retinal disease. Invest Ophthalmol Vis Sci 49:3568–3576
3. Garcia MM et al (2010) Evaluation of a behavioral method for objective vision testing and identification of achromatopsia in dogs. Am J Vet Res 71:97–102
4. Komaromy AM et al (2010) Gene therapy rescues cone function in congenital achromatopsia. Hum Mol Genet 19(13):2581–2593
5. Beltran WA et al (2012) Gene therapy rescues photoreceptor blindness in dogs and paves the way for treating human X-linked retinitis pigmentosa. Proc Natl Acad Sci U S A 109(6):2132–2137
6. Acland GM et al (2001) Gene therapy restores vision in a canine model of childhood blindness. Nat Genet 28(1):92–95
7. Occelli LM et al (2017) Gene supplementation rescues rod function and preserves photoreceptor and retinal morphology in dogs, leading the way towards treating human PDE6A-retinitis pigmentosa. Hum Gene Ther 28(12):1189–1201
8. Lheriteau E et al (2014) Successful gene therapy in the RPGRIP1-deficient dog: a large model of cone-rod dystrophy. Mol Ther 22(2):265–277
9. Petit L et al (2012) Restoration of vision in the pde6beta-deficient dog, a large animal model of rod-cone dystrophy. Mol Ther 20(11):2019–2030
10. Cideciyan AV et al (2018) Mutation-independent rhodopsin gene therapy by knockdown and replacement with a single AAV vector. Proc Natl Acad Sci U S A 115(36):E8547–E8556

Chapter 23

CRISPR Manipulations in Stem Cell Lines

Ya-Ju Chang, Xuan Cui, Sarah R. Levi, Laura A. Jenny, and Stephen H. Tsang

Abstract

Insights into genome engineering in cells have allowed researchers to cultivate and modify cells as organoids that display structural and phenotypic features of human diseases or normal health status. The generation of targeted mutants is a crucial step toward studying the biomedical effect of genes of interest. Modified organoids derived from patients' tissue cells are used as models to study diseases and test novel drugs. CRISPR-Cas9 technology has contributed to an explosion of advances that have the ability to edit genomes for the study of monogenic diseases and cancers. The generation of such mutants in human induced pluripotent stem cells (iPSCs) is of utmost importance as these cells carry the potential to be differentiated into any cell lineage. We describe recent developments that are broadening our understanding and extend DNA specificity, product selectivity, and fundamental capabilities. Furthermore, fundamental capabilities and remarkable advancements in basic research, biotechnology, and therapeutics development in cell engineering are detailed within this chapter. Using the CRISPR/Cas9 nuclease system for induction of targeted double-strand breaks, gene editing of target loci in iPSCs can be achieved with high efficiency. This chapter includes detailed protocols for the preparation of reagents to target loci of interest and transfection to genotype single cell-derived iPSC clones. Furthermore, we provide a protocol for the convenient generation of ribonucleoprotein (RNP) delivered directly to cells.

Key words Human embryonic stem cells, Human induced pluripotent stem cells, Gene editing, Loci, Ribonucleoprotein

1 Introduction

Human embryonic stem cells (ESCs) provide a sufficient cell source due to their unlimited self-renewal capacity [1]. The discovery of patient-specific induced pluripotent stem cells (iPSCs) solved both the immunogenic problem associated with the transplantation of allogeneic cells and ethical concerns [2]. Recently, considerable progress has been made to generate iPSCs from readily available cell sources like peripheral blood and the use of non-integrating vectors that express reprogramming factors [3]. However, to realize the full potential of iPSCs in regenerative medicine and disease

Stephen H. Tsang and Peter M. J. Quinn (eds.), *Retinitis Pigmentosa*,
Methods in Molecular Biology, vol. 2560, https://doi.org/10.1007/978-1-0716-2651-1_23,

modeling, disease-causing genes often need to be corrected or modified prior to conducting therapy.

Gene-mediating in ESCs was achieved decades ago, albeit at extremely low efficiencies [4]. Further studies led to a realization that early successes had exploited the cell's intrinsic repair mechanism after spontaneous genomic DNA breaks [5]. However, naturally occurring double-stranded DNA breaks (DSBs) surrounding a target locus are extremely rare, typically limiting the targeting efficiency to levels to one in a million, even with the use of homology arms (HA) extending 10 kb pairs [6]. To enhance gene targeting, tremendous effort over the past two decades has focused on creating DSBs at certain loci by targetable endonucleases. While the development of engineered endonucleases, like zinc-finger nucleases or transcription activator-like effector nucleases, have generated excitement, their limitations in design or cloning have rendered them impractical for routine laboratory use [7, 8]. The latest generation of RNA-guided endonuclease, or CRISPR-Cas9, has been widely used due to its simplicity in vector design and robustness in performance [9, 10]. CRISPR/Cas9 is an adaptive immune system that evolved in bacteria and archaea to identify and destroy invading agents such as bacteriophages or plasmids [11]. The commonly used Cas9 is from *Streptococcus pyogenes* (Sp), which we used in this study.

DSBs created by endonucleases are primarily repaired by non-homologous end joining (NHEJ) or homology-directed repair (HDR) [12]. In the absence of a template, the NHEJ pathway is utilized, introducing variable insertions or deletions (indels) at the DSB site, which may disrupt the open reading frame of the gene and generate a knockout (KO) allele. This editing approach is relatively efficient and has been widely used in genetic engineering and functional genomics research [13, 14]. In the presence of a donor template flanked with homology arms (HAs), the HDR pathway can be used to integrate the sequence between HAs to create a precise DNA deletion, substitution, or insertion, leading to the correction of pathologic genes or the targeted integration of a gene or DNA fragment of interest [15, 16]. Unfortunately, HDR-mediated knock-in (KI) using a conventional plasmid template is typically inefficient [17]. Recently, we reported a five to tenfold increase in HDR KI efficiency by using a double cut donor plasmid design, which is a conventional targeting vector flanked on either side by a Cas9 single guide RNA (sgRNA) recognition sequence [18]. We also found that HAs of 300–600 bp in length are sufficient to guide precise genome editing [18, 19]. This finding has been independently reproduced in other labs [20, 21]. A similar gene targeting strategy that takes advantage of the highly efficient double cut HDR donor design (pDonor-sg) is used in this study.

Although efficient genome editing has been achieved in many tumor cell lines [22], efforts to precisely insert a large fragment into the genome of human pluripotent stem cells (PSCs) have been challenging [23]. HDR efficiencies of 0.1–1% after creating DSBs using artificial nucleases have been reported by different labs [23, 24]. Up to 5% HDR insertion of a fluorescent protein in human iPSCs has been reported, but this is cell line-dependent [25].

The CRISPR-Cas9 system has unlocked new applications of stem cells in the treatment of human disease. To provide context, stem cells are unspecialized cells with a remarkable capacity to differentiate into any cell type in the body. In multicellular organisms, stem cells are found in embryonic stages before differentiation and also in certain adult tissues where they divide without limit to replenish worn out cells. The main difference between stem cells and other cells is their lack of specialization [1, 26, 27]. Muscle cells, brain cells, bone cells, etc. all have specific functions in the body that are not interchangeable with one another, and these specific cell types are thus differentiated. The undifferentiated property of stem cells and their ability to give rise to different specialized cell types makes them unique; as they are biology's blueprints [1]. Stem cells can be cultured in a dish by adding chemical and mechanical stimuli which stimulates them to differentiate into any cell type, allowing researchers to maintain a record the developmental process of a certain tissue from beginning to end [26]. Thus, stem cell studies could help us understand how defects accumulate during development or what biological markers are important for the process—something that cannot be achieved using other cells [27].

There are many types of stem cells: embryonic stem cells, adult stem cells, and induced pluripotent stem cells. Adult stem cells are tissue-specific stem cells that reside in certain tissues in the body. The role of adult stem cells is to continually replenish depleted cell populations. As most cells in adult tissues are differentiated, isolating adult stem cells from the mix of differentiated cells can be challenging [28]. Introduction of the CRISPR technology and the ability to grow stem cells in the lab have been among the most important breakthroughs in the disease treatments. The former is a precise gene editing tool, while the latter enables researchers to study unspecialized cells, and they differentiate into specialized ones. CRISPR and stem cells are, individually, already being tested in cell therapies; combined, these techniques have the potential to transform the field of regenerative medicine [29].

Thus, stem cell studies could help us understand how defects accumulate during development or what biological markers are important for the process—something that cannot be achieved using other cells [1, 26]. Researchers are excited to harness the potential of stem cells in cell-based therapies and regenerative medicine. As differentiated cells are not capable of dividing without limit, introducing stem cells in damaged tissues could help repair them easily [1, 10]. This has great implications in organ transplants, for instance, which is currently limited by organ donors. The ability to use the patient's own stem cells could potentially lower incidences of transplant rejection by the immune system, although several clinical trials are required before we can confirm this [30].

The CRISPR-Cas9 system has many advantages and can be used to correct many defects that occur throughout development or are present at birth, including cystic fibrosis and Huntington's disease. However, it remains unclear how we should set rules and regulations regarding which human traits are appropriate for editing. In addition, few would argue that a number of safety and efficacy concerns about CRISPR-Cas9 remain to be resolved [31]. Safety measures are needed to be executed in this technology to avoid misuse or ethical issues. Especially in light of the possibility that undesirable parties could use this technology for eugenics, it would be irresponsible to allow modification of human embryos [32]. In this respect, we must confront the need for robust regulation, even as arguments rage between the advocates of caution and progress [31, 33].

2 Materials

1. 4D-Nucleofector™ System (Lonza).
2. P3 Primary Cell 4D-Nucleofector Kit S (Lonza, #V4XP-3032).
3. mTeSR™ media (StemCell, #85850).
4. Y-27632 2HCl (Selleckchem, #129830-38-2).
5. ReLeSR™ (StemCell, #05873).
6. Dulbecco's Phosphate Buffered Saline (Thermo Fisher Scientific, #14040216).
7. Corning Matrigel Matrix (Corning, #354248).
8. gRNA (Synthego).
9. Cas9 protein (NEB #E3322S).

3 Methods

3.1 IPSC Preparation for Nucleofection

The following protocol describes the optimized conditions for the use of the Lonza/4D- Nucleofector System reagent transfection system for CRISPR-based genome editing of iPSCs cultured under mTeSR media with ROCK inhibitor (Y-27632). These steps deliver the Cas9-gRNA RNP to induce insertions and deletions through NHEJ or HDR to achieve gene editing.

3.2 Pre-nucleofection

1. Culture iPSCs in Matrigel-coated plates until they are semi-confluent.
2. Pre-treat iPSCs with ROCK inhibitor (Y-27632): Replacing the media to mTeSR media with 10-μM ROCK inhibitor (Y-27632) 1 h before nucleofection (*see* **Note 1**).
3. Each electroporation reaction will need 5.0×10^5 cells, and we typically include a reaction without plasmid as a control.

3.3 Plate and Buffer Preparation

1. Coat a new 12-well plate with Matrigel/DMEM and incubate at 37 °C for 2 h before use (*see* **Note 2**).
2. Replace coated Matrigel/DMEM to 1-mL mTeSR media with 10-μM ROCK inhibitor (Y-27632) each well. Incubate the plate at 37 °C for cell seeding after the nucleofection reaction.
3. Prepare 70-μL additional pre-warmed mTeSR with 10-μM ROCK inhibitor (Y-27632) per reaction for cell recovery after nucleofection.

3.4 Cell Preparation

1. Aliquot sufficient ReLeSR™ to passage the iPSCs. Warm reagents at room temperature (*see* **Note 3**).
2. After 1 h of ROCK inhibitor (Y-27632) pre-treatment, inspect the plate to visualize the morphology under a dissection microscope.
3. Aspirate and replace ReLeSR™ per well and incubate at 37 °C for 5 min.
4. Quench the ReLeSR™ reaction by adding 1-mL mTeSR for each well. Gently detach cells using a sterile pipette tip.
5. Dissociate the cells into a single cell suspension by pipetting the suspension carefully up and down 3–4 times.

3.5 Cell Counting

1. For nucleofection with P3 Primary Cell 4D-Nucleofector Kit S, count an aliquot of the detached cells and determine cell density.
2. Transfer the required number of cells (5.0×10^5 cells per reaction) to a new tube.
3. Centrifuge cells $100 \times g$ for 5 min at room temperature, discard the supernatant.
4. Wash cell by PBS and gently pipetting up and down, centrifuge cells $100 \times g$ for 3 min at room temperature, and discard the supernatant.
5. Resuspend cell in Lonza P3 Nucleofector solution at 20 μL/reaction. Work quickly but carefully and avoid leaving cells in Nucleofector solution for longer than 15 min. Avoid bubble formation.

3.6 Nucleofection

1. Transfer iPSC suspension to the Nucleocuvette strip (P3 Primary Cell 4D-Nucleofector Kit).
2. Transfer each cell with nucleofection buffer to each well of Nucleocuvette strip and click the lid into place (*see* **Note 4**).
3. Place the Nucleocuvette strip with closed lid into the retainer of the 4D-X core unit. Check for proper orientation of the strip.
4. Use the electroporation protocol "DS150" and press start on the display of the core unit. After run completion, the screen should display a green "+" over the wells that were meaning successfully transfected (*see* **Note 5**).
5. Aspirate recovery media (mTeSR with ROCK inhibitor Y-27632) 70 μL for each well.

3.7 Post-nucleofection

1. Transfer iPSCs from each well to the pre-incubated 12-well plate and incubate overnight in 37 °C/5% CO_2 incubator (*see* **Note 6**).
2. Change media daily with fresh mTeSR without ROCK inhibitor (Y-27632) after nucleofection.
3. Incubate the cells for 4 days then pick up the single clone iPSCs to further experiments.

3.8 Design of Targeting Components and the Use of the CRISPR Design Tool

Input target genomic DNA sequence. Use an online CRISPR design tool (benchling) that takes an input sequence (e.g., a 1-kb genomic fragment from the region of interest), identifies and ranks suitable target sites, and computationally predicts off-target sites for each intended target. Alternatively, one can manually select guide sequences by identifying the 20-bp sequence directly upstream of any 5′-NGG.

3.9 Design of the ssODN Template

Design and order custom ssODN. Purchase either the sense or antisense ssODN directly from IDT or the preferred supplier. We recommend manually designing homology arms of at least 40 nt on either side and preferably 90 nt for optimal HDR efficiency. It is not necessary to PAGE-purify the ssODN. Resuspend and dilute ssODN ultramers to a final concentration of 10 μM. Do not combine or anneal the sense and antisense ssODNs. Store them at −20 °C.

4 Notes

1. ROCK inhibitor (Y-27632) may result in a spindle-shaped cell morphology. This change will not affect the pluripotency of iPSCs; it will reverse after ROCK inhibitor removed.
2. The plates can be sealed and stored overnight at 4 °C or incubated for 2 h at 37 °C. To avoid potential sample swap, we maintain distinct lines on separate plates.

3. One hour before the cell passage, add ROCK inhibitor (Y-27632) to each plate at a final concentration of 10 uM
4. Make sure there are no bubbles in the wells; it might affect the nucleofection efficiency.
5. For different cells, different programs must be used. DS150 is a suitable program for iPS cell lines in this experiment, but other programs may be needed for other stem cell lines.
6. Because plasmid-based transfections require time for nuclear incorporation end expression, we typically wait for 24 h before further operation.

Conflict of Interest

Stephen H. Tsang receives grant support from Abeona Therapeutics, Inc and Emendo. He is also the founder of Rejuvitas and is on the scientific and clinical advisory board for Nanoscope Therapeutics and Medical Excellence Capital.

References

1. Zakrzewski W et al (2019) Stem cells: past, present, and future. Stem Cell Res Ther 10(1):68. https://doi.org/10.1186/s13287-019-1165-5
2. Volarevic V et al (2018) Ethical and safety issues of stem cell-based therapy. Int J Med Sci 15(1):36–45. https://doi.org/10.7150/ijms.21666
3. Wen W et al (2016) Enhanced generation of integration-free iPSCs from human adult peripheral blood mononuclear cells with an optimal combination of episomal vectors. Stem Cell Reports 6(6):873–884. https://doi.org/10.1016/j.stemcr.2016.04.005
4. Thomas KR, Capecchi MR (1987) Site-directed mutagenesis by gene targeting in mouse embryo-derived stem cells. Cell 51(3):503–512. https://doi.org/10.1016/0092-8674(87)90646-5
5. San Filippo J, Sung P, Klein H (2008) Mechanism of eukaryotic homologous recombination. Annu Rev Biochem 77:229–257. https://doi.org/10.1146/annurev.biochem.77.061306.125255
6. Capecchi MR (1989) Altering the genome by homologous recombination. Science 244(4910):1288–1292. https://doi.org/10.1126/science.2660260
7. Urnov FD et al (2010) Genome editing with engineered zinc finger nucleases. Nat Rev Genet 11(9):636–646. https://doi.org/10.1038/nrg2842
8. Joung JK, Sander JD (2013) TALENs: a widely applicable technology for targeted genome editing. Nat Rev Mol Cell Biol 14(1):49–55. https://doi.org/10.1038/nrm3486
9. Jinek M et al (2012) A programmable dual-RNA-guided DNA endonuclease in adaptive bacterial immunity. Science 337(6096):816–821. https://doi.org/10.1126/science.1225829
10. Cong L et al (2013) Multiplex genome engineering using CRISPR/Cas systems. Science 339(6121):819–823. https://doi.org/10.1126/science.1231143
11. Makarova KS et al (2015) An updated evolutionary classification of CRISPR-Cas systems. Nat Rev Microbiol 13(11):722–736. https://doi.org/10.1038/nrmicro3569
12. Lieber MR (2010) The mechanism of double-strand DNA break repair by the nonhomologous DNA end-joining pathway. Annu Rev Biochem 79:181–211. https://doi.org/10.1146/annurev.biochem.052308.093131
13. Wang H et al (2013) One-step generation of mice carrying mutations in multiple genes by CRISPR/Cas-mediated genome engineering. Cell 153(4):910–918. https://doi.org/10.1016/j.cell.2013.04.025
14. Hsu PD, Lander ES, Zhang F (2014) Development and applications of CRISPR-Cas9 for genome engineering. Cell 157(6):1262–1278. https://doi.org/10.1016/j.cell.2014.05.010

15. Jang HK et al (2020) Current trends in gene recovery mediated by the CRISPR-Cas system. Exp Mol Med 52(7):1016–1027. https://doi.org/10.1038/s12276-020-0466-1
16. Yamamoto Y, Gerbi SA (2018) Making ends meet: targeted integration of DNA fragments by genome editing. Chromosoma 127(4):405–420. https://doi.org/10.1007/s00412-018-0677-6
17. Paquet D et al (2016) Efficient introduction of specific homozygous and heterozygous mutations using CRISPR/Cas9. Nature 533(7601):125–129. https://doi.org/10.1038/nature17664
18. Zhang JP et al (2017) Efficient precise knockin with a double cut HDR donor after CRISPR/Cas9-mediated double-stranded DNA cleavage. Genome Biol 18(1):35. https://doi.org/10.1186/s13059-017-1164-8
19. Li XL et al (2018) Highly efficient genome editing via CRISPR-Cas9 in human pluripotent stem cells is achieved by transient BCL-XL overexpression. Nucleic Acids Res 46(19):10195–10215. https://doi.org/10.1093/nar/gky804
20. Yao X et al (2017) Homology-mediated end joining-based targeted integration using CRISPR/Cas9. Cell Res 27(6):801–814. https://doi.org/10.1038/cr.2017.76
21. Chen X et al (2017) In trans paired nicking triggers seamless genome editing without double-stranded DNA cutting. Nat Commun 8(1):657. https://doi.org/10.1038/s41467-017-00687-1
22. Hsu PD et al (2013) DNA targeting specificity of RNA-guided Cas9 nucleases. Nat Biotechnol 31(9):827–832. https://doi.org/10.1038/nbt.2647
23. Zou J et al (2009) Gene targeting of a disease-related gene in human induced pluripotent stem and embryonic stem cells. Cell Stem Cell 5(1):97–110. https://doi.org/10.1016/j.stem.2009.05.023
24. He X et al (2016) Knock-in of large reporter genes in human cells via CRISPR/Cas9-induced homology-dependent and independent DNA repair. Nucleic Acids Res 44(9):e85. https://doi.org/10.1093/nar/gkw064
25. Byrne SM et al (2015) Multi-kilobase homozygous targeted gene replacement in human induced pluripotent stem cells. Nucleic Acids Res 43(3):e21. https://doi.org/10.1093/nar/gku1246
26. Hayashi Y, Ohnuma K, Furue MK (2019) Pluripotent stem cell heterogeneity. Adv Exp Med Biol 1123:71–94. https://doi.org/10.1007/978-3-030-11096-3_6
27. De Los Angeles A et al (2015) Hallmarks of pluripotency. Nature 525(7570):469–478. https://doi.org/10.1038/nature15515
28. Montagnani S et al (2016) Adult stem cells in tissue maintenance and regeneration. Stem Cells Int 2016:7362879. https://doi.org/10.1155/2016/7362879
29. Kim EJ, Kang KH, Ju JH (2017) CRISPR-Cas9: a promising tool for gene editing on induced pluripotent stem cells. Korean J Intern Med 32(1):42–61. https://doi.org/10.3904/kjim.2016.198
30. Reisman M, Adams KT (2014) Stem cell therapy: a look at current research, regulations, and remaining hurdles. P T 39(12):846–857
31. Barman A, Deb B, Chakraborty S (2020) A glance at genome editing with CRISPR-Cas9 technology. Curr Genet 66(3):447–462. https://doi.org/10.1007/s00294-019-01040-3
32. Memi F, Ntokou A, Papangeli I (2018) CRISPR/Cas9 gene-editing: research technologies, clinical applications and ethical considerations. Semin Perinatol 42(8):487–500. https://doi.org/10.1053/j.semperi.2018.09.003
33. Shinwari ZK, Tanveer F, Khalil AT (2018) Ethical issues regarding CRISPR mediated genome editing. Curr Issues Mol Biol 26:103–110. https://doi.org/10.21775/cimb.026.103

Chapter 24

Metabolite Extraction from RPE Cells and Retinas Related to Retinitis Pigmentosa

Xuan Cui, Ya-Ju Chang, Laura A. Jenny, Sarah R. Levi, Jianhai Du, and Stephen H. Tsang

Abstract

The application of metabolomics in ophthalmology helps to identify new biomarkers and elucidate disease mechanisms in different eye diseases, as well as aiding in the development of potential treatment options. Extracting metabolites successfully is essential for potential further analysis using mass spectrometry. In this chapter, we describe how to extract metabolites from a variety of sources including (1) cells on a dish, (2) cell culture medium, and (3) tissues in vivo with and without stable isotope tracers. Samples prepared using this protocol are suitable for a range of downstream mass spectrometry analyses and are stable in solvent for weeks at −80 °C.

Key words Metabolomics, Metabolites extraction, Gas or liquid chromatography with mass spectrometric detection (GC-MS and LC-MS), RPE cells, Retina dissection

1 Introduction

The past few decades have seen an increase in the application of metabolomics, the identification and quantification of metabolites in a system, for its use in identifying new biomarkers or elucidating disease mechanisms [1]. The insights gleaned from this field of study, in turn, have proven to be critical driving forces in medicine and translational research [2, 3]. Ophthalmology is one of many fields where the use of metabolomics has expanded the scope of possible treatment options for patients. The aim of metabolomics is to identify, quantify, trace, and interpret real-time metabolite concentrations in a given biological sample [4]. The outcomes of large-scale analyses offer researchers the information needed to optimize diagnoses, identify therapeutic targets, monitor disease stage-specific biomarkers, and develop biochemical solutions to cure, slow, or prevent the progression of complex diseases [4, 5]. An understanding of the metabolome and associated pathways also

Stephen H. Tsang and Peter M. J. Quinn (eds.), *Retinitis Pigmentosa*,
Methods in Molecular Biology, vol. 2560, https://doi.org/10.1007/978-1-0716-2651-1_24,

help to improve our knowledge of the pathophysiology and mechanisms of eye diseases such as dry eyes, age-related macular degeneration, diabetic retinopathy, and inherited retinal degenerations such as retinitis pigmentosa [6]. By learning how metabolism changes during disease progression, one can bridge the knowledge gap between the clinical phenotype and molecular or cellular pathophysiology, which can be leveraged to create new strategies for drug screening or develop novel therapeutic agents.

Two main analytical platforms used for metabolite qualification and quantification are gas or liquid chromatography with mass spectrometric detection (GC-MS or LC-MS) and nuclear magnetic resonance (NMR). Compared to the lower sensitivity of NMR, MS is a highly selective and sensitive technique that aids in the identification of metabolites [7]. New methods have been developed to detect the metabolites in cells and tissues in vivo and in vitro, such as single cell metabolomics, real-time metabolomics for medium, imaging mass spectrometry, etc. While the most common method is to extract small molecules directly from cells, cell culture medium, or in vivo tissue of interest prior to MS analysis. The processing of samples is tailored based on experimental design and desired goals.

Good metabolite extraction is the key for further analysis. Here, we summarize the materials and methods necessary for the entire procedure of metabolite extraction from different sources, such as cells on dish, cell-culturing medium, and in vivo tissue. The methods in this protocol are typically used for aqueous metabolites. Samples prepared with this protocol are suitable for a range of downstream MS analyses, and the freeze-dried samples have been found to stay stable for weeks at −80 °C.

2 Materials

2.1 Basic Supplies

1. Stock 80% methanol (methanol:water = 80:20 vo/vol) stored at −20 °C. When taken out from −20 °C, 80% methanol should always be placed on dry ice. Both methanol (Cat# 34966, Sigma) and water (Cat# 14263, Sigma) should be of HPLC grade (*see* **Note 1**).
2. 0.9% NaCl (Vol/Vol) on wet ice.
3. 2 sets of prelabeled 1.5-mL tubes on wet ice.
4. 6-well plate, Corning.
5. Dry ice.
6. Homogenize.
7. Centrifuge, #5424 Eppendorf, in cold room.
8. Evaporation (*see* **Note 2**).

2.2 Materials for RPE Cell Culture

Fresh RPE culture medium could be changed one day before metabolite extraction or one day before labeling.

2.2.1 Supplies for Cell Culture

Fresh RPE culture medium could be changed one day before metabolite extraction or one day before labeling.

1. RPE culture medium [8] containing: 10% fetal bovine serum, N1-supplement (Sigma-Aldrich) 1:100 mL/mL, glutamine–penicillin–streptomycin (Sigma-Aldrich) 1:100 mL/mL, non-essential amino acid solution (Sigma-Aldrich) 1:100 mL/mL, THT 1:500 mL/mL in MEM-alpha modified medium (Sigma-Aldrich).
2. U-^{13}C glucose, #CLM-1396, Cambridge Isotope Laboratories.
3. Matrigel matrix, #356230, Corning.
4. Cell scraper, #3008, Corning.
5. Incubator.

2.2.2 Preparation of RPE Cells

The protocol for the purification and culture of fetal RPE and patient-induced pluripotent stem cell (iPSC)-derived RPE cells has been well established in the past decade. Here, we describe modified protocols that were generated by and successfully used in our lab.

1. The control cell line displayed in this protocol is fetal human RPE (hRPE) with a gestational age of 16–20 weeks. After removing the front cornea, iris, and lens of the fetal eyeball, the eyecup was dissected into four quadrants and laid flat on the dish. After removing the sensory retina, the RPE/choroid sheet was peeled off and then transferred gently into 2% (wt/vol) dispase solution for 30 min at 37 °C. After stopping the digestion with dispase, the RPE layer was peeled off from the choroid. RPE layers were collected, resuspended, and cultured in RPE culturing medium containing 15% (vol/vol) FBS on the Matrigel coated dish [9]. The medium was changed to one containing 10% FBS on the second day and then twice per week. After 4–6 weeks of maturing, the cells could be used for further study.
2. The mutant RPE cell lines were derived from the patient's skin cells. A total of 2–3 small pieces of skin minced from a skin biopsy and 1 drop of silicone grease were covered by a coverslip in a 6-well culture plate. 5 mL of biopsy-plating medium, containing 10% fetal bovine serum, 1 × Anti-Anti, and 0.1-mM β-mercaptoethanol were added into the wells slowly. The fibroblast was then transfected (5 × 10^4 fibroblast cells were plated in a 12-well plate the day before transfection) with the Sendai viruses at MOI of 3 following the manufacturer instructions. The reprogramming medium was changed every 2 days and co-cultured with feeder cells [10]. iPSC colonies were

cultured in differentiation medium containing 15% knock-out serum replacement in KO DMEM in 6-well plate pre-coated with Matrigel. Activin-A was added during days 15–28 of differentiation [11]. Eight to ten weeks later, the pigmented RPE cells were picked and transferred to new 6-well pre-coated plates, where they were then cultured with RPE culture medium for another 6–8 weeks to maturity.

2.3 Material for Retina Dissection

1. Anesthesia solution: 1 mL of 100 mg/mL ketamine, 0.1 mL of 20 mg/mL xylazine in 8.9 mL of PBS.
2. Blade, #21, VWR.
3. Tweezers, #60–529, Accuspire.
4. Liquid nitrogen.

Carry out all procedures on ice unless otherwise specified.

3 Methods

Carry out all procedures on ice unless otherwise specified.

3.1 Metabolite Extraction from Cultured RPE Cells for Liquid or Gas Chromatography-Mass Spectrometry

RPE cells directly dissected from fetal or derived from the patient's somatic cells are widely used to better understand the pathophysiology and study the in vitro phenotypes and mechanisms of eye disease.

1. Seed cells (2×10^5 per well) in 6-well plates (*see* **Note 3**).
2. Change to fresh medium 24 h before experiment. 1.5–2 mL are sufficient to cover the cells in a 6-well plate for 24 h.
3. For optimal results, stable isotope labeling identifies cell-derived compounds and provides insight into the chemical formula. If stable isotope is needed, replace with the medium containing 13C/15N/2H tracers at proper time point. The minimum wait-time needed for the best tracing effect depends on the pathway of interest (*see* **Note 3**).
4. Quickly remove medium, and add 300 μL of 80% methanol that has been precooled in each well of the plate. Scrape the plate on wet ice thoroughly (*see* **Note 4**). Then, transfer the cells with 1-mL pipette tip into 1.5-mL EP tube (*see* **Note 5**). If collecting multiple plates at short time intervals, cover the lid and leave it on dry ice. Leave the tube on dry ice until all the collection is done.
5. Shake the tubes for 5 min in cold room, and centrifuge the sample at 13,000 RPM (or the highest setting in regular benchtop centrifuge) for 15 min at 4 °C. In the meantime, label the new tubes, and precool them on an empty rack in the cold room or −20 °C freezer.

6. Take the sample carefully to the pre-chilled rack. Make sure the sample is not on the ice since that can disturb the pellet. Then, transfer the supernatant which contains the metabolites into a new tube. Take particular care to remove all the supernatant and avoid touching the pellet (*see* **Note 6**).
7. Apply **steps 2–6** to the method blank wells.
8. Store the tube containing the extracted metabolites in −80 °C until LC-MS analysis. Alternatively, freeze-dry the sample first, and then store in −80 °C until GC-MS analysis (*see* **Note 7**).

3.2 Metabolite Extraction from the Isotope-Labeled Culture Medium of RPE Cells for Liquid or Gas Chromatography-Mass Spectrometry

RPE cells are highly polarized cells, and it has been reported that metabolites are transferred to the two sides of cells separately. To test transportation of nutrition from both sides of RPE cells, extracting the metabolites in the culture medium from both sides of RPE cells on the dish offers high yield. In the following protocol, we assume that the goal is to compare different mutations in the glycolysis or TCA pathway or before and after treatment using gene editing/protein inhibitor/activator. Here, we use U-^{13}C glucose as an example.

1. Seed cells (1 × 10^5 cells per insert) onto 0.3 cm^2 cell culture inserts coated with Matrigel (*see* Subheading 3.1, **step 1**).
2. After 4–6 weeks of maturation on the transwell filters, the medium was changed to 500-μL DMEM containing 1% FBS on both sides 24 h before experiment or labeling. 5.5-mM U-^{13}C glucose was added to the medium on the basolateral side, while unlabeled glucose was added on the apical side. 20-μL medium from each side was allocated to clean tubes, which were then labeled as blank medium and stored in −80 °C (*see* Subheading 3.1, **step 3**).
3. Collect 20 μL of medium from both sides at 8 h. Different time points could be selected depending on your purpose, for example, 1 h, 4 h, 8 h, 24 h, or 48 h.
4. Apply **steps 2–3** to the method blank wells.
5. Add 80 μL of cold methanol on dry ice for 15 min to extract metabolites. Shake the tube for 5 min in cold room.
6. Centrifuge the sample at 13,000 RPM (or the highest setting in regular benchtop centrifuge) for 15 min at 4 °C (*see* Subheading 3.1, **step 5**). Store on an empty rack in the cold room or −20 °C freezer.
7. Take the sample carefully to the pre-chilled rack (not on the ice since the pellet can be disturbed) and transfer the supernatant which contains the metabolites into a new tube.
8. Repeat Subheading 3.1, **step 8**.

3.3 Metabolite Extraction from the Retina of Mice for Liquid or Gas Chromatography-Mass Spectrometry

Photoreceptor mutations are more common in humans, but there are no ideal protocols for culturing photoreceptor cells on the dish. As such, it is super important to have a protocol for collecting and extracting metabolites from neural retina. Metabolomics studies of the retina in animal models are essential to understanding the retinal metabolism and to revealing the underlying mechanisms of retinal degenerative disease. Here, we give an example of how we prepare metabolites from retinas dissected from mice.

1. Dissect the retina and process the dissection as fast as possible to protect the metabolic status in the retina. The whole procedure should take about 5 s per retina (*see* **Note 8**).
   (a) Anesthetize the mouse with mixed solution.
   (b) Sacrifice the mouse with no extra stress and as fast as possible (*see* **Note 9**). Separate the eyelids with fingers and allow lift out the eyeball from between the eyelids.
   (c) Cut the cornea into two pieces softly with a sharp and new blade (*see* **Note 10**).
   (d) Remove the lens from the eyeball using a pair of clean tweezers. Then, remove the retina by squeezing on the bottom of the eyeball (*see* **Note 11**).
   (e) Store the separated retina in a 1.5-mL Eppendorf tube, and rinse it in liquid nitrogen immediately. The tube should be transferred to −80 °C until future processing.
2. Extract the Metabolites from the Retinal Tissue.
   (a) Place the samples in the 1.5-mL tube on ice, and add 200 μL of 80% methanol on dry ice to extract the metabolites.
   (b) Homogenize the sample on wet ice with a disposable pestle for about 30–60 s, and leave the homogenized sample on dry ice for 30 min (*see* **Note 12**).
   (c) Centrifuge the sample at 13,000 RPM (or highest setting in regular benchtop centrifuge) for 15 min at 4 °C.
   (d) Take the sample carefully to the pre-chilled rack. Make sure sample is not on the ice since the pellet can be disturbed. Then, transfer the supernatant which contains the metabolites into a new tube. Take particular care to remove all the supernatant and avoid touching the pellet (*see* **Note** 7).
   (e) Clean up debris with 0.2-um syringe filter before LC. (Note: You can also clean up debris by passing the sample through filter after re-dissolving. Otherwise, add 0.2-μm filter before the column. The column life will be shortened, since this preparation is not very clean if the debris was not filtered beforehand.)
   (f) Repeat Subheading 3.1, **step 8**.

4 Notes

1. Reactions must be stopped immediately when you start to collect or process samples. Try your best to keep materials at low temperatures, as the metabolites might degrade at even slightly higher temperatures. 80% methanol is a common extraction reagent for aqueous metabolites only—such as those found in glycolysis or TCA cycle. It is not a good solvent for lipid extraction. Also, methanol is not a good solvent for extracting easily degradable or convertible molecules such as NADH, NADPH, ATP, glutathione, etc. For both cell and tissue specimens, 40:40:20 acetonitrile:methanol:water with 0.1-M formic acid (followed by neutralization with ammonium bicarbonate) is generally an effective solvent system for both quenching and extracting ATP and other high-energy phosphorylated compounds (PMID: 28654323, 17630720).
2. Some metabolites do not need to dry, like cell culture medium. Some drying may lose metabolites like SpeedVac Evaporator.
3. 35-mm plates are recommended, because the individual wells have less variability especially for time point experiments. At minimum, three wells should be used per condition. If there is a limited supply of cells, 12-well plates are also acceptable.

   Stable isotope tracer, also referred to as qualitative flux analysis, can identify cell-derived compounds and provide clarity in these situations by allowing visualization of the flow of a metabolic tracer through pathways of interest [12, 13]. It is a powerful tool to trace the dynamic metabolic reactions and reveal novel metabolic pathways within cells and between cells in the retina [13]. When labeled with stable isotope tracer, timing for collecting samples to test is variable depending on the pathway of interest and cell/tissue of interest. For example, labeled glucose goes through the glycolysis pathway in cells within minutes, while labeling of lipid pathway may take hours or even days. When the focus is tissues in vivo, the time spent on absorption and blood delivery must be taken into account. The protocol for in vivo tissue labeling would be discussed in the later part.
4. When collecting samples from the dish, remember to collect as clean and fast as possible.
5. In this protocol, we are using 1-mL pipette tips to collect RPE cells; smaller tips may get clogged with the RPE cells.
6. The pellet can be used for Western blot or protein concentration determination for normalization.
7. While evaporating the supernatant in the tubes under nitrogen gas flow is acceptable, freeze-drying is highly recommended if the instrument is available.

8. The euthanasia, dissection, and postmortem delay could impact on metabolic profile [14].

   If stable isotope tracing is needed, feed the mouse orally, do i.p. injection or i.v. injection, and then collect the samples at proper time points. Depending on the metabolites and pathways, different routes can be chosen. The advantage of bolus injection is simple and economical, but the disadvantage is you need to do multiple time points, labeling does not reach steady state, and some tracers may not be absorbed through IP. The best method is to continuous infusion through jugular vein or other vessels. For the bolus injection, tail vein is better than IP. Animals need to be fasted before this experiment.
9. The method chosen to sacrifice the mice will affect the metabolites profiles. Cervical dislocation is also recommended if permitted [14]. Studies show that CO2 exposure for 5 min dramatically degrades ATP and GTP into purine metabolites in the retina (PMID: 29727671).
10. When cutting the cornea with blade, please remember do it softly and avoid extra pressure on the eye surface. Also, the cut should be large enough so that the lens can be removed from the eyeball.
11. Remove the extra tissue, like RPE, or iris, which are black tissues.
12. To avoid extra heat produced during the process, stop several times when homogenizing the samples.

Acknowledgements

Jonas Childrens Vision Center was supported by the National Institutes of Health [grant numbers: R01EY033770 5P30CA013696, U01 EY030580, U54OD020351, R24EY028758, R24EY027285, 5P30EY019007, R01EY018213, R01EY024698, R01EY024091, R01EY12951, R01EY026682, and R21AG050437]; the Schneeweiss Stem Cell Fund; New York State [grant number SDHDOH01-C32590GG-3450000]; the Foundation Fighting Blindness New York Regional Research Center Grant [grant numbers PPA-1218-0751-COLU, and TA-NMT-0116-0692-COLU]; Nancy & Kobi Karp; the Crowley Family Funds; The Rosenbaum Family Foundation; Alcon Research Institute; the Gebroe Family Foundation; and the unrestricted funds from Research to Prevent Blindness, New York, NY, USA.

Conflict of Interest

Stephen H. Tsang receives financial support from Abeona Therapeutics, Inc and Emendo. He is also the founder of Rejuvitas and is on the scientific and clinical advisory board for Nanoscope Therapeutics and Medical Excellence Capital.

References

1. Chen L et al (2018) Recent advances in the applications of metabolomics in eye research. Anal Chim Acta 1037:28–40
2. Lains I et al (2019) Metabolomics in the study of retinal health and disease. Prog Retin Eye Res 69:57–79
3. Park KS et al (2018) Reprogramming the metabolome rescues retinal degeneration. Cell Mol Life Sci 75(9):1559–1566
4. Gowda GA et al (2008) Metabolomics-based methods for early disease diagnostics. Expert Rev Mol Diagn 8(5):617–633
5. Kosmides AK et al (2013) Metabolomic fingerprinting: challenges and opportunities. Crit Rev Biomed Eng 41(3):205–221
6. Zhang L et al (2016) Reprogramming metabolism by targeting sirtuin 6 attenuates retinal degeneration. J Clin Invest 126(12): 4659–4673
7. Dettmer K, Aronov PA, Hammock BD (2007) Mass spectrometry-based metabolomics. Mass Spectrom Rev 26(1):51–78
8. Maminishkis A et al (2006) Confluent monolayers of cultured human fetal retinal pigment epithelium exhibit morphology and physiology of native tissue. Invest Ophthalmol Vis Sci 47(8):3612–3624
9. Sonoda S et al (2009) A protocol for the culture and differentiation of highly polarized human retinal pigment epithelial cells. Nat Protoc 4(5):662–673
10. Li Y, Nguyen HV, Tsang SH (2016) Skin biopsy and patient-specific stem cell lines. Methods Mol Biol 1353:77–88
11. Li Y et al (2017) Patient-specific mutations impair BESTROPHIN1's essential role in mediating Ca(2+)-dependent Cl(−) currents in human RPE. Elife 6:e29914
12. Violante S et al (2019) Stable isotope tracers for metabolic pathway analysis. Methods Mol Biol 1978:269–283
13. Du J, Linton JD, Hurley JB (2015) Probing metabolism in the intact retina using stable isotope tracers. Methods Enzymol 561:149–170
14. Zhu S et al (2018) Impact of euthanasia, dissection and postmortem delay on metabolic profile in mouse retina and RPE/choroid. Exp Eye Res 174:113–120

Chapter 25

CRISPR-Mediated Genome Engineering in Cell Lines

Ya-Ju Chang, Joseph Ryu, Xuan Cui, and Stephen H. Tsang

Abstract

A specific targeting nuclease is a powerful tool for mediating genome alternative expression with high precision. The RNA sequence-guided Cas9 nuclease from the microbial clustered regularly interspaced short palindromic repeats (CRISPR) adaptive immune system can be used to facilitate genome engineering in cells by using a 20-nt targeting sequence. In this chapter, we describe a set of tools for Cas9-mediated genome editing via non-homologous end joining (NHEJ) or homology-directed repair (HDR) in the generation of modified cell lines for downstream functional studies. This protocol provides experimentally derived guidelines for the selection of target sites, evaluation of cleavage efficiency, and analysis of off-target activity. Beginning with target design, we will cover gene modifications and modified clonal cell lines.

Key words CRISPR, Genome engineering, Precise gene editing, Gene editing, SNP, Gene modification

1 Introduction

Gene editing is a new era of technology that is capable of modifying DNA sequences in a highly precise and specific manner. This method of genome modification lies on the therapeutic horizon of providing medical treatments for many genetic variation diseases. Clustered regularly interspaced short palindromic repeats (CRISPR) are an ideal tool for site specific genome editing [1]. It allows DNA sequences to be added, deleted, or altered at locations in the genome. Several approaches to genome editing have been developed, and a significant one is CRISPR-Cas9. The CRISPR-Cas9 system is more accurate and efficient than other existing genome editing methods. The CRISPR-Cas9 system is a microbial adaptive immune system that uses RNA-guided nucleases to cleave foreign genetic elements. It involves partially palindromic repeats separated by short stretches of DNA spacers [2–4].

Three types of the CRISPR system (I–III) has been identified across a wide range of bacterial hosts, wherein each system comprises a cluster of CRISPR-associated (*Cas*) genes, and non-coding

Stephen H. Tsang and Peter M. J. Quinn (eds.), *Retinitis Pigmentosa*,
Methods in Molecular Biology, vol. 2560, https://doi.org/10.1007/978-1-0716-2651-1_25,

RNAs. These repeats are interspaced by short variable sequences [5] derived from exogenous DNA targets known as proto-spacers, and together they constitute the CRISPR RNA (crRNA). Within the DNA target, each protospacer is associated with a protospacer adjacent motif (PAM), which can vary depending on the specific CRISPR system [6–8]. The Type II CRISPR system is one of the best characterized [9, 10] consisting of the nuclease Cas9, the crRNA array that encodes the guide RNAs, and a required auxiliary trans-activating crRNA (tracrRNA) that facilitates the processing of the crRNA array into discrete units [11]. Each crRNA unit then contains a 20-nucleotide guide sequence and a partial direct repeat, where the former directs Cas9 to a 20-bp DNA target via Watson–Crick base pairing. In the CRISPR-Cas system derived from *Streptococcus pyogenes* (which is the system used in this protocol), the target DNA must immediately precede a 5′-NGG PAM [12], whereas other Cas9 orthologs may have different PAM requirements, such as those of *S. thermophilus* (5′-NNAGAA for CRISPR1 and 5′-NGGNG for CRISPR3) and *Neisseria meningitidis* (5′-NNNNGATT) [13].

The RNA-guided nuclease function of CRISPR-Cas is reconstituted in mammalian cells through the heterologous expression of human codon-optimized Cas9 and the requisite RNA components [14–16]. Furthermore, the crRNA and tracrRNA can be fused together to create a chimeric, single-guide RNA (sgRNA). Cas9 can thus be re-directed toward almost any target of interest in immediate vicinity of the PAM sequence by altering the 20-nt guide sequence within the sgRNA.

Given its ease of implementation and multiplexing capacity, Cas9 has been used to generate engineered eukaryotic cells carrying specific mutations via both NHEJ and HDR [17]. Direct injection of sgRNA and mRNA encoding Cas9 into embryos has enabled the rapid generation of transgenic mice with multiple modified alleles [18, 19]. These results hold enormous promise for editing organisms that are otherwise genetically intractable.

Cas9 nucleases carry out strand-specific cleavage by using the conserved HNH and RuvC nuclease domains, which can be mutated and exploited for additional function. An aspartate-to-alanine (D10A) mutation in the RuvC catalytic domain allows the Cas9 nickase mutant (Cas9n) to nick rather than cleave DNA to yield single-stranded breaks, and the subsequent preferential repair through HDR can potentially decrease the frequency of unwanted indel mutations from off-target DSBs. Appropriately offset sgRNA pairs can guide Cas9n to simultaneously nick both strands of the target locus to mediate a DSB, thus effectively increasing the specificity of target recognition [20]. In addition, a Cas9 mutant with both DNA-cleaving catalytic residues mutated has been adapted to enable transcriptional regulation in *Escherichia coli* [21], demonstrating the potential of functionalizing Cas9 for diverse applications, such as recruitment of fluorescent protein labels or chromatin-modifying enzymes to specific genomic loci for reporting or modulating gene function.

Ethical concerns have been raised regarding the application of CRISPR technology in human-related studies. As was the case for stem cell research, it will take time for the safety/ethical issues to be sufficiently addressed. However, this novel technology is already in the process of being accepted in medical practice as evidenced by the increasing number of CRISPR-related clinical trials being proposed worldwide.

2 Materials

1. 4D-Nucleofector™ System (Lonza).
2. P3 Primary Cell 4D-Nucleofector Kit S (Lonza).
3. mTeSR™ media (StemCell).
4. ROCK inhibitor Y-27632 2HCl (Selleckchem).
5. ReLeSR™ (StemCell).
6. Dulbecco's Phosphate Buffered Saline (Thermo).
7. Corning Matrigel Matrix (BD).
8. gRNA (Synthego, *see* **Note 1**).
9. HifiCas9 protein (IDT, *see* **Note 2**).
10. ssODN repair template (IDT, Ultramer DNA Oligo, *see* **Note 3**).
11. 6-well plates.
12. Oligonucleotide primers (*see* **Note 4**).
13. T7 endonuclease assay (T7E1).
14. PCR Purification Kit (BioRad).

3 Methods

3.1 CRISPR gRNA Design for Gene Targeting

The design the CRISPR target site depends on the specific sequence between the position of the cut site in the genome, the specificity of the guide RNA in terms of unwanted or off-target cutting, and the activity of the Cas9 enzyme when programmed with a particular rule. When making single nucleotide changes, the position is the major factor that needs to be considered, since the frequency of introduction of mutations by HDR drops off very rapidly within a few tens of nucleotides on either side of the cut site. Design of sgRNAs can be done manually or using freely available online tools (i.e., Benchling). These tools can be used to help identify guide sequences that minimize identical genomic matches or near-matches and reduce risk of cleavage away from target sites (off-target effects). It is important to ensure that the guide sequences consist of a 20-mer ("protospacer sequence") upstream of an "NGG" sequence ("protospacer adjacent motif" or PAM) at the genomic recognition site. sgRNA-A's protospacer sequence and PAM happen to fall on the bottom (Crick) strand, while sgRNA-B's protospacer sequence and PAM fall on the top (Watson) strand. However, DSB will occur independent of orientation of the protospacer sequence/PAM relative to the top or bottom strand.

As such, take care to determine the reverse complement of each guide sequence. Obtain 24- or 25-mer oligos for each guide and its associated reverse complement including additional nucleotides for cloning and expression purposes.

3.2 Cell Culture (iPSC as Sample Here)

We routinely use the patient-derived induced pluripotent stem cell (iPSC) line for editing. The cell line should be derived from a single cell to maximize homogeneity within the population. Additionally, it should be cultured under feeder-free conditions typically on 10-cm tissue culture dishes in mTeSR medium on Matrigel coating plate. Cells should be routinely passaged 1:5 every week. Cells should be cultured in a humidified incubator at 37 °C and 5% CO_2.

1. Remove spent medium and wash cell layer once with DPBS.
2. Incubate with ReLeSR medium (1 mL/10 cm dish) for 1 min, and discard the medium. Wait for 5 min at 37 °C and 5% CO_2.
3. Aspirate Gentle Cell Dissociation Reagent and add 5 mL mTeSR medium.
4. Slightly pipette the cell to manually detach dissociated colonies from the culture surface (*see* **Note 5**).
5. Transfer 0.2-mL cell suspension into a fresh 10-cm dish containing an additional 8 mL mTeSR medium.

3.2.1 Gene Targeting by Nucleofection

Rehydrate sgRNA (Synthego)

1. Briefly centrifuge tubes containing sgRNA oligos to ensure sgRNA pellets are collected at the bottom.
2. Carefully rehydrate sgRNA in an appropriate nuclease-free buffer (1X TE buffer, 10-mM Tris–HCl, 1-mM EDTA, pH 8.0) and pulse vortex for 30 s to ensure complete mixing. The final concentration of the sgRNA will be 100 μM (100 pmol/μL).
3. Store rehydrated sgRNA at −20 °C. It will be stable for up 6 months.
4. Dilute sgRNA (Synthego).
5. Add 6 μL of 100-μM sgRNA to 14 μL of nuclease-free water to make a 30-μM sgRNA (30 pmol/μL).

6. Use diluted sgRNA immediately or store at −20 °C for up to 3 month or more to 6 months (*see* **Note 6**).
7. Form RNP complexes.
8. Dilute Cas9 2NLS to 20 μM (20 pmol/μL) in a suitable buffer.
9. Form sgRNA: Cas9 RNP (1:3–1:6 depends on the cell type) complexes in a sterile micro-centrifuge tube for the RNP delivery.
10. Incubate at room temperature for 10 min to assemble the RNP complexes.
11. RNP complexes are stable at room temperature for up to 1 h and at 4 °C for up to 1 week.

iPS Collection for Nucleofection

1. Remove the medium from 10-cm dish and wash once with DPBS.
2. Add 5 mL of ReLeSR for 1 min and discard the ReLeSR. Keep the dish for reaction for 5 min at 37 °C incubator.
3. Stop the reaction by adding 1 mL mTeSR with ROCK inhibitor.
4. Slightly mix the cell to create a single cell suspension.
5. Count the cells and aliquot 1×10^6 into a sterile tube.
6. Centrifuge at 300 g for 10 min to pellet.
7. Resuspend in 30-μL complete P3 buffer.
8. To make base changes by HDR, add 500 pmol of purified ssDNA oligonucleotide (5 μL of 100-μM stock) to the RNP complex.
9. Transfer cells into nucleofection well, dispensing carefully between the electrodes to avoid formation of bubbles.
10. Electroporate with the 4D-Nucleofector on program DS150 (the program depend on each cell line, should test before CRISPR experiment).
11. Transfer cells from the electrode well to 6-well plate containing 3 mL of mTeSR with 10-μM ROCK inhibitor. Take care to pipette the cell gently as cells are very fragile at this point (*see* **Note 7**).
12. Incubate for 24 h, and then exchange medium for mTeSR without ROCK inhibitor.
13. Change medium daily until cells reach approximately 70% confluence for sub-culturing. At this stage, it is recommended that CRISPR activity is confirmed using, e.g., T7E1 or TIDE analysis (*see* **Note 8**). This is an important step before continuing with sub-culturing since many guide RNAs (~20–25%) have very low activity, and it is possible to eliminate these at this stage.

3.3 Screening CRISPR/Cas9 Clones for Deletions and Clone Selection

For suspension cells, transfer all clones to a single 96-well plate that already contains 50-μL cell culture media per well for a final volume of 150 μL. This facilitates screening by allowing a multichannel pipette to be used for the remainder of the steps. Transfer 50 μL from each well (leaving 100 μL in each well) to a 96-well PCR plate using a multichannel pipette. Centrifuge PCR plate at 400 × g for 5 min, and remove supernatant by flicking the PCR plate over a sink. Add 50 μL of DNA extraction solution per well and resuspend. Continue the step for suspension cells.

For adherent cells, aspirate media. Add 20 μL of 0.05% trypsin-EDTA to each well with a clone present. Resuspend cells in 200 μL of media. Pipette mix to detach cells. Place 100 μL each into two separate 96-well flat-bottom plates. Keep one plate to allow for clones to grow and use the other plate to screen each clone for deletions. Add an additional 100 μL to each well for a total volume of 200 μL. Wait 24–72 h to allow cells to grow. Aspirate media. Add 50-μL DNA extraction solution per well, resuspend and transfer to 96-well PCR plate. Extract the gDNA from clones. Run sample in thermocycler: 65 °C for 6 min and 98 °C for 2 min to extract gDNA.

Screen each clone using the same PCR primers and reaction conditions optimized on the bulk cells. Select the clones identified with the desired deletion and move to larger plate or flask for growth.

1. For a single, confluent well of a 6-well plate, prepare 1 mL of lysis buffer and supplement it with 20 μL Proteinase K.
2. Aspirate medium from the well and wash cell layer with PBS, aspirating again.
3. Add the lysis buffer mixture to the well and allow to stand for 30–60 s.
4. Collect the lysate in a microfuge tube and incubate at 60 °C for at least 1 h to overnight (*see* **Note 9**).
5. Inactivate the proteinase K by incubating the lysate at 95 °C for 10 min.
6. Dilute the lysate 1:10 with nuclease-free water.
7. Use the diluted lysate to prepare a 20 μL PCR mix according to the set of primers designed to generate a 500 bp product (500_F/R).
8. Run the PCR with the cycling protocol described in **Note 10** (*see* **Note 10**).
9. To 10 μL of the PCR product, add 1.5 μL NEBuffer 2 and 1.5 μL Nuclease-free H2O. Include a second control reaction which will receive no T7E1.

10. Form the hetero-duplexes by heat-cooling the mixture in a thermal cycler using the protocol described in **Note 10**.
11. Add 2 μL of T7E1 (diluted in NEBuffer 2 to a final concentration of 1 U/μL). For control digests, use 2 μL NEBuffer 2.
12. Incubate at 37 °C for 1 h.
13. Add an appropriate volume of loading dye to the samples.
14. Run the samples on a 2.5% agarose gel at 70 V for 45 min.

3.3.1 Colony Picking

Single cell-derived colonies should be manually picked from the culture surface approximately 8–10 days after subcloning. At this point, colonies should be 1–2 mm in size, uniform, and round in appearance with bright borders (*see* **Note 11**). Prior to picking, equal numbers of 96-well plates should be prepared with Matrigel substrate at a concentration of 5 μg/cm^2. Each well should be prefilled with 150-μL mTeSR medium supplemented with rock inhibitor.

1. Aspirate the medium from the 10-cm dish of colonies.
2. Wash once in PBS.
3. Add 5 mL of gentle cell dissociation buffer and incubate at 37 °C for 3 min (*see* **Note 12**).
4. Aspirate the Gentle Cell Dissociation Reagent taking care not to disrupt the colonies.
5. Add 10 mL mTeSR medium.
6. Using a dissection microscope and a P20 pipette (set to 10 μL), manually pick individual colonies by scraping from the culture surface and collecting in the pipette.
7. Transfer the cells to a 96-well plate Matrigel-containing 100 μL mTeSR medium supplemented with rock inhibitor. Use a fresh tip per colony to prevent cross contamination.
8. Colonies are usually picked in batches of 96 which can be processed for genotyping as whole plates. Once sufficient numbers of colonies have been picked, triturate the cells 5–6 times to break colonies into smaller fragments (*see* **Note 13**) and transfer 50 μL into one Matrigel and the other 50 μL into one Matrigel-coated plate, thereby creating two duplicate 96-well plates of colonies (*see* **Note 14**).
9. Cells should be cultured for approximately 5 days (or until wells are confluent) with daily 200-μL mTeSR medium changes, before freeing/lysing (*see* **Note 15**).

3.3.2 Sanger Sequencing

When designing a genotyping strategy, it is important to consider its ability to identify mixed or mosaic clones (i.e., those colonies deriving from multiple different edited cells), and its scalability to the large number of clones that often must be screened to obtain the cell line of interest. Here, we present a high-throughput sequencing based strategy that involves a three-step PCR from crude cell lysates that are easily prepared from 96-well plates, followed by sequencing on an Illumina MiSeq instrument that allows screening of tens of plates on a single run. It is also highly sensitive to detect each individual allele in a mixed population down to <1% of the total alleles, making identification of mixed clones simple and accurate. Colonies growing on Matrigel-coating plate can be lysed 2–4 days post picking. Lysate plates are used for genotyping of edited clones and are generated in a similar way to the lysates used in the T7E1 assay.

1. Remove spent medium.
2. Wash cells once in PBS.
3. Incubate with 100-μL lysis buffer supplemented with 2-μL proteinase K/well at 60 °C from 1 h to overnight (*see* **Note 10**).
4. Inactivate the proteinase K at 95 °C for 10 min.
5. Store lysates at 20 °C or use directly for PCR.
6. Dilute lysates 1:10 in nuclease-free H_2O.
7. Prepare 10-μL PCR reaction for each well, using the set of primers designed to generate a 500-bp product (500_F/R).
8. Run PCR thermocycler program.
9. Recommended: run 3 μL of product on a 1.5% gel, made up to 20 μL in ddH 2 0 to ensure PCR was successful, with 10-μL gel low range quantitative DNA ladder combined with 10-μL H_2O.
10. Assemble PCR as in **step 7** using instead the 200_F/R primers and 0.5 μL of the round one 500-bp product as template.
11. Run PCR thermocycler program mentioned in **step 8**. Recommended annealing temperature of 60 °C.
12. Recommended: run 3 μL of product on a 1.5% gel, as in **step 9**.

3.3.3 PCR Program

Purified PCR produce should be prepared for sequencing via column purification. Concentration for sequencing is 1-μL PCR product and 15 μL of 5 pM primer. Program is as follows:

1. 1 min at 96 °C (1×).
2. 30 s at 96 °C.
3. 15 s at 50 °C.

4. 4 min at 60 °C (30×).
5. 1 min incubation at 4 °C (1×).
6. Samples were analyzed by an applied biosystems DNA Analyzer.

3.3.4 TIDE Method for Quantitative of Genome Editing

User quality control should be ensured by visualizing deviating signal and decomposition yielding the spectrum of indels and frequencies. Inference of the base composition prediction of +1 insertion, a pool of iPS cells without editing (control) and with editing (sample) were analyzed by TIDE.

4 Notes

1. Synthemax is prepared by dissolving 10-mg powder in 10-mL sterile distilled water to make a 1-mg/mL stock and stored in aliquots at 4 °C. Further dilution in water 1:40 and 1:100 make a working dilution for coating plates at a concentration of 5 μg/cm^2 and 2 μg/cm^2, respectively.
2. We find that full length synthetic, chemically modified guides from Synthego or Sigma are highly effective and, in most cases, superior to the crRNA:tracrRNA hybrid. We use the same molar amounts and concentrations as for the crRNA:tracrRNA hybrid, namely, an approximately twofold molar excess of guide RNA compared to Cas9 protein.
3. HDR ssDNA oligonucleotides can be ordered from many suppliers, but we typically use Ultramer oligos from IDT, due to the higher proportion of full-length products with the correct sequence that are obtained. We find that simple desalted purification is sufficient, but HPLC or PAGE purified oligonucleotides work equally effectively.
4. Recent results suggest that the predominant repair mechanism when using a ssODN is the annealing of the oligo to the resected 5' ends of the DNA that are formed after a double strand break, and its use as a template for DNA polymerases.
5. Cells adhere to Synthemax very well, so cell scrapers need to be used to manually detach colonies which have not dislodged during incubation with gentle cell dissociation reagent. Do not use excessive trituration to dislodge attached colonies since this will result in cell clusters which are too small for routine passaging, leaving cells vulnerable to poor growth/colony compaction during onward culture. Continual passaging of pluripotent cells as single cells has also been shown to increase accumulation of karyotypic abnormalities.

6. When diluting Cas9 protein, DTT should be added fresh from a frozen, 0.1-M stock solution immediately before use.
7. Cells are very delicate following nucleofection; therefore, handling of cells should be minimized. Transfer from cuvette to culture dish using a wide bore Pasteur pipette and disperse over the culture surface using a gentle swirling/back-and-forth movement. Work quickly once mixing the RNP complex, template, buffer, and cells together, minimizing the length of exposure of the cells to these components. The Accutase treatment duration time is somewhat cell line specific and can be reduced to increase viability, but not so much as to compromise obtaining single cells.
8. An alternative to the T7E1 assay is to send PCR products from the 500-bp amplification for sequencing and analyze sequencing traces with TIDE [16] (https://tide-calculator.nki.nl/) or ICE (https://ice.synthego.com/#/). Note that a WT sequencing read is also required to calibrate such software.
9. Lysis is usually performed for 1 h at 60 °C; however, incubation times can be increased to overnight if necessary.
10. If during the preparation of 500-bp PCR product, PCR is unsuccessful, it is likely to be due to inhibition of the PCR by the lysate, low DNA concentration, or ineffective primers. Primers can be optimized by trying a range of annealing temperatures or adding DMSO to the reaction mix (5% v/v final concentration). Inhibition by components in the lysate can be improved by diluting it or lysing cells in a larger volume of lysis buffer. If the DNA concentration is too low, try lysing in a smaller volume of lysis buffer or not diluting the DNA before adding to the PCR. Genomic DNA can also alternatively be obtained using a column-based system, such as Qiagen DNeasy Blood & Tissue Kit (69504).
11. It is important to seed single cells during subcloning to ensure colonies arise from single cells. hiPSCs do not grow well from single cells and will often survive better as small clumps of cells. It can be difficult to identify colonies generated from single cells but the size and shape of the colonies relative to others on the plate can be a good indicator of success. Try to avoid picking colonies which are growing close to each other or touching.
12. Incubation in cell dissociation reagent serves simply to aid breaking apart of the colony during trituration and splitting into Matrigel/Synthemax plates. It is not intended to detach and break apart colonies from the plate before picking.
13. If colonies are breaking into very small clumps (~5–10 cells) during colony picking, reduce the incubation time with gentle cell dissociation reagent. If colonies too dissociated at this

stage, there is a high risk of cells floating off into the picking medium, which can result in the cross contamination of colonies.

14. Matrigel plates serve as the freezing plates in which cell stocks will be bulked up and frozen (*see* Subheading 3.3.1, **step 7**) for storage until genotyping confirms successful editing. The Synthemax plates will be grown up and lysed for genotyping analysis to identify suitable edited clones (*see* Subheading 3.3.1, **step 8**).
15. If cells are picked out of the tissue culture hood or with the front of the hood open, Penicillin and Streptomycin solution (Thermo 15140122) can be added for 24 h to help prevent contamination.

Acknowledgments

National Cancer Institute Core (5P30CA013696), Foundation Fighting Blindness (TA-NMT-0116-0692-COLU), and New York State (C029572).

Conflict of Interest

Stephen H. Tsang receives grant support from Abeona Therapeutics, Inc and Emendo. He is also the founder of Rejuvitas and is on the scientific and clinical advisory board for Nanoscope Therapeutics and Medical Excellence Capital.

References

1. Hsu PD, Lander ES, Zhang F (2014) Development and applications of CRISPR-Cas9 for genome engineering. Cell 157(6):1262–1278
2. Deveau H, Garneau JE, Moineau S (2010) CRISPR/Cas system and its role in phage-bacteria interactions. Annu Rev Microbiol 64: 475–493
3. Horvath P, Barrangou R (2010) CRISPR/Cas, the immune system of bacteria and archaea. Science 327(5962):167–170
4. Garneau JE et al (2010) The CRISPR/Cas bacterial immune system cleaves bacteriophage and plasmid DNA. Nature 468(7320):67–71
5. Makarova KS et al (2011) Evolution and classification of the CRISPR-Cas systems. Nat Rev Microbiol 9(6):467–477
6. Marraffini LA, Sontheimer EJ (2008) CRISPR interference limits horizontal gene transfer in staphylococci by targeting DNA. Science 322(5909):1843–1845
7. Brouns SJ et al (2008) Small CRISPR RNAs guide antiviral defense in prokaryotes. Science 321(5891):960–964
8. Barrangou R et al (2007) CRISPR provides acquired resistance against viruses in prokaryotes. Science 315(5819):1709–1712
9. Sapranauskas R et al (2011) The Streptococcus thermophilus CRISPR/Cas system provides immunity in Escherichia coli. Nucleic Acids Res 39(21):9275–9282
10. Magadan AH et al (2012) Cleavage of phage DNA by the Streptococcus thermophilus CRISPR3-Cas system. PLoS One 7(7):e40913
11. Gasiunas G et al (2012) Cas9-crRNA ribonucleoprotein complex mediates specific DNA cleavage for adaptive immunity in bacteria.

Proc Natl Acad Sci U S A 109(39):E2579–E2586

12. Jinek M et al (2012) A programmable dual-RNA-guided DNA endonuclease in adaptive bacterial immunity. Science 337(6096): 816–821
13. Zhang Y et al (2013) Processing-independent CRISPR RNAs limit natural transformation in Neisseria meningitidis. Mol Cell 50(4): 488–503
14. Cong L et al (2013) Multiplex genome engineering using CRISPR/Cas systems. Science 339(6121):819–823
15. Mali P et al (2013) RNA-guided human genome engineering via Cas9. Science 339(6121):823–826
16. Jinek M et al (2013) RNA-programmed genome editing in human cells. elife 2:e00471
17. Hwang WY et al (2013) Efficient genome editing in zebrafish using a CRISPR-Cas system. Nat Biotechnol 31(3):227–229
18. Wang H et al (2013) One-step generation of mice carrying mutations in multiple genes by CRISPR/Cas-mediated genome engineering. Cell 153(4):910–918
19. Shen B et al (2013) Generation of gene-modified mice via Cas9/RNA-mediated gene targeting. Cell Res 23(5):720–723
20. Ran FA et al (2013) Double nicking by RNA-guided CRISPR Cas9 for enhanced genome editing specificity. Cell 154(6): 1380–1389
21. Qi LS et al (2013) Repurposing CRISPR as an RNA-guided platform for sequence-specific control of gene expression. Cell 152(5): 1173–1183

Chapter 26

CRISPR Off-Target Analysis Platforms

Christine L. Xu, Merry Zhechao Ruan, Sara D. Ragi, and Stephen H. Tsang

Abstract

The clustered regularly interspaced short palindromic repeats (CRISPR)-Caspase9 (Cas9) system provides a programmable technology that may be used to edit the eukaryotic genome and epigenome. CRISPR/Cas9 includes a guide RNA targeted to a gene of interest which hybridizes to a nucleotide sequence next to a protospacer-adjacent motif (PAM) which guides the Cas9 endonucleases to the target site for cleavage via double-strand breaks. A caveat of the CRISPR/Cas9 system is the creation of off-target double-strand breaks (DSBs) which may result in anomalous insertions, deletions, and translocations. Thus, assays for the sensitive detection and analysis of off-target editing are critical. Here, we describe currently available CRISPR technologies, CRISPR applications, and current analysis platforms to detect off-target effects including genome-wide, unbiased identification of DSBs enabled by sequencing (GUIDE-Seq), high-throughput genomic translocation sequencing (HTGTS), breaks labeling, enrichments on streptavidin and next-generation sequencing (BLESS), and in vitro nuclease-digested genome sequencing (Digenome-seq).

Key words CRISPR/Cas9, Off-target effects, GUIDE-Seq, HTGTS, BLESS, Digenome-seq

1 Introduction

The clustered regularly interspaced short palindromic repeats (CRISPR)/CRISPR associated (cas) system is part of the adaptive immune system in bacteria and archaea. It cleaves and silences foreign nucleic acids using CRISPR RNA. In 2012, CRISPR/Cas9 was engineered into a powerful and easy-to-use genome editing tool [1], which contains a guide RNA (gRNA) designed for the gene of interest. This ~20 nt gRNA can be easily synthesized in vitro. When introduced into the cell, the gRNA hybridizes with a nucleotide sequence next to a protospacer-adjacent motif (PAM) and guides the Cas9 endonucleases to the target site for cleavage via double-strand breaks. Since the development of the first Cas9 from *Streptococcus pyogenes*, Cas9 from other bacterial strains have been engineered and utilized to meet specific editing needs. These bacteria include *Neisseria meningitidis*, *Staphylococcus aureus*,

Stephen H. Tsang and Peter M. J. Quinn (eds.), *Retinitis Pigmentosa*,
Methods in Molecular Biology, vol. 2560, https://doi.org/10.1007/978-1-0716-2651-1_26,

Streptococcus thermophilus, and *Treponema denticola*. The various strains of CRISPR/Cas9 have different requirements in gRNA design as well as different PAM sequences. However, all of the existing CRISPR/Cas9 systems can introduce off-target double-strand breaks (DSBs) that differ by up to several nucleotides from the on-target sites. These DSBs in off-target locations can produce insertions, deletions, and translocations [2]. Effective genome editing for both research and clinical purposes requires accurate prediction and detection of off-target effects.

2 How Off-Targeting Effects of CRISPR-Cas9 Occur and Why They Matter

In theory, sgRNA are engineered so that CRISPR/Cas9 carry out seamless genome editing in an efficient and specific manner. In reality, however, CRISPR/Cas9 can also induce unwanted off-target effects at sites other than the designated target location. The optimal PAM site for SpCas9 is 5'-NGG, and albeit with less efficiency, SpCas9 has also been known to cleave sites with PAM sites that are 5'-NAG or 5'-NGA [3]. Furthermore, CRISPR/Cas9 can tolerate a few nucleotide mismatches between the sgRNA and the target sequence, especially when the mismatches are in the region distal to the PAM sequence [4]. If the DNA or sgRNA generates a bulge during their binding interaction due to a DNA insertion or deletion relative to the sgRNA, CRISPR/Cas9 still possesses the ability to cleave the off-target site. Not only could off-target mutagenesis result in local mutations such as indels, frameshift, missense, and nonsense mutations, but also more severe chromosomal rearrangements such as deletions, inversions, and translocations [5]. These chromosomal rearrangements are especially worrisome, because they could lead to the activation of oncogenes.

3 Detecting Off-Target Mutations

In response to the discovery that CRISPR/Cas9 could lead to off-target mutations, various methods were developed. Sanger sequencing can detect off-target sites with great precision, but this method is both costly and time-consuming [4]. High-throughput sequencing can measure the frequencies of indels at high volumes (hundreds of sites at a time) with high accuracy and sensitivity. Polymerase chain reaction artifacts that lead to false-positive sequences, however, limit the reliability of using high-throughput sequencing for analyzing off-target effects [5]. Restriction fragment length polymorphism analysis (RFLP) has conventionally been used to detect mutations generated by programmable nucleases [6]. Unfortunately, the limited availability of restriction sites usable by RFLP in target DNA sites make this method undesirable for analyzing CRISPR/Cas9 off-target effects.

In recent years, four methods have been generated to overcome the obstacles of off-target site analysis posed by methods such as Sanger sequencing, high-throughput sequencing, and RFLP analysis: (1) genome-wide, unbiased identification of DSBs enabled by sequencing (GUIDE-Seq); (2) high-throughput genomic translocation sequencing (HTGTS); (3) breaks labeling, enrichments on streptavidin, and next-generation sequencing (BLESS); and (4) in vitro nuclease-digested genome sequencing (Digenome-seq) [7]. In the following sections, we will discuss these off-targeting analysis platforms in detail.

3.1 HTGTS

High-throughput genome-wide translocation sequencing (HTGTS) was introduced in 2011 to identify genome-wide translocation junctions of yeast I-SceI meganuclease-generated double-strand breaks (DSBs), including off-target translocation junctions [8].

In 2014, Frock et al. combined HTGTS with linear amplification-mediated PCR (LAM-PCR), developing this technology into a general method for detecting on-target and off-target double-strand breaks introduced by engineered nucleases [9]. This technology first clones "bait–prey" junctions from genome DNA using LAM-PCR, ligating them to adapters of known sequences for library amplification. Then, sequences of interest ("prey") are identified with a bioinformatic pipeline [10]. LAM-HTGTS with different Cas9::sgRNA revealed off-target hotspots numbering from none to dozens or more, and it also led to the discovery of translocations between bona fide nuclease targets on homologous chromosomes for the first time [9].

The biggest advantage of LAM-HTGTS is that it detects potential off-target sites as well as collateral damage as a consequence of unspecific cleavages (recurrent translocations). However, the detection rate is limited by the scarcity of translocation events and strong dependence on the 3D genome organization [10].

3.2 GUIDE-Seq

In 2015, Joung et al. introduced another technology to detect off-target cleavage activities of CRISPR RNA-guided nucleases (RGNs) called genome-wide, unbiased identification of DSBs enabled by sequencing (GUIDE-seq) [11]. This method transfects edited cells with small, modified double-stranded oligonucleotides (dsODNs) that are incorporated into existing double-strand breaks. These ODNs are used as tags for amplification before sequencing. Later, double-stranded breaks are identified by mapped amplified sequences. The authors tested their method on 13 RGNs in 2 human cell lines and identified non-canonical PAMs, including previously described NGA, NAA, NGT, NGC, and NCG sequences, as well as new off-target sites not detected in silico or by chromatin immunoprecipitation sequencing (ChIP-seq) [11].

GUIDE-seq is a highly sensitive method as it can detect off-target sites occurring at a frequency of 0.1% in a cell population. In addition, this method is highly precise because dsODN capture can directly map off-target sites. The number of reads at a given site also correlates with the frequency of CRISPR/Cas9-RNA generated double-stranded breaks. However, GUIDE-seq is limited by the transfection efficiency of target cells and may be difficult to apply in certain cell types [10].

3.3 BLESS

Breaks labeling, enrichments on streptavidin, and next-generation sequencing (BLESS) was introduced to the scientific community by Crosetto et al. in 2013 [12]. It involves off-target analysis using in situ labeling in cells that are fixed and permeable. Cells are fixed prior to DNA analysis in order to stabilize the chromatin and to prevent artificial DSBs and false positives from skewing the data. Then, cells are incubated with proteinase K for purification of the intact nuclei. DNA with DSBs are ligated and bound to linkers and biotin before being extracted, fragmented, and captured on streptavidin beads. Linkers are ligated and digested with endonucleases, and then the DNA strands undergo PCR and sequencing.

Although BLESS offers an unbiased way to analyze off-target mutations, a significant drawback is that it can miss off-target sites due to the fact that it only captures DSBs at one fixed moment in time [13]. Furthermore, it is prone to cell fixation artifacts and the difficulties latent in optimizing the cell harvesting time [11].

3.4 Digenome-Seq

In vitro digested genome sequencing (Digenome-seq) utilizes cell-free DNA to detect off-target effects [7]. Cas9 digests the DNA in vitro, yielding DNA fragments that have the same 5′ end at the cleavage sites. Then, by using the Integrative Genomics Viewer (IGV) computer program and whole genome sequencing, all of these sequence reads sharing the same 5′ end can be aligned and identified. Digenome-seq has been shown to detect CRISPR/Cas9 off-target effects genome-wide at a frequency of 0.1% or lower. It is also unbiased and does not capture DSBs that were generated randomly. Since Digenome-seq analyzes cell-free DNA, the DSBs generated by Cas9 are not disrupted by DSB repair machinery. Furthermore, Digenome-seq can be used to analyze multiplex gene editing, since it has the ability to analyze DSBs generated by CRISPR/Cas9 for up to 10 sgRNAs [14]. Since PCR is not involved in this method, Digenome-seq does not fall prey to PCR artifacts that can result from amplification of DNA [4]. This advantage is not shared by GUIDE-seq, HTGTS, or BLESS, because these other methods rely on PCR.

Despite its efficiency at detecting CRISPR off-target mutations, Digenome-seq also has its disadvantages. Using in vitro cell-free conditions avoids problems by DSB repair machinery, but Digenome-seq also could generate false-positive or false-negative results, due to differences in Cas9's activity and specificity in vivo versus in vitro [14]. Additionally, Digenome-seq can be costly when off-targeting analysis must be done on Cas9's DSBs generated by one sgRNA. Even though Digenome-seq is able to analyze multiple cut sites due to multiplex gene editing, the sequencing depth can be challenging when used to test more than one sgRNA.

4 Reducing Off-Target Effects

In light of recent discoveries that CRISPR/Cas9 can yield harmful and worrisome off-target mutations, researchers have been developing methods in order to reduce them. In 2014, Cho et al. demonstrated that choosing a 20-nucleotide (nt) long target sequences which differs from other genomic locations by a minimum of 2–3 nt would reduce off-target effects [5]. Cas9 is particularly efficient at detecting target mismatches when they are in the PAM sequence or in the area upstream of the PAM sequence [4]. Web-based tools such as ChopChop (http://chopchop.re.fas.harvard.edu), CRISPR Design (http://crispr.mit.edu), and Cas-OFFinder (http://www.rgenome.net/casoffinder) have been developed to aid researchers in choosing the best possible combination of target site and sgRNA.

Researchers have found that making modifications to the sgRNA can also reduce off-target effects. Adding two additional guanines at the 5′ end of the sgRNA have shown superior specificity than traditional sgRNAs when used for CRISPR in human cells [5]. Alternatively, truncating the conventional 20-nt long sgRNA into a shorter 17-nt sgRNA (tru-sgRNA) have also demonstrated increased specificity, including more sensitivity to target mismatches due to less binding energy in the sgRNA DNA interaction [4]. A downside of using tru-sgRNAs, however, is that there are not as many unique sites of 17-nt stretches in the genome that differ from other 17-nt long sequences by at least 2–3 nt.

Modifications to Cas9 have also yielded useful results in reducing off-target effects. When one of the two nuclease domains in Cas9 are mutated, it becomes a Cas9 nickase [5, 15–17]. Pairing two Cas9 nickases together have been used to generate single-stranded breaks on opposite DNA strands instead of one double-stranded cut, and this method has been shown to double CRISPR's specificity. A drawback of this method, however, is that two sgRNAs must be made (one for each Cas9 nickase) and two PAMs must be selected, limiting the flexibility of experimental design when using paired nickases.

Delivering Cas9 as a ribonucleoprotein (RNP) rather than within a plasmid has also been used as a method for reducing off-target effects [4]. Delivery of Cas9 RNPs into the cell can be achieved via protein transduction, lipofection, or electroporation [18–20]. Unlike plasmids encoding Cas9 and sgRNAs, which can be expressed continuously, Cas9-sgRNA RNPs are expressed shortly after cell delivery and degraded by proteases endogenous to the cell [4]. Plasmid fragments can be randomly integrated into the genome, but this is not a possibility for Cas9 RNPs.

5 Future Directions and Conclusions

CRISPR-Cas9-based technology has developed rapidly since its debut, with multiple clinical trials in the pipeline. In addition, the US Department of Agriculture has recently introduced regulations for agricultural products in the market which are generated by CRISPR-Cas9 [21]. These developments demonstrate how CRISPR-Cas9 lies at the cutting edge of genome editing, with an ever-expanding repertoire of applications. As more CRISPR-Cas9 research is conducted, investigators will shine light on how to improve on-target specificity and better detect off-target effects.

Conflicts of Interest

Stephen H. Tsang receives financial support from Abeona Therapeutics, Inc and Emendo. He is also the founder of Rejuvitas and is on the scientific and clinical advisory board for Nanoscope Therapeutics.

References

1. Jinek M et al (2012) A programmable dual-RNA-guided DNA endonuclease in adaptive bacterial immunity. Science 337(6096): 816–821
2. Sander JD, Joung JK (2014) CRISPR-Cas systems for editing, regulating and targeting genomes. Nat Biotechnol 32(4):347–355
3. Hsu PD et al (2013) DNA targeting specificity of RNA-guided Cas9 nucleases. Nat Biotechnol 31(9):827–832
4. Koo T, Lee J, Kim JS (2015) Measuring and reducing off-target activities of programmable nucleases including CRISPR-Cas9. Mol Cells 38(6):475–481
5. Cho SW et al (2014) Analysis of off-target effects of CRISPR/Cas-derived RNA-guided endonucleases and nickases. Genome Res 24(1):132–141
6. Urnov FD et al (2005) Highly efficient endogenous human gene correction using designed zinc-finger nucleases. Nature 435(7042): 646–651
7. Kim D et al (2015) Digenome-seq: genome-wide profiling of CRISPR-Cas9 off-target effects in human cells. Nat Methods 12(3):237–243. 1 p following 243
8. Chiarle R et al (2011) Genome-wide translocation sequencing reveals mechanisms of chromosome breaks and rearrangements in B cells. Cell 147(1):107–119
9. Frock RL et al (2015) Genome-wide detection of DNA double-stranded breaks induced by engineered nucleases. Nat Biotechnol 33(2):179–186
10. Martin F et al (2016) Biased and unbiased methods for the detection of off-target cleavage by CRISPR/Cas9: an overview. Int J Mol Sci 17(9):1507
11. Tsai SQ et al (2015) GUIDE-seq enables genome-wide profiling of off-target cleavage

by CRISPR-Cas nucleases. Nat Biotechnol 33(2):187–197
12. Crosetto N et al (2013) Nucleotide-resolution DNA double-strand break mapping by next-generation sequencing. Nat Methods 10(4):361–365
13. Zhang XH et al (2015) Off-target effects in CRISPR/Cas9-mediated genome engineering. Mol Ther Nucl Acids 4:e264
14. Zischewski J, Fischer R, Bortesi L (2017) Detection of on-target and off-target mutations generated by CRISPR/Cas9 and other sequence-specific nucleases. Biotechnol Adv 35(1):95–104
15. Kim E et al (2012) Precision genome engineering with programmable DNA-nicking enzymes. Genome Res 22(7):1327–1333
16. Ran FA et al (2013) Double nicking by RNA-guided CRISPR Cas9 for enhanced genome editing specificity. Cell 154(6):1380–1389
17. Mali P et al (2013) CAS9 transcriptional activators for target specificity screening and paired nickases for cooperative genome engineering. Nat Biotechnol 31(9):833–838
18. Kim S et al (2014) Highly efficient RNA-guided genome editing in human cells via delivery of purified Cas9 ribonucleoproteins. Genome Res 24(6):1012–1019
19. Zuris JA et al (2015) Cationic lipid-mediated delivery of proteins enables efficient protein-based genome editing in vitro and in vivo. Nat Biotechnol 33(1):73–80
20. Ramakrishna S et al (2014) Gene disruption by cell-penetrating peptide-mediated delivery of Cas9 protein and guide RNA. Genome Res 24(6):1020–1027
21. Waltz E (2018) With a free pass, CRISPR-edited plants reach market in record time. Nat Biotechnol 36(1):6–7

Chapter 27

Generation of Human iPSC-Derived Retinal Organoids for Assessment of AAV-Mediated Gene Delivery

Amy Tso, Bruna Lopes da Costa, Alexandra Fehnel, Sarah R. Levi, Laura A. Jenny, Sara D. Ragi, Yao Li, and Peter M. J. Quinn

Abstract

Human retinal organoids derived from induced pluripotent stem cells (iPSCs) serve as a promising preclinical model for testing the safety and efficacy of viral gene therapy. Retinal organoids recapitulate the stratified multilayered epithelium structure of the developing and maturating human retina. As such, retinal organoids are unique tools to model retinal disease and to test therapeutic interventions toward their amelioration. Here, we describe a method for the generation of human iPSC-derived retinal organoids and how they can be utilized for the assessment of recombinant adeno-associated viral (rAAV)-mediated gene delivery.

Key words Adeno-associated virus (AAV), 3D retinal organoids, Retinal pigment epithelium (RPE), Induced pluripotent stem cells (iPSCs), AMASS (agarose microwell array seeding and scraping), Transgene expression assay, Gene therapy, Cell tropism

1 Introduction

Successful translation of safe and effective viral gene therapy from preclinical models to human clinical trials depends on a model's ability to recapitulate human biology. Human induced pluripotent stem cell (iPSC)-derived retinal organoids can recapitulate human retinogenesis and thus mimic, in part, the structure and function of the developing and maturating human retina. Retinal organoids not only host all the major neuronal and glial retinal cell types but also reflect the multilayered structure of the human retina [1–3]. Organoids and engineered microfluidic organo-on-chips are sensitive, quantitative, and scalable phenotypic assays, acting as clinically relevant surrogates for the evaluation of therapeutics [4]. Human iPSC-derived retinal organoids can serve as alternatives or replacements for existing preclinical models in order to expedite the drug development

Stephen H. Tsang and Peter M. J. Quinn (eds.), *Retinitis Pigmentosa*,
Methods in Molecular Biology, vol. 2560, https://doi.org/10.1007/978-1-0716-2651-1_27,

timeline and save resources. Preclinical models, such as two-dimensional (2D) cell cultures and animal models, are unable to fully recapitulate the complex cellular interactions and molecular mechanisms of the healthy and diseased human retina to the same extent as human retinal organoids [5, 6].

Patient iPSC-derived retinal organoids have been utilized to model a plethora of human retinal diseases, including retinitis pigmentosa (RP) and Leber congenital amaurosis (LCA). To a point, patient iPSC-derived retinal organoids mimic the in vivo pathophysiology of the patient's retinal disease in vitro (for review, *see* [6]) [7–17]. This is significant as disease progression and phenotypes can differ from patient to patient due to individual genetics and exposure to varying environmental factors. The patient iPSC-derived retinal organoids inherently account for personal genetic factors that influence disease pathology, while environmental stressors can be added to the culture media [5]. Healthy iPSC-derived retinal organoids from age- and sex-matched donors without retinal diseases are used as controls. Nonetheless, the generation of isogenic controls to circumvent genetic variations should be considered. As such, teams are going beyond studying disease pathogenesis by using CRISPR/Cas9 technology to correct the patient mutations in iPSCs to test whether the differentiated organoids would restore healthy phenotypes [18–20].

However, for the development of translational therapies, targeting treatment to post-mitotic retinal cell types would be ideal. Recombinant adeno-associated virus (rAAV) vectors are the leading platform for in vivo delivery of gene therapies to human retinal cell types. The clinical success of rAAV-mediated gene therapeutics for the eye can be partly attributed to rAAVs low immunogenicity and cytotoxicity profile; the relatively limited amount of rAAV needed for transduction of the retina and retinal pigment epithelium (RPE); and the immune-privileged status of the eye. Furthermore, both dividing and non-dividing cells, such as photoreceptors, can be transduced by rAAV [2, 21]. Human retinal organoids are being widely implemented to assess cell tropism, transduction efficiency, and transgene expression levels of rAAV-mediated gene therapy vectors, testing various serotype/promoter combinations [10, 15, 22–26]. Previously, the Wijnholds Lab hypothesized that photoreceptor cell transduction by AAV5, AAV9, and ShH10Y445F occurs once photoreceptor segments have sufficiently matured. Therefore, cell tropism would be based on the bioavailability of receptors for AAV uptake [15]. More recently, Garita-Hernandez et al. tested the early transduction efficiency of several AAV serotypes in retinal organoids and found that transduction efficiency was correlated with the expression of the AAVs corresponding cell surface receptor [22]. Here, we used AAV8(Y733F)-CMV-GFP and found limited peripheral expression in early retinal organoids. However, in older retinal organoids, we found expression of both the inner and outer nuclear layers by AAV8(Y733F)-CMV-GFP.

In this chapter, we describe the differentiation of iPSCs to form embryoid bodies, followed by their development to neuroepithelium, and ultimately maturating retinal organoids. Thereafter, the retinal organoids are infected with rAAV, fixed, embedded, and immunostained to assess the cell tropism, transduction efficiency, and transgene expression level of the viral vector.

2 Materials

2.1 Cell Culture and Reagents

1. iPSCs (*see* **Note 1**).
2. Matrigel.
3. mTeSR plus (StemCell Technologies).
4. ReLeSR (StemCell Technologies).
5. CryoStor CS10 (StemCell Technologies).
6. mTeSR plus/blebbistatin: 0.4-μL blebbistatin add to 2 mL mTeSR plus. The final concentration should be 10 μM diluted from a 50 mM (−)-blebbistatin stock in DMSO (*see* **Note 2**).
7. DMEM/F12: L-glutamine, sodium bicarbonate.
8. DMEM: D-glucose, L-glutamine, sodium pyruvate.
9. F12: L-glutamine.
10. FBS (Fetal Bovine Serum), ES Cell Qualified.
11. NIM1 (neural induction medium 1) (50 mL): 48.99-mL DMEM/F12, 10-μL 10-mg/mL heparin (final concentration, 2 μg/mL), 0.5-mL Media-Non-Essential Amino Acids (100×, MEM NEAA), 0.5-mL N2 supplement (100×), sterile filter; store at 4 °C ≤ 1 month.
12. NIM2 (neural induction medium 2) (50 mL): 48-mL DMEM/ F12 (3:1), 0.5-mL MEM NEAA, 1-mL B27 Supplement (50×, minus vitamin A), 0.5-mL Penicillin-Streptomycin (P/S, 10,000 U/mL), sterile filter; store at 4 °C ≤ 1 month.
13. RLM1 (retinal lamination medium 1) (50 mL): 42.9-mL DMEM/ F12 (3:1), 0.1-mL taurine (100-μM final concentration), 5-mL FBS, 1-mL B27, 0.5-mL MEM NEAA, 0.5-mL P/S, sterile filter; store at 4 °C ≤ 1 month.
14. RLM2 (retinal lamination medium 2) (50 mL): RLM1 supplemented with 0.1 μL per mL of 10 mM retinoic acid.
15. RLM3 (retinal lamination medium 3) (50 mL): RLM1 without B27, replaced with N2 supplement and retinoic acid reduced to 0.05 μL per mL.
16. DPBS (Dulbecco's phosphate buffered saline).

17. 15% and 30% (wt/vol) sucrose solution in PBS.
18. 4% Paraformaldehyde (PFA) solution in PBS.
19. OCT compound.
20. Poly-HEMA (Poly 2-hydroxyethyl methacrylate) coated plates (50 mL): Add 1 g of poly-HEMA to 50-mL 95% EtOH and dissolve at 65 °C with agitation overnight (20 mg/mL solution). Cool and store at room temperature. Add 700 μL per well of solution for a 6-well plate and dry overnight in laminar flowhood. Plates can be stored long term at room temperature when Parafilm wrapped.
21. Agarose.
22. Agarose microwell arrays: Add 2 g of agarose to 100-mL ddH_20 and dissolve in autoclave (2% agarose w/v solution). Keep warm, and in a laminar flowhood add 500 μL of solution to each "MicroTissues 3D Petri Dish micro-mold spheroids" mold. After agarose microwell array molds solidify, transfer each mold to a well each to a 12-well plate. Add 1.5-μL mTeSR medium per well with agarose microwell array mold. Agarose microwell arrays can be stored for several weeks in plates at 4 °C when Parafilm wrapped.

2.2 Equipment

1. Incubator (humidified, 37 °C, 5% CO_2).
2. Laminar flow hood, class II.
3. 37 °C bead bath/water bath.
4. Inverted light microscope.
5. Fluorescent microscope.
6. Cryovials.
7. 10 × 10 × 5 mm Specimen Cryomold® Biopsy.
8. Sterile filters 0.22 μm.
9. Serological pipettes.
10. Filter tips.
11. Centrifuge tubes.
12. 6-well plates.
13. 24-well plates.
14. 96-well plates.
15. Curved tweezers.
16. Cryostat.
17. MicroTissues 3D Petri Dish micro-mold spheroids (Sigma-Aldrich).
18. Cell counter.

3 Methods

3.1 Human Pluripotent Stem Cell Culture (See Note 2)

All iPSC lines should be checked for their genome integrity (karyotype), pluripotency, and ability to form all three germ layers (ectoderm, mesoderm, endoderm) before beginning the differentiation protocol (*see* Fig. 1).

3.1.1 Matrigel Coating

1. Thaw one aliquot of Matrigel on ice (*see* **Note 3**).
2. Pre-cool 50-mL falcon tube, 1-mL and 10-mL serological pipette tips in −20 °C.
3. Transfer 25 mL of 4 °C DMEM/F12 to the pre-cooled 50-mL falcon tube.
4. Transfer 1 mL of the 25-mL 4 °C DMEM/F12 to Matrigel aliquot and then transfer entire contents back to the 50-mL falcon tube. Briefly vortex.
5. Using the pre-cooled 10-mL serological pipette, quickly add 1 mL per well of a 6-well plate.
6. Incubate at room temperature for 1 h before use (*see* **Note 4**).
7. Remove excess Matrigel DMEM/F12 mix from well before adding mTeSR plus medium and seeding iPSCs.

3.1.2 Cell Thawing

1. Prewarm mTeSR plus medium to room temperature.
2. Thaw cells quickly in a 37 °C bead bath with occasional gentle mixing.
3. When only a very small amount of ice is left, transfer to 15-mL conical tube and dilute with 10 mL of prewarmed mTeSR plus medium.
4. Centrifuge the suspension of cells for 5 min at 300 × g at room temperature.
5. Aspirate medium without disturbing cell pellet and resuspend in 2-mL mTeSR plus medium with rock inhibitor Y27632 with a final concentration of 1 μM per 1 mL (*see* **Note 5**).
6. Transfer 2 mL to a Matrigel-coated well of a 6-well plate. Distribute iPSC aggregates by agitating the plate in a side-to-side and back-to-front motion in the incubator. Incubate the plate at 37 °C, 5% CO_2.

3.1.3 Cell Passaging

1. Prewarm mTeSR plus medium and Matrigel-coated 6-well plates to room temperature.
2. Aspirate medium from each well and add 1 mL of DPBS to wash cells.
3. Aspirate DPBS from each well and add 1 mL of ReLeSR.
4. Aspirate ReLeSR after 1 min, leaving a thin film over the induced pluripotent colonies.

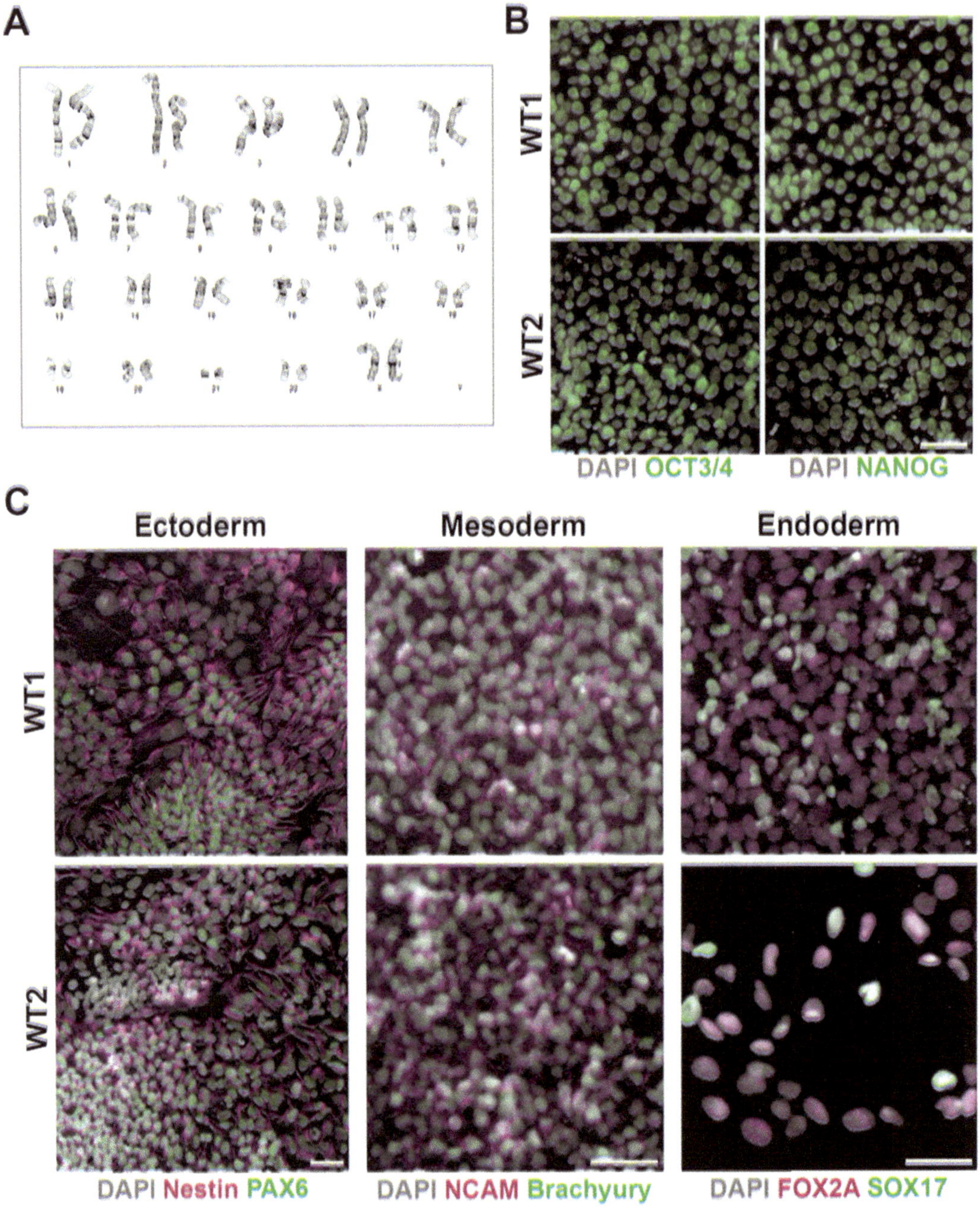

Fig. 1 Verification of induced pluripotent stem cell (iPSC) genome integrity, pluripotency, and germ layer formation. To verify genome integrity, iPSC lines were analyzed by G-band karyotyping (Cell Line Genetics) (**a**). Pluripotency of iPSC lines was confirmed by immunohistochemistry using markers Oct3/4 and Nanog (**b**). Germ layer potential of iPSC was confirmed by immunohistochemistry: ectoderm (Nestin and Pax6), mesoderm (Brachyury and NCAM), and endoderm (FOX2A and Sox17) (**c**). Scale bars, 50 μm

5. Incubate cultures at 37 °C for 6 min (*see* **Note 6**).
6. Add 1 mL per well of prewarmed mTeSR plus medium.
7. Detach colonies by tapping the side of the plate while firmly gripping the plate with opposite hand. Tap for approximately 30–60 s to dislodge colonies; differentiated cells will remain attached to well (*see* **Note** 7).
8. Transfer the dislodged iPSC aggregates to a 15-mL tube using a 5-mL serological pipette. Pipette gently to get ideal aggregate size of between 50 and 200 μm.
9. Plate aggregates at desired density, typically 1 in 10 to 1 in 50. Distribute aggregates by agitating the plate in a side-to-side and back-to-front motion in the incubator. Incubate the plate at 37 °C, 5% CO_2.
10. Leave the plate in the incubator and do not disturb the next day. Subsequently, continue with normal medium changing and monitor cell growth.

3.1.4 Cryopreservation

1. Spin down iPSC aggregates from **step 8** of Subheading 3.1.3 in the 15-mL conical tube for 5 min at 300 × g at room temperature.
2. Aspirate medium without disturbing cell pellet.
3. Add 1 mL of cold CryoStor CS10, gently flick tube to resuspend pellet, and transfer suspension to a cryovial.
4. Incubate cells in cryovial for 10 min at 2–8 °C.
5. Cryopreserve cells using an isopropanol freezing container and place in −80 °C overnight.
6. For long-term storage, move to −135 °C liquid nitrogen storage container.

3.2 Retinal Organoid Differentiation and Long-Term Culture

Retinal organoid differentiation from human iPSCs was performed as previously described with minor modifications (*see* Fig. 2a) [3, 15, 25]. Some technical modifications were also introduced for mechanical dissociation of iPSCs into evenly sized fragments (*see* Subheading 3.2.1) and for retinal organoid detachment (*see* Subheading 3.2.3) [27, 28]. Additionally, we describe our implementation of agarose microwell array seeding and scraping (AMASS) method for embryoid body generation and retinal organoid detachment [27].

3.2.1 Day 0: Embryoid Body Production

1. Prewarm mTeSR plus medium, add blebbistatin for a final concentration of 10 μM.
2. Using 90% confluent iPSCs (*see* **Note 8**), create an approximately 1–1.5 mm^2 checkerboard-scrapping pattern with a 200-μl pipette tip (*see* **Notes 9** and **10** and Fig. 2b).
3. Use a cell scraper to lift the iPSC colony fragments (*see* Fig. 2c) and transfer to a 15-mL conical tube to sink by gravity. Aspirate medium.

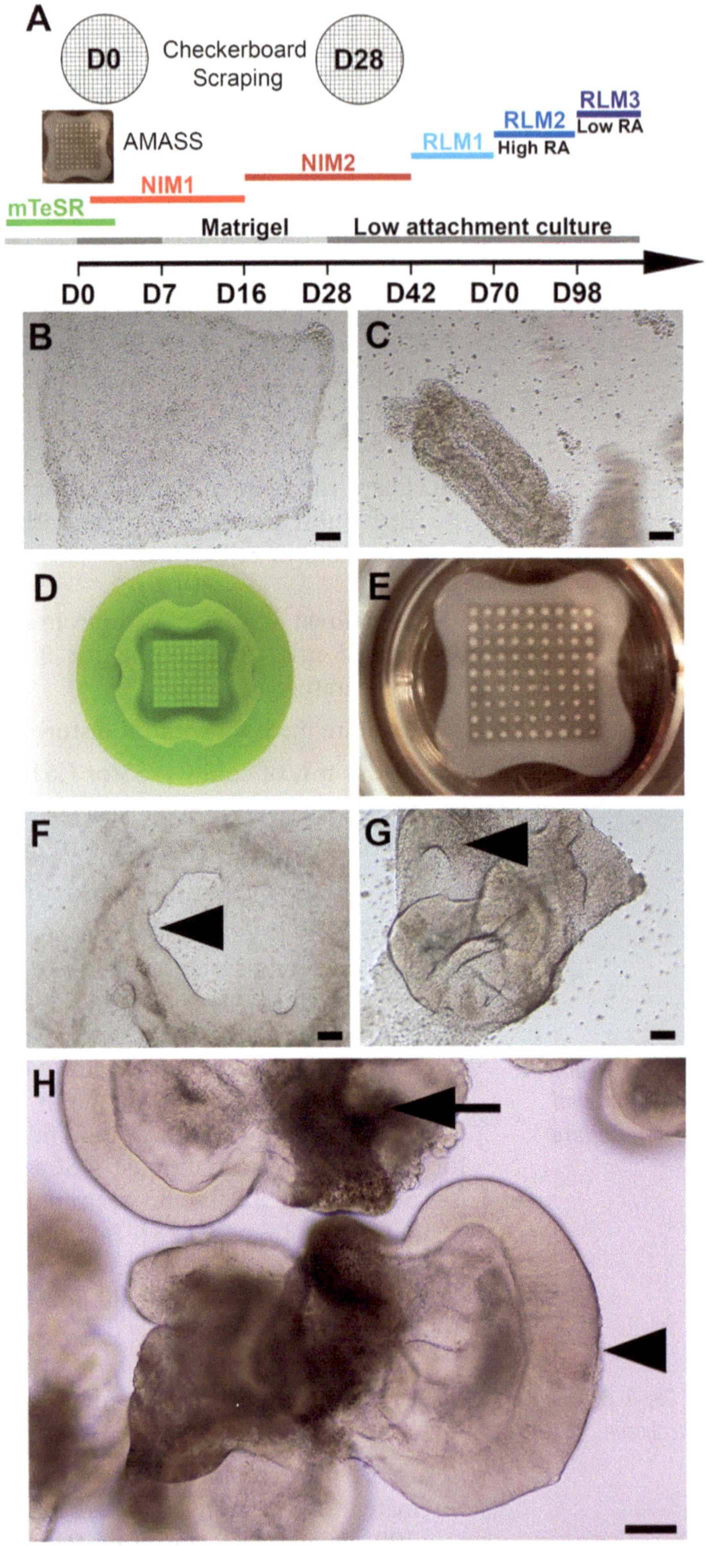

Fig. 2 Timeline of differentiation from human induced pluripotent stem cells (hiPSCs) to retinal organoid models (**a**). hiPSCs cultured on Matrigel are

4. Add 2 mL of blebbistatin/mTeSR plus medium and plate in 1 well of a poly-HEMA coated 6-well plate. Incubate the plate at 37 °C, 5% CO_2 overnight.
5. Exchange one third of medium with NIM1 on day 1. Incubate the plate at 37 °C, 5% CO_2 overnight.
6. Exchange one third of medium with NIM1 on day 2. Incubate the plate at 37 °C, 5% CO_2 overnight.
7. Transfer embryoid bodies to a 15-mL conical tube to sink by gravity and aspirate medium. Add 2 mL of NIM1 medium and plate in 1 well of a poly-HEMA coated 6-well plate (*see* **Note 11**).
8. Exchange half of medium daily until day 7 (*see* Fig. 2a).

3.2.2 Alternative Embryoid Body Production Method: AMASS (Agarose Microwell Array Seeding and Scraping)

1. Prewarm agarose microwell arrays made from micro-molds (*see* Fig. 2d) in 12-well plates in incubator at 37 °C and aspirate medium before cell seeding.
2. Prewarm mTeSR plus medium, add blebbistatin for a final concentration of 10 mM.
3. Using 90% confluent iPSCs (*see* **Note 8**) use ReLeSR (*see* Subheading 3.1.3) to dislodge iPSC aggregates and transfer to 15-mL tube for cell counting.
4. Seed cells (at 1000 to 3000 cells per microwell) onto agarose microwell arrays by transferring 150 μL of blebbistatin/mTeSR plus medium into the top of each agarose micro-mold in a 12-well plate.
5. Incubate at 37 °C, 5% CO_2, for 30 min to allow the cells to settle in the microwells.

Fig. 2 (continued) checkerboard scraped at day 0 (**b**), lifted with a cell scraper (**c**), and upon addition of blebbistatin form embryoid bodies (EBs) in low attachment conditions. Alternatively, EBs can be generated using the agarose microwell array seeding and scraping (AMASS) method using micro-molds (**d**, **e**). During the initial 3 days, they are transitioned from mTeSR plus, day 0, to neural induction medium 1 (NIM1), day 3, by performing one third medium exchanges on days 1 and 2. At day 7, the EBs are plated on Matrigel-coated wells and differentiated toward neuroepithelium; medium is changed to NIM2 on day 16. On day 28, clear neuroepithelium (arrowheads) have formed (**f**), checkerboard scrapping and lifting with a cell scraper is performed (**g**). From this point forward, retinal organoids are cultured under low attachment conditions. Between days 30 and 40, retinal organoids are sorted from other cellular debris and organoid structures to leave retinal organoids (arrowhead) with attached retinal pigment epithelium (arrow) (**h**). At day 42, retinal lamination medium (RLM1) is used to encourage further maturation, and subsequently, at day 70 (RLM2) and day 98 (RLM3), different amounts of retinoic acid are used to promote photoreceptor cell type specification. Scale bars: 100 μm

6. Add 1.5 mL of blebbistatin/mTeSR plus medium per well in 12-well plate to completely cover each cell seeded agarose mold. Incubate the plate at 37 °C, 5% CO_2 overnight (*see* Fig. 2e).
7. Exchange one third of medium with NIM1 on day 1. Incubate the plate at 37 °C, 5% CO_2 overnight.
8. Exchange one third of medium with NIM1 on day 2. Incubate the plate at 37 °C, 5% CO_2 overnight.
9. Exchange majority of medium with NIM1 on days 3, leave enough not to disturb embryoid bodies, and subsequently exchange half of medium daily until day 7 (*see* Fig. 2a). Incubate the plate at 37 °C, 5% CO_2.

3.2.3 Day 7: Transfer Embryoid Bodies to Matrigel-Coated Plates

1. Transfer embryoid bodies to a 15-mL conical tube to sink by gravity and aspirate medium.
2. Resuspend embryoid bodies in 500 μL and transfer to Matrigel-coated 6-well plates that contain 2 mL of NIM1 per well.
3. Adequately distribute the embryoid bodies evenly in the 6-well plate wells (*see* **Note 12**) and incubate the plate at 37 °C, 5% CO_2. Exchange medium daily (*see* **Note 13**).
4. On day 16, change from NIM1 to NIM2 medium, and incubate at 37 °C, 5% CO_2. Exchange medium daily until day 28 (*see* Fig. 2a).

3.2.4 Day 28: Retinal Organoid Detachment and Sorting

1. Perform checkerboard scrapping (*see* **Note 14**), as in **step 2** of Subheading 3.1.1, on the neuroepithelium structures attached to Matrigel-coated wells (*see* Fig. 2f).
2. Use a cell scraper to lift the entire contents (*see* Fig. 2g) of 1-well of a 6-well plate and transfer to a 15-mL conical tube to sink by gravity.
3. Aspirate medium and wash three times with PBS, letting contents sink by gravity each time.
4. Resuspend contents with 2 mL of NIM2 and plate on 1-well of a Poly-HEMA coated 6-well plate and incubate the plate at 37 °C, 5% CO_2.
5. Change NIM2 medium every other day and incubate the plate at 37 °C, 5% CO_2.
6. Between days 30 and 40, phase-bright and stratified neuroepithelium, typically with attached RPE, should be sorted from other structures and debris using an inverted light microscope (*see* Fig. 2h).

3.2.5 Day 42: Retinal Organoid Maturation and Maintenance (See **Notes 15** and **16**)

From the maturation stage, a Monday, Wednesday, Friday medium changing schedule can be utilized. Retinal organoids can be double fed for over the weekend cell culture.

1. On day 42, switch to retinal lamination medium 1 (RLM1).
2. On day 70, switch to RLM2.
3. On day 98, switch to RLM3 (*see* Fig. 2a).

3.3 AAV Transduction of Retinal Organoids and Accompanying Retinal Pigment Epithelium

The use of adeno-associated virus (AAV) for labeling off or delivery to retinal cells is also amenable in retinal organoids. A number of serotypes have been successfully used including AAV2/2, AAV2/5, AAV2-7 m8, AAV2/8, AAV2/9, and AAV6 variant serotype ShH10Y445F for infection of photoreceptors or Müller glial cells [15, 23, 24]. AAV expression levels will vary depending on the capsid used and should be optimized for your choice of capsid and retinal organoid differentiation stage. In our example, we infected day 44 and day 140 retinal organoids with AAV8 (Y733F)-CMV-GFP and analyzed GFP expression 21 days and 16 days later, respectively (*see* Figs. 3). Furthermore, we infected day 44 RPE spheroids with AAV8(Y733F)-CMV-GFP and analyzed GFP expression 21 days (*see* Figs. 4).

1. Thaw purchased or prepared AAV construct.
2. Add your AAV to 50 μL of media; chose medium suitable for the retinal organoids age. Use a final concentration of at least 1×10^{10} genome copies.
3. Transfer two retinal organoids to one well of a 96-well plate and aspirate medium.
4. Resuspend retinal organoid with the 50 μL of virus/medium suspension from **step 2** and incubate at 37 °C, 5% CO_2 for 24 h.
5. Transfer both retinal organoids to a 15-mL conical tube to sink by gravity. Aspirate medium and wash three times using 5-mL DPBS per wash.
6. Resuspend in 2 mL of retinal organoid age appropriate medium and transfer to an agarose coated well of a 24-well plate.
7. Change medium according to medium schedule for retinal organoid age.
8. If using an AAV which express GFP, expression levels can be monitored using a fluorescent microscope. When AAV infected organoids have reach desired stage, they can be harvested for immunohistochemistry or other desired downstream analysis.

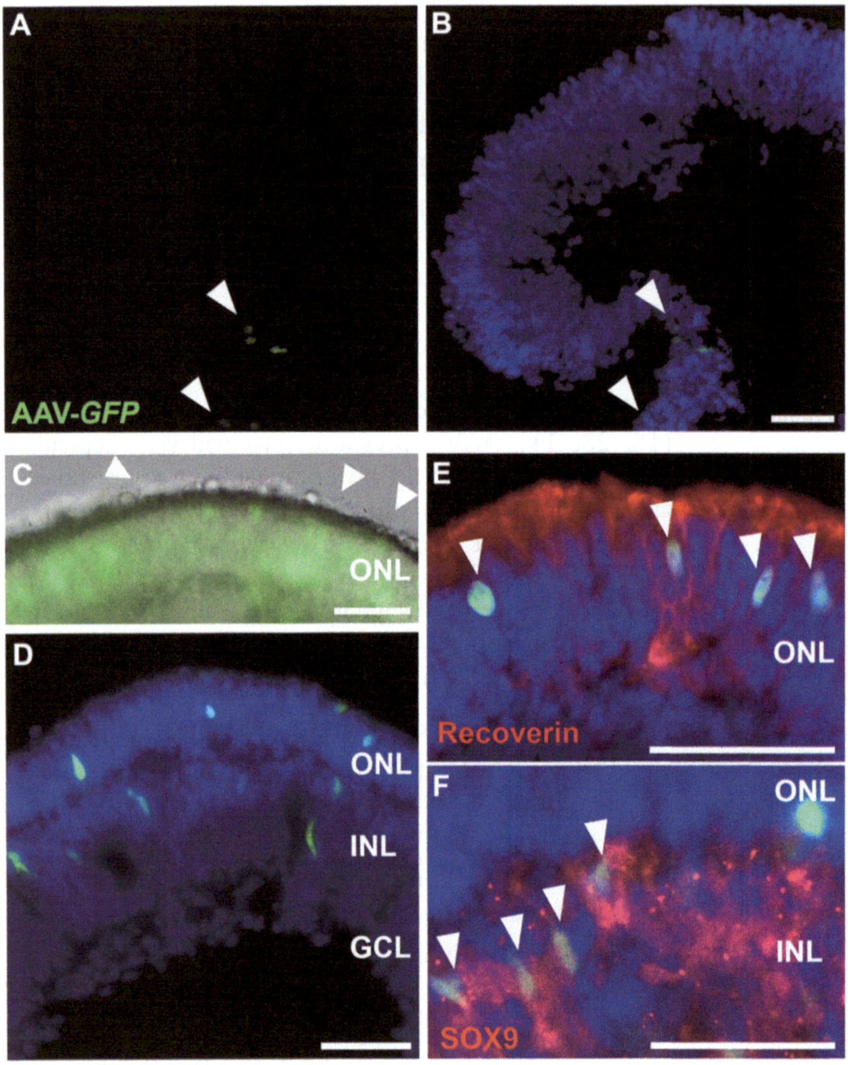

Fig. 3 Adeno-associated virus (AAV) infected human induced pluripotent stem cell (hiPSC)-derived retinal organoids. Retinal organoids infected with AAV8(Y733F)-CMV-GFP (green) at differentiation day 44 (**a**, **b**) analyzed 21 days later (DD65) and at differentiation day 140 (**c**–**f**) analyzed 16 days later (DD156). The GFP expression (**a**) overlaps with the periphery of the early retinal organoid (arrowheads **b**). Bright-field image showing GFP expression in late retinal organoid; segments can be detected (arrowheads, **c**). GFP expression is found in both the outer nuclear layer (ONL) and inner nuclear layer (INL) (**d**). GFP expression overlaps with recoverin staining (red) in the ONL, arrowheads (**e**). GFP expression overlaps with Sox9 staining (red) in the INL (arrowheads, **f**). ONL, outer nuclear layer; INL, inner nuclear layer; GCL, ganglion cell layer. Scale bars: 50 μm

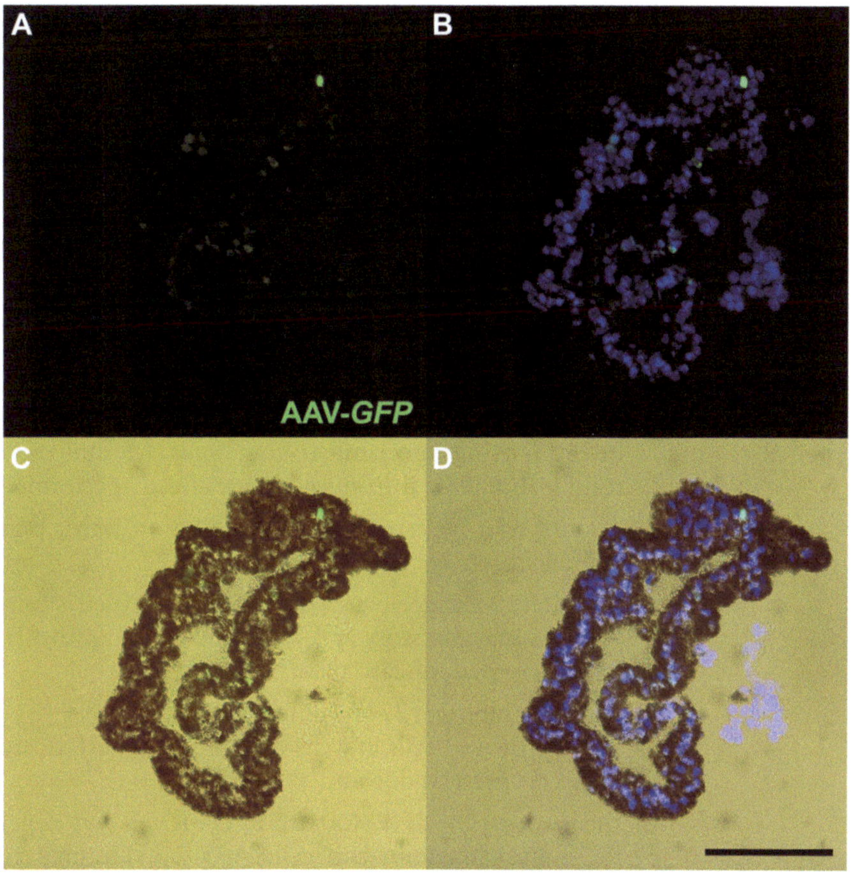

Fig. 4 Adeno-associated virus (AAV) infected human induced pluripotent stem cell (hiPSC)-derived retinal pigment epithelium (RPE). RPE infected with AAV8(Y733F)-CMV-GFP at differentiation day 44 and analyzed 21 days later (DD65). The GFP expression (**a**) overlaps with several pigmented RPE cells (**b–d**). Scale bar: 100 μm

3.4 Harvesting Retinal Organoids for Immunohistochemistry

1. Transfer desired number of retinal organoids to a 15-mL conical tube and aspirate medium.
2. Wash three times with 5 mL DPBS.
3. Fix retinal organoids in 1 mL of 4% PFA for 30 min at room temperature and subsequently wash once with 5-mL DPBS.
4. Aspirate DPBS and incubate retinal organoids in 1 mL of 15% sucrose for 30 min. Retinal organoids should sink to the bottom of the tube.
5. Aspirate 15% sucrose and incubate retinal organoids in 1 mL of 30% sucrose for 30 min. Retinal organoids should sink to the bottom of the tube.
6. Transfer retinal organoids in minimal amount of 30% sucrose to cryomold. Aspirate 30% sucrose (*see* **Note 17**).
7. Add OCT to cryomold, and using curved tweezer, gently mix and then position central and to the bottom of cryomold the retinal organoids.

8. Freeze retinal organoids over dry ice and store at −20 °C until ready for sectioning. For longer-term storage, place in −80 °C. Cut section on cryostat at 8–10 μm.

4 Notes

1. In this protocol, we used two previously validated and published wild-type iPSC lines [29, 30].
2. Perform all iPSC, medium and retinal organoid handling using a laminar flow hood except if stipulated. Follow sterile technique whiles culturing to prevent contamination, i.e., wipe down all medium bottles and plastic ware with 70% ethanol before moving into laminar flow hood. Monthly mycoplasma testing should be introduced if not already performed.
3. Aliquot Matrigel stock based on dilution factor provided by manufacturer.
4. If coated Matrigel plates are not to be used straight away, Parafilm seal and store at 4 °C for up to 3 months. If medium has evaporated, discard plate.
5. ROCK inhibitor Y27632 enhances iPSC survival [31]. Typical start up thawed cells in wells with the same surface area as they were cryopreserved from.
6. Incubation time of iPSCs with ReLeSR will vary depending on the culture medium and cell line used. Optimal conditions should be investigated prior to differentiation procedure.
7. Alternatively, a plate vortexer can be used if available.
8. Prior to start of the experiment, remove any differentiated areas by scraping with a pipette tip.
9. The mechanical method of embryoid body generation under static conditions using ROCK inhibitor Y27632 has been identified to lead to consistent formation of laminated retinal neuroepithelium with photoreceptors that exhibit mature electrophysiological responses [28]. In this protocol, we use blebbistatin instead of Y27632; blebbistatin acts downstream of ROCK inhibition.
10. Alternatively, a stem cell passaging tool may be utilized for scoring colonies leading to evenly sized fragments [27].
11. Commercial, poly-HEMA or agarose-coated well low attachment plates can be used.
12. Even distribution can be achieved by agitating the plate in a side-to-side and back-to-front motion.
13. Full medium change is not required; leave a small amount of medium in well.
14. Checkerboard scrapping used as alternative to microdissection using a needle point or 1000-μl pipette tip. The procedure is

faster than manual microdissection; non-neuroepithelium debris is removed during the sorting procedure [27].

15. Recent publications have highlighted the use of reagents such as 9-cis-retinal, 11-cis-retinal, levodopa, triiodothyronine, and DAPT for the generation of retinal organoids enriched for photoreceptor subtypes [32, 33].
16. Retinal organoid number per 1 well of a poly-HEMA coated 6-well plate should be optimized to limit retinal organoid merging in early stage lifted and sorted retinal organoids.
17. It is important to remove all excess 30% sucrose as remaining water content may cause freezing artifacts in retinal organoid tissue.

Acknowledgement

B.L.D.C. is a recipient of the Capes PhD scholarship. Jonas Children's Vision Care is supported by the National Institute of Health 5P30CA013696, U01 EY030580, U54OD020351, R24EY028758, R24EY027285, 5P30EY019007, R01EY018213, R01EY024698, R01EY026682, R21AG050437, the Schneeweiss Stem Cell Fund, New York State [SDHDOH01-C32590GG-3450000], the Foundation Fighting Blindness New York Regional Research Center Grant [TA-NMT-0116-0692-COLU], Nancy & Kobi Karp, the Crowley Family Funds, The Rosenbaum Family Foundation, Alcon Research Institute, the Gebroe Family Foundation, the Research to Prevent Blindness (RPB) Physician-Scientist Award, unrestricted funds from RPB, New York, NY, USA. P.M.J.Q. is the current recipient of a Curing Retinal Blindness Foundation (CRBF) grant, a Knights Templar Eye Foundation (KTEF) Career Starter grant, the International Retinal Research Foundation (IRRF) Loris and David Rich Postdoctoral Scholar Award and a New York Stem Cell Foundation (NYSCF)—Druckenmiller Fellowship.

Conflicts of Interest

Peter M.J. Quinn receives research support from Rejuvitas, Inc.

References

1. Capowski EE et al (2019) Reproducibility and staging of 3D human retinal organoids across multiple pluripotent stem cell lines. Development 146(1):dev171686
2. Quinn PMJ, Wijnholds J (2019) Retinogenesis of the human fetal retina: an apical polarity perspective. Genes (Basel) 10(12):987
3. Zhong X et al (2014) Generation of three-dimensional retinal tissue with functional photoreceptors from human iPSCs. Nat Commun 5:4047
4. Manafi N et al (2021) Organoids and organ chips in ophthalmology. Ocul Surf 19:1–15

5. Aasen DM, Vergara MN (2020) New drug discovery paradigms for retinal diseases: a focus on retinal organoids. J Ocul Pharmacol Ther 36(1):18–24
6. Artero Castro A et al (2019) Deciphering retinal diseases through the generation of three dimensional stem cell-derived organoids: concise review. Stem Cells 37(12):1496–1504
7. Arno G et al (2016) Mutations in REEP6 cause autosomal-recessive retinitis pigmentosa. Am J Hum Genet 99(6):1305–1315
8. Gao ML et al (2020) Patient-specific retinal organoids recapitulate disease features of late-onset retinitis pigmentosa. Front Cell Dev Biol 8:128
9. Guo Y et al (2019) Modeling retinitis pigmentosa: retinal organoids generated from the iPSCs of a patient with the USH2A mutation show early developmental abnormalities. Front Cell Neurosci 13:361
10. Lane A et al (2020) Modeling and rescue of RP2 retinitis pigmentosa using iPSC-derived retinal organoids. Stem Cell Rep 15(1):67–79
11. Li G et al (2019) Generation and characterization of induced pluripotent stem cells and retinal organoids from a Leber's congenital Amaurosis patient with novel RPE65 mutations. Front Mol Neurosci 12:212
12. Lukovic D et al (2020) Retinal organoids derived from hiPSCs of an AIPL1-LCA patient maintain cytoarchitecture despite reduced levels of mutant AIPL1. Sci Rep 10(1):5426
13. Megaw R et al (2017) Gelsolin dysfunction causes photoreceptor loss in induced pluripotent cell and animal retinitis pigmentosa models. Nat Commun 8(1):271
14. Parfitt DA et al (2016) Identification and correction of mechanisms underlying inherited blindness in human iPSC-derived optic cups. Cell Stem Cell 18(6):769–781
15. Quinn PM et al (2019) Human iPSC-derived retinas recapitulate the fetal CRB1 CRB2 complex formation and demonstrate that photoreceptors and Muller glia are targets of AAV5. Stem Cell Rep 12(5):906–919
16. Sharma TP et al (2017) Patient-specific induced pluripotent stem cells to evaluate the pathophysiology of TRNT1-associated retinitis pigmentosa. Stem Cell Res 21:58–70
17. Shimada H et al (2017) In vitro modeling using ciliopathy-patient-derived cells reveals distinct cilia dysfunctions caused by CEP290 mutations. Cell Rep 20(2):384–396
18. Bohrer LR et al (2019) Correction of NR2E3 associated enhanced S-cone syndrome patient-specific iPSCs using CRISPR-Cas9. Genes (Basel) 10(4):278.
19. Deng WL et al (2018) Gene correction reverses ciliopathy and photoreceptor loss in iPSC-derived retinal organoids from retinitis pigmentosa patients. Stem Cell Rep 10(4): 1267–1281
20. Huang KC et al (2019) Morphological and molecular defects in human three-dimensional retinal organoid model of X-linked juvenile retinoschisis. Stem Cell Rep 13(5):906–923
21. Wang D, Tai PWL, Gao G (2019) Adeno-associated virus vector as a platform for gene therapy delivery. Nat Rev Drug Discov 18(5): 358–378
22. Garita-Hernandez M et al (2020) AAV-mediated gene delivery to 3D retinal organoids derived from human induced pluripotent stem cells. Int J Mol Sci 21(3)
23. Gonzalez-Cordero A et al (2018) Assessment of AAV vector tropisms for mouse and human pluripotent stem cell-derived RPE and photoreceptor cells. Hum Gene Ther 29(10): 1124–1139
24. Khabou H et al (2018) Noninvasive gene delivery to foveal cones for vision restoration. JCI Insight 3(2): e96029.
25. Quinn PM et al (2018) Production of iPS-derived human retinal organoids for use in transgene expression assays. Methods Mol Biol 1715:261–273
26. Tornabene P et al (2019) Intein-mediated protein trans-splicing expands adeno-associated virus transfer capacity in the retina. Sci Transl Med 11(492):eaav4523
27. Cowan CS et al (2020) Cell types of the human retina and its organoids at single-cell resolution. Cell 182(6):1623–1640. e34
28. Mellough CB et al (2019) Systematic comparison of retinal organoid differentiation from human pluripotent stem cells reveals stage specific, cell line, and methodological differences. Stem Cells Transl Med 8(7):694–706
29. Ji C et al (2019) Investigation and restoration of BEST1 activity in patient-derived RPEs with dominant mutations. Sci Rep 9(1):19026
30. Li Y et al (2017) Patient-specific mutations impair BESTROPHIN1's essential role in mediating Ca(2+)-dependent Cl(-) currents in human RPE. elife 6:e29914.
31. Baharvand H et al (2010) An efficient and easy-to-use cryopreservation protocol for human ES and iPS cells. Nat Protoc 5(3):588–594
32. Kaya KD et al (2019) Transcriptome-based molecular staging of human stem cell-derived retinal organoids uncovers accelerated photoreceptor differentiation by 9-cis retinal. Mol Vis 25:663–678
33. Zerti D et al (2020) Developing a simple method to enhance the generation of cone and rod photoreceptors in pluripotent stem cell-derived retinal organoids. Stem Cells 38(1):45–51

Chapter 28

Culture of Human Retinal Explants for Ex Vivo Assessment of AAV Gene Delivery

Wen-Hsuan Wu, Amy Tso, Mark P. Breazzano, Laura A. Jenny, Sarah R. Levi, Stephen H. Tsang, and Peter M. J. Quinn

Abstract

Due to the clinically established safety and efficacy profile of recombinant adeno-associated viral (rAAV) vectors, they are considered the "go to" vector for retinal gene therapy. Design of a rAAV-mediated gene therapy focuses on cell tropism, high transduction efficiency, and high transgene expression levels to achieve the lowest therapeutic treatment dosage and avoid toxicity. Human retinal explants are a clinically relevant model system for exploring these aspects of rAAV-mediated gene delivery. In this chapter, we describe an ex vivo human retinal explant culture protocol to evaluate transgene expression in order to determine the selectivity and efficacy of rAAV vectors for human retinal gene therapy.

Key words Adeno-associated virus (AAV), Cell tropism, Gene therapy, Human retinal explant culture

1 Introduction

Human retinal explants serve as a clinically relevant model for translational research, having been employed for diverse studies including gene expression, angiogenesis, regenerative medicine, and gene therapy [1]. Recombinant adeno-associated virus (AAV)-mediated gene therapy has proven a successful platform toward the amelioration of retinal disease. Luxturna (voretigene neparvovec-rzyl) was the first FDA- and EMA- approved AAV gene therapy for retinitis pigmentosa (RP) and Leber congenital amaurosis (LCA) patients. It restores the production of the RPE65 enzyme to transduced retinal pigment epithelium (RPE) cells [2, 3]. To date, there are several ongoing clinical trials for RP and other retinal disorders, including achromatopsia (*CNGA3, CNGB3*), X-linked retinoschisis (RS1), and choroideremia (*REP1, CHM*) [4].

Stephen H. Tsang and Peter M. J. Quinn (eds.), *Retinitis Pigmentosa*,
Methods in Molecular Biology, vol. 2560, https://doi.org/10.1007/978-1-0716-2651-1_28,

Design of rAAV-mediated gene therapy focuses on cell tropism, transduction efficiency, and transgene expression levels for effective, safe, and on-target gene therapy. Cell tropism, or cell specificity, is crucial as toxicity can occur if the virus enters and enables transgene expression in off-target cells. Promoter choice regulates cell tropism due to the cell-type specificity of promoters; broadly active promoters can induce toxicity [5, 6]. Little is understood about which cellular determinants or AAV structures govern cell tropism. AAV entry receptor (AAVR) and G protein-coupled receptor 108 (GPR108) are essential AAV entry determinants [7, 8]. Furthermore, capsid pseudotype also affects cell tropism due to difference in capsid-specific sugar moieties [9, 10]. AAV vectors should be designed for the smallest number of virions possible to elicit the most effective therapeutic response in a patient. Although the eye is a relatively immune-privileged organ, there have been reports of inflammation and immunogenicity from high doses of AAV vectors during clinical trials [11, 12]. High transduction efficiency and transgene expression levels, coupled with cellular specificity, can lower the dosage needed for therapeutic treatment. Transgene expression levels can be elevated by incorporating *cis*-acting elements, such the bovine growth hormone polyA (bGHpA), SV40 late signal sequences, or the Woodchuck hepatitis virus posttranscriptional regulatory element (WPRE), which enhance transgene expression and prevents transgene silencing [13, 14].

Over the last several years, many AAV gene therapy clinical trials for retinal disorders have failed to reproduce the same levels of efficacy observed in animal models. This translational gap between animal models and human patients can be attributed to species-specific differences in the anatomy and physiology of the eye [1]. The ability of human retinal explants to recapitulate the in vivo conditions of the human retina enables them to serve as a preclinical model capable of evaluating rAAVs and bridging the translational gap from bench to bedside. Preservation, however, of the complex architecture of the retina in vitro is an essential consideration when utilizing this organotypic system, as the explants undergo progressive degeneration in culture [15–17]. Human retinal explants have been widely implemented to validate cell tropism, transduction efficiency, and transgene expression levels of rAAV-mediated gene therapy vectors, testing various serotype/promoter combinations [18–24]. Recently, human retinal explant cultures were used to verify the photoreceptor-specific tropism and transduction efficiency of EDIT-101, a gene-editing therapy for LCA type 10 [25]. EDIT-101 is now undergoing phase I/II clinical trials in 18 LCA type 10 patients [26].

In this chapter, we describe a free-floating organotypic culture system for the ex vivo assessment of rAAV-mediated gene delivery to human retinal biopsy punches. The human retina is extracted from post-retinectomy or post-mortem donor eyes; biopsy punches are made and subsequently preserved in an ex vivo culture media. The retinal biopsy punches are transduced with rAAV vectors carrying a fluorescent reporter gene (i.e., GFP), allowing transduction efficiency, cell tropism, and transgene expression levels to be detected or measured through fluorescence microscopy. Subsequently, switching of the reporter gene with the therapeutic transgene will facilitate the expression of the healthy gene to the target cells of interest.

2 Materials

2.1 Cell Culture and Reagents

1. Retinal Explant Culture Medium (50 mL): 43-mL Neurobasal-A media, 5-mL FBS (Fetal Bovine Serum), ES Cell Qualified, 1-mL B27 Supplement (50×, minus vitamin A), 0.5-mL N2 supplement (100×), 0.5-mL Penicillin-Streptomycin (P/S, 10,000 U/mL), sterile filter; store at 4 °C $\leq$ 2 weeks.
2. DPBS (Dulbecco's phosphate buffered saline).
3. 15% and 30% (wt/vol) sucrose solution in PBS.
4. 4% Paraformaldehyde (PFA) solution in PBS.
5. OCT compound.

2.2 Equipment and Supplies

1. 3-mm-diameter dissecting trephine.
2. Incubator (humidified, 37 °C, 5% CO_2).
3. Laminar flow hood, class II.
4. 37 °C bead bath/water bath.
5. Inverted light microscope.
6. Fluorescence microscope.
7. 10 × 10 × 5 mm Specimen Cryomold® Biopsy.
8. Sterile filters 0.22 μm.
9. Pipette gun and serological pipettes.
10. 15-mL conical tubes.
11. Sterile blade.
12. Sterile scissors.
13. Sterile curved and straight tweezers.
14. Dry ice.
15. Cryotome.
16. Pipettes and filter tips.
17. Filter paper.
18. Petri dish.
19. 24-well plates.
20. 48-well plates.

3 Methods

3.1 Isolation of Human Retina from Eye Cup

These studies are approved by the Columbia University Institutional Review Board (IRB-AAAB6560) and adhere to the guidelines in the Declaration of Helsinki. Donor human eyes were obtained within 16-h post mortem from the Eye-Bank for Sight Restoration, Inc. or within 2 h from patients undergoing enucleation surgery under the auspices of the Department of Pathology in Columbia University Medical Center (*see* **Note 1**).

1. Place the eye in a petri dish.
2. Remove the lens and iris of the donor eye carefully by making a circumferential incision at the pars plana (*see* **Note 2**).
3. Cut small incisions in the peripheral retina to make the eyecup flat. Remove the vitreous as much as possible, with careful attention to minimize traction on the retina (*see* **Note 3**).
4. Detach the retina from the eyecup by cutting the optic nerve. Place the cut between the retina and the RPE (*see* Fig. 1a).

3.2 Culture of Human Retinal Biopsy Punches

As previously described, retinal explant punches are cultured as free-floating preparations being immersed in culture medium with their retinal ganglion cell side facing up [16].

1. Transfer freshly extracted human retinal tissue to a petri dish containing DPBS.
2. Using a 3-mm-diameter dissecting trephine, excise the desired number of punches for downstream analysis (*see* Fig. 1b) (*see* **Notes 4** and **5**).

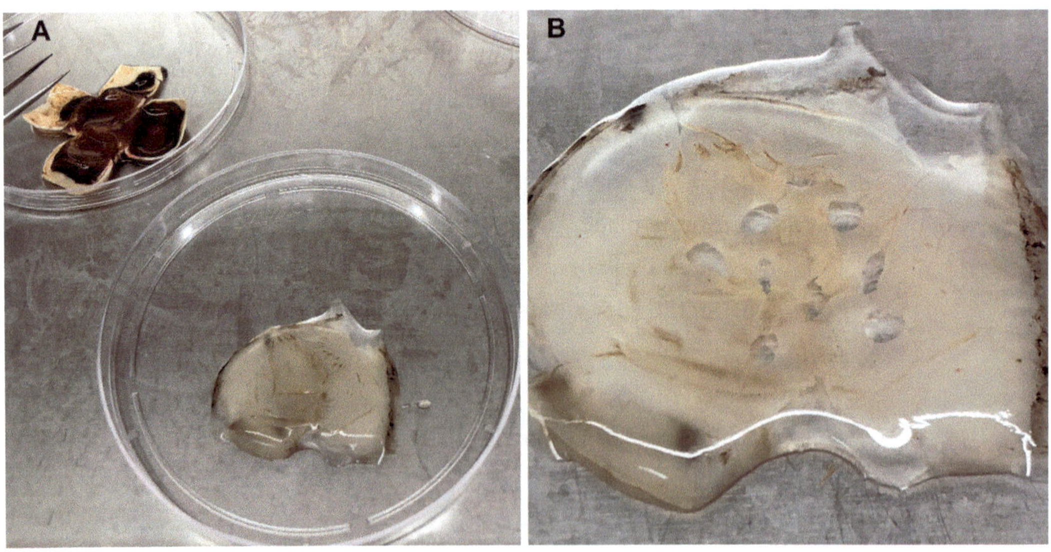

Fig. 1 Isolation of retinal biopsy punches. (**a**) Open and butterfly the eye (top left). Make an excision at the optic nerve between the retina and retinal pigment epithelium to free the tissues. (**b**) Using a 3-mm punch, collect the desired number of retinal biopsies. Group biopsies for cell culture by localization, e.g. central to peripheral

3. Cut a P1000 pipette tip with sterile scissors to allow for a large bore size (*see* **Note 6**).
4. Transfer, using modified P1000 pipette tip, 3-mm retinal explant punches to a 24-well plate and aspirate medium.
5. Resuspend retinal explants with the 500 μL retinal explant medium and incubate at 37 °C, 5% CO_2.
6. Make sure retinal explants are freely floating and immersed in retinal explant medium with ganglion cell side facing up (*see* **Note 7**).
7. Retinal explants are ready for downstream analysis (*see* **Note 8**).

3.3 AAV Transduction of Human Retinal Explants

1. Thaw purchased or prepared AAV construct on ice directly before use.
2. Centrifuge viral suspension and then add the AAV to 200 μL of retinal explant medium. Use a final concentration of at least 1×10^{10} genome copies (*see* **Note 9**).
3. Cut a P1000 pipette tip with sterile scissors to allow for a large bore size (*see* **Note 6**).
4. Transfer two 3-mm retinal explant punches to a 48-well plate and aspirate medium.
5. Resuspend retinal explants with the 200 μL of virus/medium suspension from **step 2** and incubate at 37 °C, 5% CO_2 for 24 h.
6. Transfer both retinal explants to a 15-mL conical tube to sink by gravity using modified P1000 pipette tip. Aspirate medium and wash three times using 5-mL DPBS per wash.
7. Resuspend in 2 mL of retinal explant medium and transfer to a low attachment well of a 24-well plate (*see* **Note 10**).
8. A Monday, Wednesday, Friday medium changing schedule can be utilized (*see* **Note 11**). Retinal explants can be double fed for over the weekend cell culture.
9. If using an AAV that expresses GFP, expression levels can be monitored using a fluorescent microscope (*see* Fig. 2). When the AAV-infected retinal explants have reached the desired stage, they can be harvested for immunohistochemistry or other desired downstream analysis.

3.4 Harvesting Human Retinal Explants for Immunohistochemistry

1. Attach the retinal explants, ganglion side down, to 3-mm filter paper circular punches (*see* **Note 12**).
2. Cut a P1000 pipette tip with sterile scissors to allow for a large bore size (*see* **Note 6**).
3. Transfer the retinal explants, using the modified pipette tip, to a 15-mL conical tube and carefully aspirate medium.

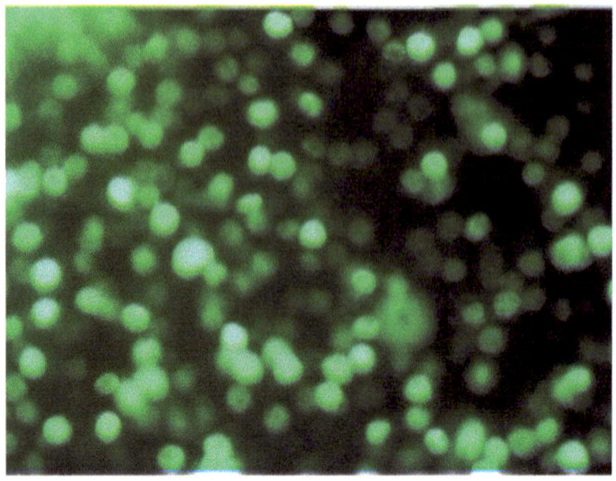

Fig. 2 Live-cell image of retinal biopsy punch transduced with AAV8(Y733F)-CMV-GFP at 7 days post-transfection

4. Fix the retinal explants in 1 mL of 4% PFA for 30 min at room temperature and subsequently wash once with 5-mL DPBS.
5. Aspirate DPBS and incubate the retinal explants in 1 mL of 15% sucrose for 30 min.
6. Aspirate 15% sucrose and incubate the retinal explants in 1 mL of 30% sucrose for 30 min.
7. Transfer retinal explants in a minimal amount of 30% sucrose to the cryomold. Aspirate excess 30% sucrose from the cryomold (*see* **Note 13**).
8. Add OCT to cryomold, and using curved tweezer, gently move the retinal explant in to a central position (*see* **Note 14**).
9. Freeze retinal explants over dry ice and store at −20 °C until ready for sectioning. For longer-term storage, place in −80 °C.
10. Remember to correctly orientate for your needs the frozen retinal explants on the specimen disk. Cut sections on a cryostat at 8–10 μm in thickness and attach to microscope slides.
11. Slides can be stored at −20 °C or −80 °C until needed to for immunohistochemistry.

4 Notes

1. In the human retina, a negative correlation between time after post-mortem and protein abundance has been indicated [27, 28]. It is therefore vital to minimize the time between post-mortem and start of retinal explant culture.
2. Care should be made to minimize collateral trauma to the eye by stabilizing the globe. A sawing-motion for the incision can also help.

3. The posterior hyaloid is often still attached in younger eyes with particularly adherent vitreomacular attachments [29].
4. Note the location from which retinal biopsy punches are excised, e.g., central or peripheral retina.
5. Punches can be collected starting from the fovea and moving out toward the peripheral retina.
6. Make sure the cut is a straight clean cut, and there are no frayed edges that tissue could get caught on.
7. Identification of the retinal ganglion cell side should be straight forward as it will not have the remnants of the retinal pigment epithelium layer attached.
8. Collect an untreated retinal explant prior to continuing with AAV transduction. This control will allow assessment of the extent of retinal degeneration over the 7–14-day culture period post-AAV transduction. Staining of outer segments is a good indication of retinal explant health.
9. AAV serotypes have different transduction efficiencies, also depending on the titer used. These conditions should be optimized for the desired experimental outcome.
10. Commercial, poly-HEMA or agarose coated well low attachment plates can be used. They prevent any sticking of explants to the base of the well.
11. Do not remove all media, to create conditioned medium changes.
12. Attaching the retinal explant to filter paper will minimize tissue folding and therefore improve cryostat sectioning.
13. It is important to remove all excess 30% sucrose as remaining water content may cause freezing artifacts in the retinal explant.
14. When manipulating retinal explant, use filter paper covered side to reduce damage.

Acknowledgement

S.H.T. and Jonas Children's Vision Care is supported by the National Institute of Health 5P30CA013696, U01 EY030580, U54OD020351, R24EY028758, R24EY027285, 5P30EY019007, R01EY018213, R01EY024698, R01EY026682, R21AG050437, the Schneeweiss Stem Cell Fund, New York State [SDHDOH01-C32590GG-3450000], the Foundation Fighting Blindness New York Regional Research Center Grant [TA-NMT-0116-0692-COLU], Nancy & Kobi Karp, the Crowley Family Funds, The Rosenbaum Family Foundation, Alcon Research Institute, the Gebroe Family Foundation, the

Research to Prevent Blindness (RPB) Physician-Scientist Award, unrestricted funds from RPB, New York, NY, USA. P.M.J.Q. is the current recipient of a Curing Retinal Blindness Foundation (CRBF) grant, a Knights Templar Eye Foundation (KTEF) Career Starter grant, the International Retinal Research Foundation (IRRF) Loris and David Rich Postdoctoral Scholar Award and a New York Stem Cell Foundation (NYSCF)—Druckenmiller Fellowship.

Conflict of Interest

Stephen H. Tsang receives financial support from Abeona Therapeutics, Inc and Emendo. He is also the founder of Rejuvitas and is on the scientific and clinical advisory board for Nanoscope Therapeutics. Peter M.J. Quinn receives research support from Rejuvitas, Inc.

References

1. Murali A et al (2019) Retinal explant culture: a platform to investigate human neuro-retina. Clin Exp Ophthalmol 47(2):274–285
2. FDA approves novel gene therapy to treat patients with a rare form of inherited vision loss. 2017 [cited 2020 04-25-2020]; Available from: https://www.fda.gov/news-events/press-announcements/fda-approves-novel-gene-therapy-treat-patients-rare-form-inherited-vision-loss
3. New gene therapy for rare inherited disorder causing vision loss recommended for approval. 2018 [cited 2020 04-25-2020]; Available from: https://www.ema.europa.eu/en/news/new-gene-therapy-rare-inherited-disorder-causing-vision-loss-recommended-approval
4. Alves, C. and J. Wijnholds, AAV-mediated gene therapy for CRB1-hereditary retinopathies.. Intechopen, 2018
5. Castle MJ et al (2016) Controlling AAV tropism in the nervous system with natural and engineered capsids. Methods Mol Biol 1382: 133–149
6. Le Bras A (2019) A look at AAV toxicity in the mouse. Lab Animal 48,142.
7. Pillay S et al (2016) An essential receptor for adeno-associated virus infection. Nature 530(7588):108–112
8. Dudek AM et al (2020) GPR108 is a highly conserved AAV entry factor. Mol Ther 28(2): 367–381
9. Wu Z et al (2006) Alpha2,3 and alpha2,6 N-linked sialic acids facilitate efficient binding and transduction by adeno-associated virus types 1 and 6. J Virol 80(18):9093–9103
10. Kaludov N et al (2001) Adeno-associated virus serotype 4 (AAV4) and AAV5 both require sialic acid binding for hemagglutination and efficient transduction but differ in sialic acid linkage specificity. J Virol 75(15):6884–6893
11. Bainbridge JW et al (2015) Long-term effect of gene therapy on Leber's congenital amaurosis. N Engl J Med 372(20):1887–1897
12. Rabinowitz J, Chan YK, Samulski RJ (2019) Adeno-associated virus (AAV) versus immune response. Viruses 11(2):102.
13. Powell SK, Rivera-Soto R, Gray SJ (2015) Viral expression cassette elements to enhance transgene target specificity and expression in gene therapy. Discov Med 19(102):49–57
14. Patricio MI et al (2017) Inclusion of the woodchuck hepatitis virus posttranscriptional regulatory element enhances AAV2-driven transduction of mouse and human retina. Mol Ther Nucl Acids 6:198–208
15. Fernandez-Bueno I et al (2012) Time course modifications in organotypic culture of human neuroretina. Exp Eye Res 104:26–38
16. Osborne A et al (2016) Human organotypic retinal cultures (HORCs) as a chronic experimental model for investigation of retinal ganglion cell degeneration. Exp Eye Res 143:28–38

17. Murali A et al (2020) Characterisation and validation of the 8-fold quadrant dissected human retinal explant culture model for pre-clinical toxicology investigation. Toxicol In Vitro 63:104716
18. Fradot M et al (2011) Gene therapy in ophthalmology: validation on cultured retinal cells and explants from postmortem human eyes. Hum Gene Ther 22(5):587–593
19. Tolmachova T et al (2013) Functional expression of Rab escort protein 1 following AAV2-mediated gene delivery in the retina of choroideremia mice and human cells ex vivo. J Mol Med (Berl) 91(7):825–837
20. De Silva SR et al (2016) Single residue AAV capsid mutation improves transduction of photoreceptors in the Abca4(−/−) mouse and bipolar cells in the rd1 mouse and human retina ex vivo. Gene Ther 23(11):767–774
21. Hickey DG et al (2017) Tropism of engineered and evolved recombinant AAV serotypes in the rd1 mouse and ex vivo primate retina. Gene Ther 24(12):787–800
22. Quinn PM et al (2019) Human iPSC-derived retinas recapitulate the fetal CRB1 CRB2 complex formation and demonstrate that photoreceptors and Muller glia are targets of AAV5. Stem Cell Rep 12(5):906–919
23. Khabou H et al (2018) Noninvasive gene delivery to foveal cones for vision restoration. JCI Insight 3(2): e96029.
24. Wiley LA et al (2018) Assessment of adeno-associated virus serotype tropism in human retinal explants. Hum Gene Ther 29(4):424–436
25. Maeder ML et al (2019) Development of a gene-editing approach to restore vision loss in Leber congenital amaurosis type 10. Nat Med 25(2):229–233
26. Single ascending dose study in participants with LCA10. Allergan 2020; Available from: Editas Medicine, Inc.
27. Cabral T et al (2017) Dissection of human retina and RPE-choroid for proteomic analysis. J Vis Exp (129): 56203.
28. Hughes JM et al (2010) Active HIF-1 in the normal human retina. J Histochem Cytochem 58(3):247–254
29. Breazzano MP et al (2016) Vitreomacular attachment ultrastructure and histopathological correlation. Curr Eye Res 41(8): 1098–1104

Chapter 29

Prime Editing for the Installation and Correction of Mutations Causing Inherited Retinal Disease: A Brief Methodology

Yi-Ting Tsai, Bruna Lopes da Costa, Nicholas D. Nolan, Salvatore Marco Caruso, Laura A. Jenny, Sarah R. Levi, Stephen H. Tsang, and Peter M. J. Quinn

Abstract

Inherited retinal diseases (IRDs) encompass a large heterogeneous group of rare blinding disorders whose etiology originates from mutations in the 280 genes identified to date. Clustered regularly interspaced short palindromic repeats (CRISPR)/CRISPR-associated (Cas) systems represent a promising avenue for the treatment of IRDs, as exemplified by FDA clinical trial approval of EDIT-101 (AGN-151587), which removes a deep intronic variant in the *CEP290* gene that causes Leber congenital amaurosis (LCA) type 10. Prime editing is a novel double-strand break (DSB) independent CRISPR/Cas system which has the potential to correct all 12 possible transition and transversion mutations in addition to small deletions and insertions. Here, as a proof-of-concept study, we describe a methodology using prime editing for the in vitro installation and correction of the classical *Pde6b*^{rd10} c.1678C > T (p.Arg560Cys) mutation which causes autosomal recessive retinitis pigmentosa (RP) in mice.

Key words *Rd10*, *Pde6b*, Ophthalmology, Gene editing, Prime editing, Inherited retinal diseases (IRDs), Retinal degeneration, CRISPR/Cas9 systems, Retinitis pigmentosa (RP)

1 Introduction

Sight is considered our most valued and dominant sense with vision impairment or blindness severely impacting the quality of life [1, 2]. Inherited retinal diseases (IRDs) are caused by mutations in 280 identified genes with limited treatment options available (RetNet, Retinal Information Network; https://sph.uth.edu/

Yi-Ting Tsai, Bruna Lopes da Costa, Nicholas D. Nolan and Salvatore M. Caruso contributed equally.

Stephen H. Tsang and Peter M. J. Quinn (eds.), *Retinitis Pigmentosa*,
Methods in Molecular Biology, vol. 2560, https://doi.org/10.1007/978-1-0716-2651-1_29,

retnet/; accessed in August 2020). Gene augmentation has been at the forefront for developing IRD treatment options, with Luxturna (voretigene neparvovec-rzyl) becoming the first Food and Drug Administration (FDA)- and European Medicines Association (EMA)-approved gene therapy for patients with mutations in the RPE65 gene [3]. While gene augmentation holds great promise for the treatment of IRDs, it is restricted to the amelioration of loss-of-function mutations and is unsuitable for treating mutations that lead to dominant-negative or gain-of-function effects [4, 5]. Further, achieving physiologically relevant levels of your transgene in the diseased retina, through optimized combinations of promoter and *cis*-acting elements, can be difficult to obtain for effective, safe, and on-target gene augmentation. As an example, ubiquitous promoters can produce strong and stable expression levels but can additionally induce toxicity. In this regard, native promoters may allow for more favorable cell type-specific expression profiles [6–8]. Lastly, large IRD genes are not amenable to conventional single AAV-mediated gene augmentation strategies and would require a gene-editing or split intein approach [9, 10].

Genome surgery can overcome several of the aforementioned hurdles by allowing for the in situ correction or disruption of a patient's specific mutation. Gene editing utilizing clustered regularly interspaced short palindromic repeats (CRISPR)/CRISPR-associated (Cas) systems have revolutionized gene therapeutics. The Cas9 nuclease in conjunction with a guide RNA (gRNA) can precisely disrupt DNA at the targeted locus in the patient's genome, introducing double-strand breaks (DSBs). Subsequent DNA repair processes can help favor gene disruption through non-homologous end-joining (NHEJ) (independent of cell cycle phase) of DSBs or precisely edit the patient's gene through incorporating a donor DNA repair template using homology-directed repair (HDR) pathway (S and G2 phase of the cell cycle) [11–13]. However, despite HDRs' ability to incorporate precise edits, this process is inefficient and leads to frequent formation of insertions/deletions (indels) at the edited locus. The development of DSB independent CRISPR/Cas systems, such as base and prime editing, that greatly reduce the introduction of indels at the editing locus hold great promise for the future of IRD therapeutics [14, 15]. Currently, the success of retinal genome surgery is now epitomized by EDIT-101 (AGN-151587) for the treatment of LCA10. EDIT-101 uses dual gRNAs in conjunction with Cas9 ortholog from *Staphylococcus aureus* for the removal of the aberrant splice donor created by the IVS26 mutation in the *CEP290* gene and is now undergoing phase I/II clinical trials in 18 LCA10 patients [16, 17]. For a recent and detailed overview of CRISPR/Cas-based gene editing approaches for the treatment of IRDs, please see Gallego et al. (2020) [18].

In this chapter, we describe the use of the DSB independent "search-and-replace" prime editing approach that, unlike base editing, has the potential to correct all 12 possible transition (interchanges of purines or of pyrimidines) and transversion (interchanges of purine for pyrimidine bases, or vice versa) point mutations in addition to small deletions, insertions, and combinations of these. Prime editing is a valuable alternative to base editing when there is no suitably positioned PAM to the target mutation or when the target window has multiple adenines or cytosines present. Further, prime editing can precisely edit the human genome but contrary to the prototypical CRISPR-Cas9-mediated HDR is DSB and donor DNA repair template free [15]. The prime editor consists of the H840A *Streptococcus pyogenes* Cas9 (spCas9) nickase linked to an optimized Moloney murine leukemia virus (M-MLV) reverse transcriptase (RT) in conjunction with a prime editing guide RNA (pegRNA). The pegRNA is extended at the 3′ of the sgRNA to include a primer binding sequence (PBS) and a RT template (RTT) that encodes the desired edit. In brief, the prime editor is directed to nick the PAM-containing strand of DNA, at the specified locus in the genome, by the protospacer of the pegRNA. Subsequently, the PBS can hybridize with the 3′ end of the nicked DNA, thus allowing the M-MLV RT to extend the nicked DNA according to the RTT by reverse transcription. Following reverse transcription, flap equilibration will take between the 3′-flap (contains edit) and the 5′ flap (lacks edit). Due to the susceptibility of the 5′ flap to excision by endonucleases, the edited strand is more likely to be incorporated. Lastly, after the 3′ flap is ligated and a heteroduplex is formed, endogenous mismatch repair mechanisms determine if the edited or unedited strand is incorporated. The incorporation of the edited strand can be enhanced by nicking the unedited strand with a nicking sgRNA (nsgRNA), the PE3 system [15].

Here, as a proof-of-concept study on the applicability of prime editing for the correction of mutations that lead to IRDs, we install and correct the classical *Pde6b*^{rd10} c.1678C > T (p.Arg560Cys) mutation in the Neuro-2a (N2a) mouse neuroblastoma cell line. This *Pde6b* mutation causes autosomal recessive retinitis pigmentosa (RP) in the retinal degeneration 10 (Rd10) mouse model and is amenable to correction using CRISPR/Cas9-mediated homology-directed repair (HDR) [19]. In Fig. 1, we provide a schematic of the installation and correction strategy for the *Pde6b*^{rd10} c.1678C > T (p.Arg560Cys) mutation. In Figs. 2 and 3, we give an overview of our assembly strategy. Lastly, in Figs. 4 and 5, we provide Sanger sequencing and next-generation sequencing data showing the successful installation and correction of the Pde6brd10c.1678C > T (p.Arg560Cys) mutation.

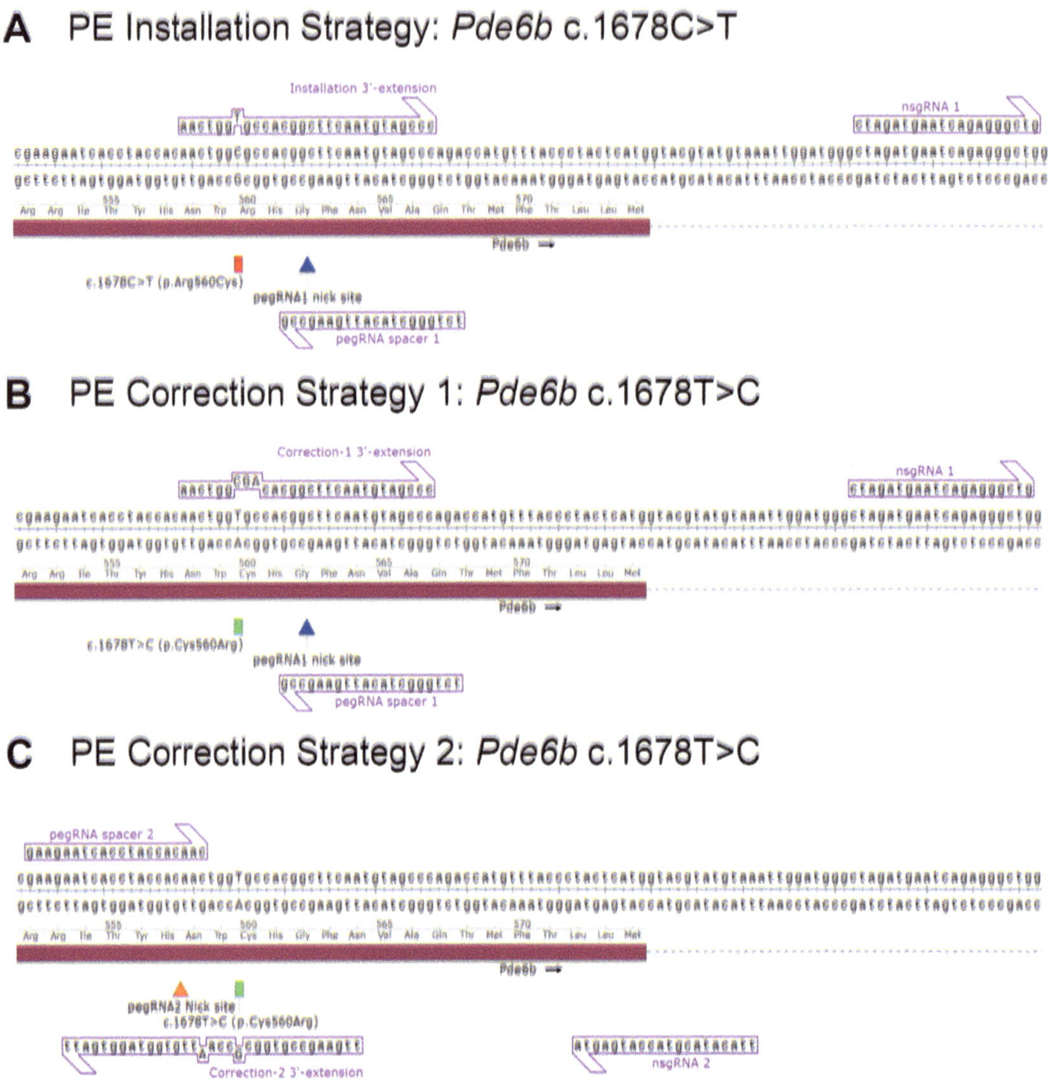

Fig. 1 Schematic of prime editing strategy for the *Pde6b*^{rd10} c.1678C > T (p.Arg560Cys) mutation. (**a**) The prime editing strategy for the installation of the *Pde6b*^{rd10} c.1678C > T mutation. (**b**) The prime editing strategy 1 for the correction of the *Pde6b*^{rd10} c.1678C > T mutation. (**c**) The prime editing strategy 2 for the correction of the *Pde6b*^{rd10} c.1678C > T mutation. (Images from: "SnapGene software (from Insightful Science; available at snapgene.com)")

2 Materials

2.1 pegRNA and nsgRNA Assembly

1. pegRNA spacer 1 oligos *Pde6b*^{rd10} locus (Integrated DNA Technologies (IDT) Custom DNA oligos).

   Top strand oligonucleotide: 5′-CACCGtctgggctacattgaagccg GTTTC-3′.

   Bottom strand oligonucleotide: 5′-CTCTGAAACcggcttcaatg tagcccagaC-3′

2. pegRNA spacer 2 oligos *Pde6b*^{rd10} locus (IDT Custom DNA oligos).

   Top strand oligonucleotide: 5′-CACCgaagaatcacctaccacaac GTTTC-3′.

   Bottom strand oligonucleotide: 5′-CTCTGAAACgttgtggtagg tgattcttc-3′

3. Installation 3′-extension oligos *Pde6b*^{rd10} locus (IDT Custom DNA oligos).

   Top strand oligonucleotide: 5′-GTCCaactggtgccacggcttcaatg tagccc.

   Bottom strand oligonucleotide: 5′-CGCGgggctacattgaagccg tggcaccagtt

4. Correction-1 3′-extension oligos *Pde6b*^{rd10} locus (IDT Custom DNA oligos).

   Top strand oligonucleotide: 5′-GTCCaactggcgacacggcttcaatg tagccc.

   Bottom strand oligonucleotide: 5′-CGCGgggctacattgaagccgtg tcgccagtt

5. Correction-2 3′-extension oligos *Pde6b*^{rd10} locus (IDT Custom DNA oligos).

   Top strand oligonucleotide: 5′-GTCCttgaagccgtggcgccaattg tggtaggtgatt.

   Bottom strand oligonucleotide: 5′-CGCGaatcacctaccacaattgg cgccacggcttcaa

6. pegRNA scaffold oligos (IDT Custom DNA oligos) [19].

   Top strand oligonucleotide: 5′-agagctaagaaattagcaagttgaaataa ggctagtccgttatcaacttgaaaaagtgggaccgagtcg-3′.

   Bottom strand oligonucleotide: 5′-ggaccgactcggtcccactttt caagttgataacggactagccttatttcaacttgctaatttcttag-3′

7. nsgRNA 1 oligos *Pde6b*^{rd10} locus (IDT Custom DNA oligos).

   Top strand oligonucleotide: 5′-CACCGctagatgaatcagagggctg-3′.

   Bottom strand oligonucleotide: 5′-AAACcagccctctgattcatctagC-3′

8. nsgRNA 2 oligos *Pde6b*^{rd10} locus (IDT Custom DNA oligos).

   Top strand oligonucleotide: 5′-CACCGttacatacgtaccatgagta-3′.

   Bottom strand oligonucleotide: 5′-AAACtactcatggtacgtatgt aaG-3′

9. pU6-pegRNA-GG-Vector plasmid (Addgene plasmid ID: 132777).

10. pU6-spacer-acceptor plasmid (Homemade, available upon request).
11. BsaI-HFv2 (New England Biolabs).
12. 10× CutSmart Buffer.
13. ddH_2O.
14. 10× T4 DNA ligase buffer (New England Biolabs).
15. T4 PNK.
16. T4 DNA ligase (New England Biolabs).
17. Lysogeny Broth (LB) medium supplemented with 100 μg/mL ampicillin. Prepare from a 100 mg/mL ampicillin stock.
18. 100 mm LB agar plates supplemented with 100-μg/ml ampicillin.
19. Stellar Competent Cells.
20. Plasmid screening primers.
21. QIAprep or other Spin Miniprep Kit.
22. U6-Forward screening primer: 5′-aaatggactatcatatgcttaccg-3′.

2.2 Additional Plasmid Constructs

1. pCMV-PE2-P2A-GFP plasmid (Addgene plasmid ID: 132776).

2.3 Cell Culture and Reagents

1. Cell Transfection: DMEM: Dulbecco's Modified Eagle's medium supplemented with 10% fetal calf serum (FCS) and 1% Glutamax.
2. Cell Maintenance: DMEM: Dulbecco's Modified Eagle's medium supplemented with 10% fetal calf serum (FCS), 1% Glutamax, and 1% v/v penicillin/streptomycin (PS).
3. N2A cells: Neuro-2a mouse neuroblastoma cell line (CCL-131, ATCC).
4. Dulbecco's phosphate-buffered saline (DPBS) without $Ca2^+$ and $Mg2^+$ (Life Technologies).
5. 0.25% Trypsin-EDTA: 0.25% Trypsin-EDTA (Life Technologies) containing phenol red.
6. Lipofectamine 2000 (Life Technologies).
7. Opti-MEM® I reduced serum medium (Life Technologies).
8. Incubator (humidified, 37 °C, 5% CO_2).
9. Laminar flow hood, class II.

2.4 Equipment and Plasticware

1. Inverted light microscope.
2. Fluorescent microscope.
3. Cell Counter.

4. Nanodrop.
5. T25.
6. 24-well culture plates.
7. Parafilm.
8. Serological pipettes.
9. 15-mL conical tubes.
10. 1.5-mL Eppendorf's.
11. PCR strip tubes.
12. P10, P200, and P1000 pipette tips.

2.5 DNA Extraction, PCR Reagents, and Sample Preparation

1. Proteinase K, 20 mg/Ml stock.
2. Dulbecco's phosphate-buffered saline (DPBS) *with* $Ca2^+$ and $Mg2^+$ (Life Technologies).
3. Sanger sequencing primers $Pde6b^{rd10}$ locus (IDT Custom DNA oligos).

   Forward primer: 5′-atgtactctgctccccaggtc-3′.

   Reverse primer: 5′-acacaattggcatccttgggc-3′.
4. Primers for Amplicon-EZ of $Pde6b^{rd10}$ locus contain the partial Illumina adapter sequences (IDT Custom DNA oligos).

   Forward primer: 5′-acactctttccctacacgacgctcttccgatctatgtactct gctccccaggtc-3′.

   Reverse primer: 5′-gactggagttcagacgtgtgctcttccgatctacacaatt ggcatccttgggc-3′.
5. 2.5 mM dNTP mix.
6. ddH_2O.
7. DMSO.
8. 5X Phire Green Reaction Buffer (Thermo Scientific).
9. Phire Hot Start II DNA Polymerase (Thermo Scientific).
10. 5X Phusion HF Buffer (Thermo Scientific).
11. Phusion Hot Start II High-Fidelity DNA Polymerase (Thermo Scientific).
12. QIAquick or other PCR purification kit.

3 Methods

3.1 Prime Editing Guide RNA (pegRNA) and Nicking Single Guide RNA (nsgRNA) Design

1. Use a prime editing design tool to develop your pegRNA and nsgRNA sequences. There are many software options and websites available. We have used the following Web-based pegRNA and nsgRNA design programs which provide detailed instructions on their use.
   (a) pegFinder: http://pegfinder.sidichenlab.org/ [20]
   (b) PrimeDesign: https://primedesign.pinellolab.partners.org/ [21]
   (c) Prime Editing Design Tool: https://primeedit.nygenome.org/

3.2 pegRNA and nsgRNA Construction

Here we modified the pU6-pegRNA-GG-acceptor into a pU6-spacer-acceptor that allows for cloning of nsgRNAs with BsaI. We generated a 2694-bp linearized vector from the pU6-pegRNA-GG-acceptor using the forward primer: 5′-tcaagtcagaggtggcgaaac-3′ and the reverse primer: 5′-gagttcgaaatcgaaggtgaaggt-3′. We ordered by gBlocks™ Gene Fragments (Integrated DNA Technologies) a 418-bp double-stranded DNA fragment (*see* Table 1) that contained the gRNA scaffold and subsequent termination sequence. This was amplified by PCR using the forward primer: 5′-ttcgatttcgaactcgtgaccg-3′ and reverse primer: 5′-ccacctctgacttgagcgtc-3′. The linearized vector and fragment were then annealed using In-Fusion cloning to create the pU6-spacer-acceptor plasmid. Use your desired 5′-3′ spacer sequence for the top strand oligonucleotide (including a 5' CACC overhang) and use the reverse complement of the target sequence for the bottom strand oligonucleotide (including a 5' AAAC overhang). For efficient transcript ion initiation spacer as well as nsgRNA sequences must begin with a G nucleotide.

Table 1
gBlocks™ gene fragment sequence for pU6-spacer-acceptor

5′-ttcgatttcgaactcgtgaccgttaacggaaccttccatacgaactttgaaacgcatgaactctttgataac gtcttcgctactcgccatagatcctttctcctctttcagatccgtgctcagtatctctatcactgatagggat gtcaatctctatcactgatagggaggtctcggtttcagagctaagaaattagcaagttgaaataaggcta gtccgttatcaacttgaaaaagtgggaccgagtcggtcctttttttaagcttgggccgctcgaggtacct ctctacatatgacatgtgagcaaaaggccagcaaaaggccaggaaccgtaaaaaggccgcgttgctgg cgtttttccataggctccgcccccctgacgagcatcacaaaaatcgacgctcaagtcagaggtgg-3’

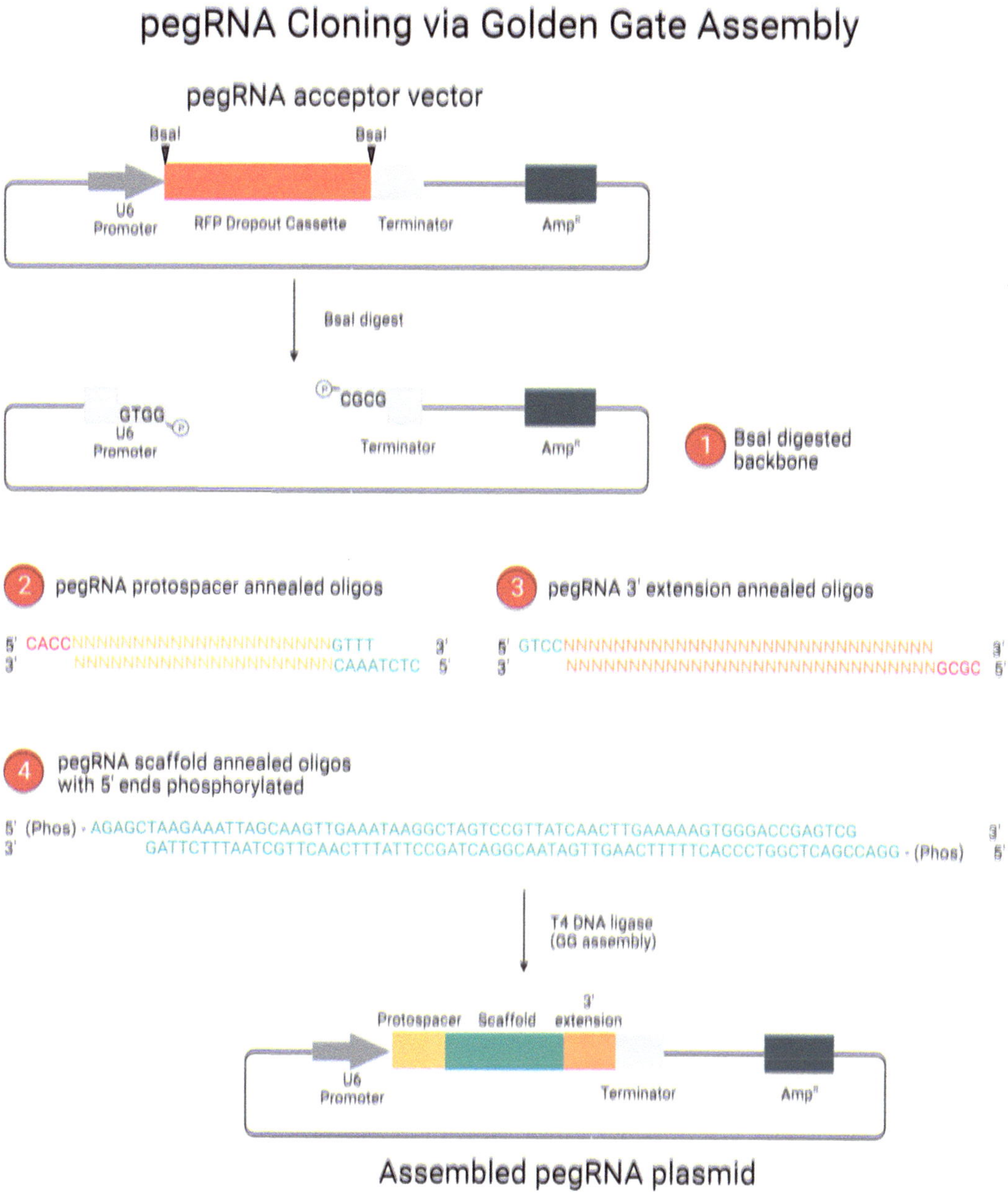

Fig. 2 Schematic of pegRNA cloning method by Golden Gate assembly. First, the pegRNA acceptor vector is linearized by restriction enzyme BsaI. *E. coli* transformed with non-digested plasmid will appear red during subsequent growth. Next the pegRNA protospacer, scaffold, and 3′ extension annealed oligos are added to the linearized backbone mixture and ligated with T4 DNA ligase. The resultant assembled plasmid contains the entire pegRNA sequence and when transformed into *E. coli* will appear white, enabling a preliminary screening of successfully transformed constructs

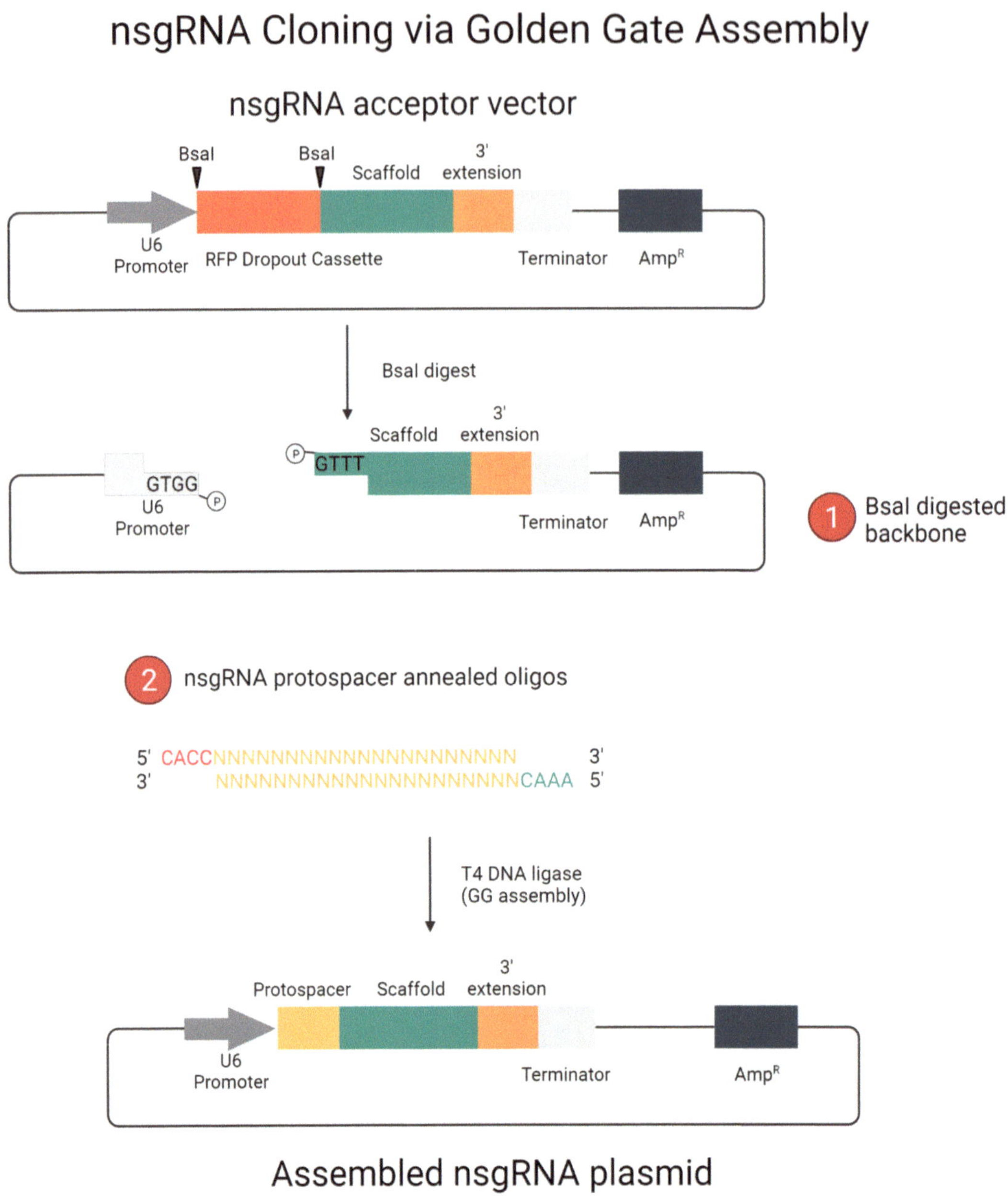

Fig. 3 Schematic of nsgRNA cloning method by Golden Gate assembly. First, the nsgRNA acceptor vector, which contains the scaffold and 3′ termination sequence, is linearized by restriction enzyme BsaI. *E. coli* transformed with non-digested plasmid will appear red during subsequent growth. Next the nsgRNA protospacer is added to the linearized backbone mixture and ligated with T4 DNA ligase. The resultant assembled plasmid contains the nsgRNA sequence and when transformed into *E. coli* will appear white, enabling a preliminary screening of successfully transformed constructs

3.2.1 Digest pU6-pegRNA-GG-Vector and pU6-Spacer-Acceptor Plasmids

1. Digest 1 μg of the pU6-pegRNA-GG-Vector plasmid with BsaI-HFv2 overnight at 37 °C:

1 μg	pU6-pegRNA-GG-Vector plasmid
1.0 μL	BsaI-HFv2
5.0 μL	10× CutSmart buffer
X μL	*ddH_20*
50.0 μL	Total reaction volume

2. Digest 1 μg of the pU6-spacer-acceptor plasmid with BsaI-HFv2 overnight at 37 °C:

1 μg	pU6- spacer-acceptor plasmid
1.0 μL	BsaI-HFv2
5.0 μL	10× CutSmart buffer
X μL	*ddH_20*
50.0 μL	Total reaction volume

3. Use QIAquick PCR purification kit and elute in ddH_20. Nanodrop and dilute digested plasmid to a final concentration of 30 ng/μl using ddH_20 (*see* **Note 1**). The digested and purified pU6-pegRNA-GG-Vector and pU6- spacer-acceptor are now ready for pegRNA and nsgRNA assembly, respectively.

3.2.2 Anneal Oligonucleotides

1. Dilute your desired complementary pegRNA spacer, pegRNA extension, phosphorylated pegRNA scaffold oligonucleotide, and nsgRNA pairs to 100-μM stock using ddH_20 (*see* **Note 2**).
2. Combine 1 μL of the top oligonucleotide (100 μM) and 1 μL of the bottom oligonucleotide (100 μM) to 23 μL of ddH_20 and anneal in a thermocycler by heating at 95 °C for 3 min and then cooling gradually (0.1 °C/s) to 22 °C.
3. Dilute the annealed oligonucleotide pair 1:4 by adding 75 μl of ddH_20 for a final concentration of 1 μM. Annealed oligonucleotides are now ready for pegRNA and nsgRNA assembly.

3.2.3 pegRNA and nsgRNA Assembly

1. pegRNA assembly combine and, in a thermocycler, start the PCR program protocol:

   16 °C for 5 min and 37 °C for 5 min and repeat for a total of 8 cycles (*see* **Note 3**).

1.0 μL	Digested pU6-pegRNA-GG-Vector plasmid, 30 ng/μL stock
1.0 μL	Annealed pegRNA spacer, 1 μM stock

(continued)

1.0 μL	Annealed pegRNA extension, 1 μM stock
1.0 μL	Annealed phosphorylated pegRNA scaffold, 1 μM stock
0.25 μL	BsaI-HFv2
0.50 μL	T4 DNA ligase
1.0 μL	10× T4 DNA ligase buffer
4.25 μL	*ddH_20*
10.0 μL	Total reaction volume

2. nsgRNA combine and, in a thermocycler, start the PCR program protocol:
   16 °C for 5 min and 37 °C for 5 min and repeat for a total of 8 cycles (*see* **Note 3**).
3.

1.0 μL	Digested pU6-spacer-acceptor plasmid, 30 ng/μL stock
1.0 μL	Annealed nsgRNA spacer, 1-μM stock
0.25 μL	BsaI-HFv2
0.50 μL	T4 DNA ligase
1.0 μL	10× T4 DNA ligase buffer
6.25 μL	ddH_20
10.0 μL	Total reaction volume

4. Post incubation place assemblies in a thermocycler: 15 min at 37 °C, then 15 min at 80 °C, then hold at 12 °C.

3.2.4 Transformation of Assembled Plasmids

1. Take competent cells out of −80 °C and thaw on ice.
2. Remove premade agar plates with ampicillin (100 μg/mL) from 4 °C storage, warm to room temperature, and then incubate in 37 °C incubator.
3. Add 1 μL of the 10-μL assembly reaction (*see* **Note 4**), from **step 3** of Subheading 3.2.3, into 20 μL of competent cells. Gently mix by flicking the bottom of the tube with your finger, leave on ice for 1 min.
4. Heat shock the transformation by submerging the bottom 1/2 of the tube into a 42 °C water bath for 45 s.
5. Place your tube back into ice for 2 min.

6. Take 3 μL of the heat-shocked transformation and spread on 1/8th of a 100-mm LB agar plate and incubate in 37 °C incubator overnight.
7. The following morning (18 h of incubation) remove the plate from the incubator and leave at room temperature until late afternoon (24 h of incubation in total).
8. Pick 1–2 white colonies per pegRNA and nsgRNA assembly and inoculate into 3 mL of LB medium with 100 μg/mL of ampicillin. Incubate at 37 °C and shake overnight.
9. Following the manufacturer's instructions, isolate the plasmid using the QIAprep Spin Miniprep Kit.
10. Use the U6 promoter forward screening primer: 5′-aaatggactatcatatgcttaccg-3′ to verify the sequence by Sanger sequencing. Assembled pegRNA and nsgRNA vectors are now ready for in vitro validation.

3.3 In Vitro Validation of Prime Editing Strategy

3.3.1 Seeding Cells the Day Before Transfection

1. Prewarm the cell maintenance medium to room temperature.
2. Aspirate medium and wash twice with DPBS without $Ca2^+$ and $Mg2^+$ to remove dead cells. Check under an inverted microscope to ensure all cell debris is removed.
3. Add 3 mL of Trypsin-EDTA T25 flask of N2A cells and incubate at 37 °C for 10 min. Check under the microscope to make sure all cells are lifted.
4. Add 5 mL of cell transfection medium and resuspend cells; spin down the cells at 300 × g for 3 min.
5. Resuspend the cells in 1 mL of cell maintenance medium and use a cell counter to quantify.
6. Seed cells in a 24-well plate at 5×10^4 cells per well with 500 μL of growth medium in each well.
7. Incubate cells overnight at 37 °C.

3.3.2 Cell Transfection of N2A Cells

1. Prewarm the cell transfection medium to room temperature.
2. One hour before transfection, refresh the medium on the seeded 24-well plate with cell transfection medium, 500 μL per well.
3. Follow the standard Lipofectamine 2000 protocol. Below, we describe the amounts for 1 well of a 24-well plate.
4. Combine 30 μL of Opti-MEM with 1.5 μL of Lipofectamine 2000 reagent in a PCR tube.
5. In a separate PCR tube combine 30 μL of Opti-MEM with a total of 1.5 μg of DNA. Use a molar ratio of 1:1.63:0.55 for

pCMV-PE2-P2A-GFP: pU6-pegRNA-GG-Vector: pU6-spacer-acceptor. For 1.5 μg, this is 1038 ng of pCMV-PE2-P2A-GFP, 345 ng of pU6-pegRNA-GG-Vector and 115 ng of the pU6-spacer-acceptor.

6. Add the diluted DNA to the diluted Lipofectamine 2000 reagent and incubate for 25 min at room temperature.
7. The 60 μl of DNA-lipid complex can be added dropwise to 1 well of a 24-well plate.
8. Incubate cells for at 37 °C for 3 days and then isolate DNA (*see* **Note 5**).

3.3.3 DNA Isolation

1. Prewarm N2A medium to room temperature.
2. Aspirate medium and wash twice with DPBS without $Ca2^+$ and $Mg2^+$ to remove dead cells. Check under an inverted microscope to ensure all cell debris is removed.
3. Add 50 μL of Trypsin-EDTA in each well of a 24-well plate and incubate at 37 °C for 10 min. Check under the microscope to make sure all cells are lifted.
4. Add 150 μL of DPBS with $Ca2^+$ and $Mg2^+$ and transfer the full 200 μL to a PCR strip tube. Check under the microscope to confirm that the majority of the cells were collected.
5. Spin down the cells for 1 min at a low speed and carefully remove 100 μL, leaving around 100 μL to resuspend the cells.
6. In a thermocycler start the DNA extraction protocol: 20 min at 95 °C, 1 h at 56 °C, 30 min at 95 °C.
7. Pause the program before the start of the second step (1 h at 56 °C) and add 10 μL of proteinase K.
8. The samples are ready to use as template for PCR reactions: Subheadings 3.4.1 and 3.4.2. For long-term storage, the sample should be preserved in a -20 °C freezer.

3.4 Analysis of Prime Editing Efficiency

3.4.1 Sanger Sequencing

1. Use the forward primer: 5′-atgtactctgctccccaggtc-3′ and reverse primer: 5′-acacaattggcatccttgggc-3′ for PCR.
2. Run PCR in a thermocycler: use Phusion Hot Start II High-Fidelity DNA Polymerase with the following recipe:

5.0 μL	5X Phusion HF Buffer (Thermo Scientific)
2.0 μL	2.5-mM dNTP
1.25 μL	DMSO
0.1 μL	Forward primer (100 mM)
0.1 μL	Revere primer (100 mM)
0.2 μL	Phusion DNA polymerase (Thermo Scientific)

(continued)

5.0 μL	5X Phusion HF Buffer (Thermo Scientific)
15.35 μL	ddH_20
1.0 μL	DNA sample from 3.4.3.
25.0 μL	Total reaction volume

3. In a thermocycler start, the PCR program protocol: 3 min at 95 °C, repeat cycles of 5 s at 95 °C, 5 s at 57C, 20s at 72 °C, then 10 min at 72 °C.
4. Use 3 μL to run the PCR product in a 1.5% agarose gel. The product should be a single 218-bp band.
5. Send for Sanger sequencing. Programs such as Synthego's ICE analysis tools can be used for a rough estimation of efficiency. We strongly recommend to use a next-generation sequencing approach.

3.4.2 Next-Generation Sequencing: Amplicon-EZ

1. Use the forward primer: 5′-acactctttccctacacgacgctcttccgatct atgtactctgctccccaggtc-3′ and reverse primer: 5′-gactggagtt cagacgtgtgctcttccgatctacacaattggcatccttgggc-3′, which cont ain the partial Illumina adapter sequences, for PCR (*see* **Note 6**).
2. Run PCR in a thermocycler: use Phusion Hot Start II High-Fidelity DNA Polymerase with the following recipe:

5.0 μL	5X Phusion HF Buffer (Thermo Scientific)
2.0 μL	2.5-mM dNTP
1.25 μL	DMSO
0.1 μL	Forward primer (100 mM)
0.1 μL	Revere primer (100 mM)
0.2 μL	Phusion DNA Polymerase (Thermo Scientific)
15.35 μL	ddH_20
1.0 μL	DNA sample from 3.4.3.
25.0 μL	Total reaction volume

3. In a thermocycler, start the PCR program protocol: 3 min at 95 °C, repeat cycles of 5 s at 95 °C, 5 s at 57C, 20s at 72 °C, then 10 min at 72 °C.
4. Verify the PCR product produces a single band by running on a gel (1.5% wt/vol agarose gel with 0.5X TBE buffer).
5. Use the QIAquick PCR purification kit to purify the rest of the amplicon.

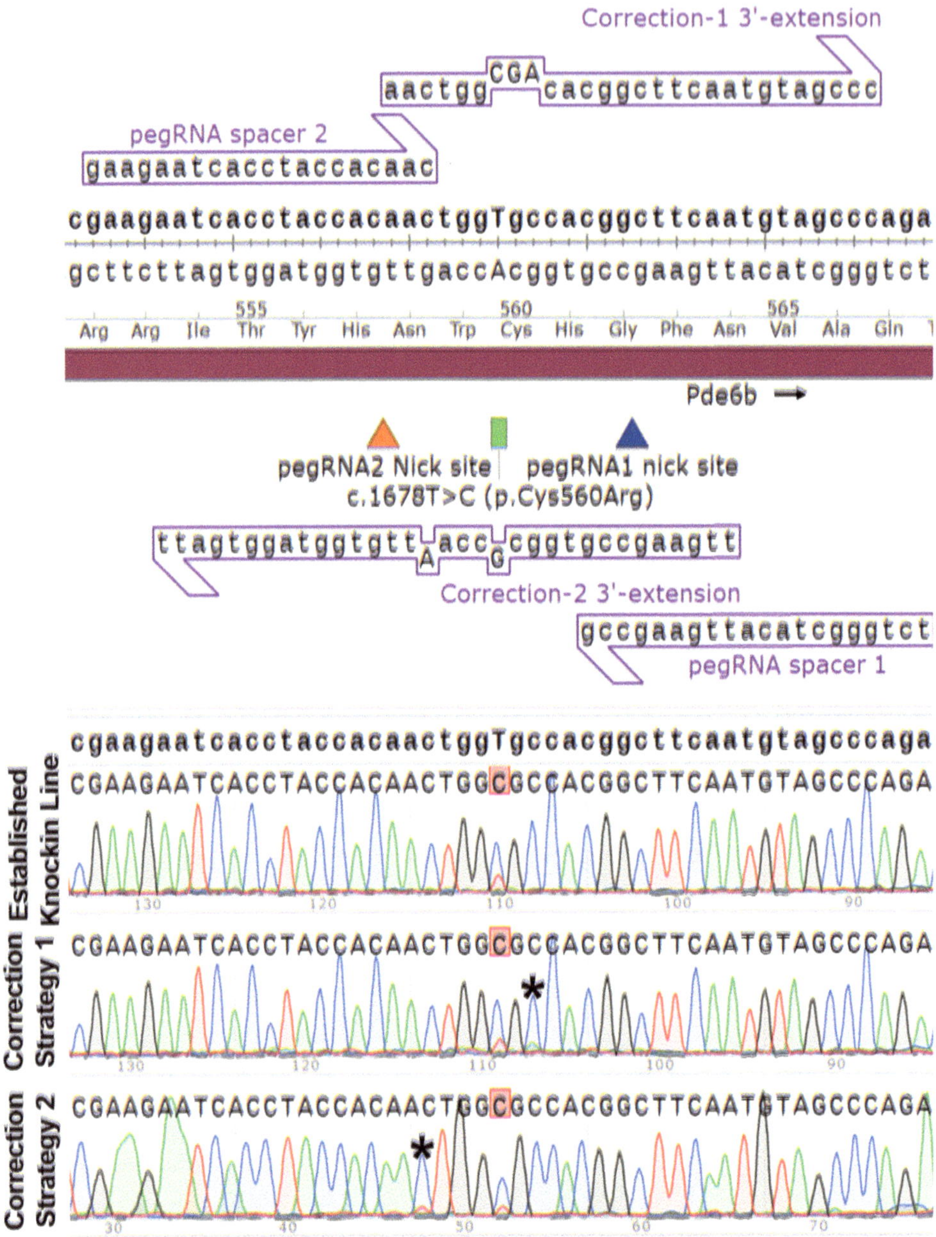

Fig. 4 Example Sanger sequencing of the installation and correction of the *Pde6b*^{rd10} c.1678C > T (p. Arg560Cys) mutation. Sanger sequencing traces of the established knockin line from a single N2A clone with the installed *Pde6b*^{rd10} c.1678C > T mutation (the N2A cells are triploid at this genomic locus (*see* **Note 7**)). The Sanger sequencing traces for prime editing correction strategies 1 and 2 represent a mixed edited population from a bulk of cells. In the prime editing correction strategy 1, alongside the correction of the p. Arg560Cys back to the Arg codon, there is insertion of a silent mutation as specified in the Correction-1 3′-extension. This changes codon 560 from cysteine (TGC) back to arginine (CGA, wild-type codon is CGC). In the prime editing correction strategy 2, alongside the correction of the p.Arg560Cys back to the wild-type Arg codon, there is insertion of a silent mutation as specified in the Correction-2 3′-extension. This changes codon 558 asparagine (AAC) to asparagine (AAT) in addition to changing codon 560 from cysteine (TGC) back to arginine (CGC). (Images from: "SnapGene software (from Insightful Science; available at snapgene.com)")

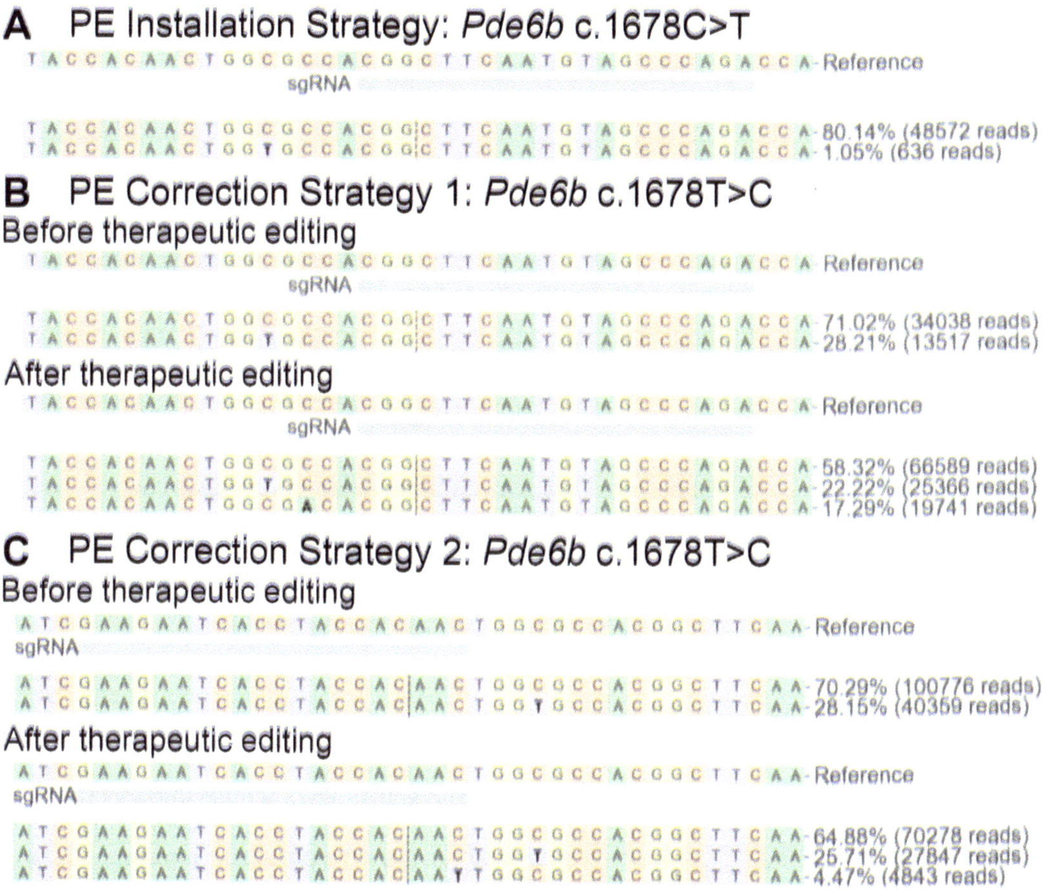

Fig. 5 Next-generation sequencing of the installation and correction of the *Pde6b*^{rd10} c.1678C > T (p. Arg560Cys) mutation. (**a**) Successful installation of the *Pde6b*^{rd10} c.1678C > T in 1.05% of N2A cells. We subsequently found an error in the sequence of the scaffold used for this experiment; therefore, editing efficiency may be higher. (**b**) PE correction strategy 1 leads to repair of the c.1678C > T mutation in addition to incorporating the silent mutation c.1680C > A. (**c**) PE correction strategy 2 leads to repair of the c.1678C > T mutation in addition to incorporating the silent mutation c.1674C > T. (Images from CRISPResso2 analysis [21])

6. Measure the concentration of your sample and normalize to 20 ng/μL prior to submission.
7. Send at least 500 ng of double-stranded DNA (25 μL of 20 ng/μL stock) for sequencing.
8. Data analysis:

   Upload the .fastq or .fastq.gz files to:

   8.1 CRISPResso2: https://crispresso.pinellolab.partners.org/submission [22]

   8.2 Cas-analyzer: http://www.rgenome.net/cas-analyzer/# [23]

4 Notes

1. In our protocol, we have found it unnecessary to gel purify the vector backbones.
2. Oligonucleotides can be heated to 55 °C for 1–5 min to aid reconstitution.
3. Alternatively, the pegRNA and nsgRNA assemblies can be combined and incubated for 10 min at room temperature.
4. Incubating the cell/construct mix for 20–30 min here can improve cloning efficiency moderately.
5. The pCMV-PE2-P2A-GFP allows for monitoring of cell transfection efficiency by GFP fluorescence.
6. Amplicon size excluding adapters must be between 150–500 bp.
7. N2A cells have an unstable karyotype within a stemline range of 94 to 98 chromosomes. See characteristics section: https://www.atcc.org/products/ccl-131#.

Acknowledgement

B.L.D.C. is a recipient of the Capes PhD scholarship. S.H.T. and Jonas Children's Vision Care is supported by the National Institute of Health 5P30CA013696, U01 EY030580, U54OD020351, R24EY028758, R24EY027285, 5P30EY019007, R01EY018213, R01EY024698, R01EY026682, R21AG050437, the Schneeweiss Stem Cell Fund, New York State [SDHDOH01-C32590GG-3450000], the Foundation Fighting Blindness New York Regional Research Center Grant [TA-NMT-0116-0692-COLU], Nancy & Kobi Karp, the Crowley Family Funds, The Rosenbaum Family Foundation, Alcon Research Institute, the Gebroe Family Foundation, the Research to Prevent Blindness (RPB) Physician-Scientist Award, unrestricted funds from RPB, New York, NY, USA. P.M.J.Q. is the current recipient of a Curing Retinal Blindness Foundation (CRBF) grant, a Knights Templar Eye Foundation (KTEF) Career Starter grant, the International Retinal Research Foundation (IRRF) Loris and David Rich Postdoctoral Scholar Award and a New York Stem Cell Foundation (NYSCF)—Druckenmiller Fellowship.

Conflicts of Interest

Stephen H. Tsang receives financial support from Abeona Therapeutics, Inc and Emendo. He is also the founder of Rejuvitas and is on the scientific and clinical advisory board for Nanoscope Therapeutics. Peter M.J. Quinn receives research support from Rejuvitas, Inc.

References

1. Enoch J et al (2019) Evaluating whether sight is the most valued sense. JAMA Ophthalmol 137(11):1317–1320
2. Vu HT et al (2005) Impact of unilateral and bilateral vision loss on quality of life. Br J Ophthalmol 89(3):360–363
3. Maguire AM et al (2021) Clinical perspective: treating RPE65-associated retinal dystrophy. Mol Ther 29(2):442–463
4. Tsai YT et al (2018) Clustered regularly interspaced short palindromic repeats-based genome surgery for the treatment of autosomal dominant retinitis pigmentosa. Ophthalmology 125(9):1421–1430
5. Christie KA et al (2020) Mutation-independent allele-specific editing by CRISPR-Cas9, a novel approach to treat autosomal dominant disease. Mol Ther 28(8): 1846–1857
6. Mussolino C et al (2011) AAV-mediated photoreceptor transduction of the pig cone-enriched retina. Gene Ther 18(7):637–645
7. Buck TM, Wijnholds J (2020) Recombinant adeno-associated viral vectors (rAAV)-vector elements in ocular gene therapy clinical trials and transgene expression and bioactivity assays. Int J Mol Sci 21(12)
8. Wu W et al (2021) Molecular and therapeutic strategies for retinitis pigmentosa: culture of human retinal explants for ex vivo assessment of AAV gene delivery, in methods in molecular biology, W. JM, editor. Humana Press, New York
9. Fry LE, McClements ME, MacLaren RE (2021) Analysis of pathogenic variants correctable with CRISPR base editing among patients with recessive inherited retinal degeneration. JAMA Ophthalmol 139(3):319–328
10. Tornabene P et al (2019) Intein-mediated protein trans-splicing expands adeno-associated virus transfer capacity in the retina. Sci Transl Med 11(492)
11. Gasiunas G et al (2012) Cas9-crRNA ribonucleoprotein complex mediates specific DNA cleavage for adaptive immunity in bacteria. Proc Natl Acad Sci U S A 109(39):E2579–E2586
12. Jinek M et al (2012) A programmable dual-RNA-guided DNA endonuclease in adaptive bacterial immunity. Science 337(6096): 816–821
13. Mao Z et al (2008) DNA repair by nonhomologous end joining and homologous recombination during cell cycle in human cells. Cell Cycle 7(18):2902–2906
14. Komor AC et al (2016) Programmable editing of a target base in genomic DNA without double-stranded DNA cleavage. Nature 533(7603):420–424
15. Anzalone AV et al (2019) Search-and-replace genome editing without double-strand breaks or donor DNA. Nature 576(7785):149–157
16. Maeder ML et al (2019) Development of a gene-editing approach to restore vision loss in Leber congenital amaurosis type 10. Nat Med 25(2):229–233
17. Single ascending dose study in participants with LCA10. Allergan 2020; Available from: Editas Medicine, Inc.
18. Gallego C, Goncalves M, Wijnholds J (2020) Novel therapeutic approaches for the treatment of retinal degenerative diseases: focus on CRISPR/Cas-based gene editing. Front Neurosci 14:838
19. Vagni P et al (2019) Gene editing preserves visual functions in a mouse model of retinal degeneration. Front Neurosci 13:945
20. Chow RD et al (2021) A web tool for the design of prime-editing guide RNAs. Nat Biomed Eng 5(2):190–194
21. Hsu JY et al (2021) PrimeDesign software for rapid and simplified design of prime editing guide RNAs. Nat Commun 12(1):1034
22. Clement K et al (2019) CRISPResso2 provides accurate and rapid genome editing sequence analysis. Nat Biotechnol 37(3):224–226
23. Park J et al (2017) Cas-analyzer: an online tool for assessing genome editing results using NGS data. Bioinformatics 33(2):286–288

Chapter 30

Large-Scale Single-Nucleus RNA Sequencing Compatible with Complex Archived Samples

Chao-Yu Liu and Hsu-Hsin Chen

Abstract

Transcriptome profiling at single-cell resolution allows us to identify and assess functional cell types and cellular states, including those within degenerating ocular tissues in retinitis pigmentosa. The technology is particularly valuable when studying tissues with high cellular heterogeneity, or when specific cell types are of interest. In this chapter, we introduce a detailed protocol of a medium-throughput single-nucleus RNA sequencing technique that utilizes frozen tissue as input sample. This protocol can be executed by any researcher with basic training in molecular biology techniques. With this protocol, a single experimenter can easily process two samples per day up to cDNA amplification, and library preparations can be done in batches of 8. Routinely we can obtain ~20 K nuclei per eye from 3 to 4 library preparations.

Key words Gene expression profiling, Deep sequencing, Parallel mRNA analysis, Single-cell transcriptomics, sNuc-seq

1 Introduction

All physical features we manifest are influenced by genes, but genomic sequences alone are not sufficient to decode the molecular identities of tissue composition, nor the molecular basis underlying healthy versus diseased tissue. While all of our somatic cells share nearly identical genome, their drastic variations in morphology and function are dictated by the expression of different subsets of the shared genome. As a result, analyzing the expressed genome (the transcriptome), in particular the messenger RNAs that accounts for a large portion of the variations, is thus a common first step toward understanding biological functions of cells and tissues.

The resolution of transcriptome profiling is an important aspect for data interpretation. Within the same tissue, gene expression patterns are highly dependent on cell types and subtypes, and even within the same cell type/subtype, considerable gene expression variability due to cell states has been observed in various tissues

Stephen H. Tsang and Peter M. J. Quinn (eds.), *Retinitis Pigmentosa*,
Methods in Molecular Biology, vol. 2560, https://doi.org/10.1007/978-1-0716-2651-1_30,

[1–3], including the retina (see below). Thus, differential expression analysis from traditional bulk RNA sequencing, in which heterogeneous cell populations are mixed in each sample, could mask meaningful signal from rarer populations in tissue and accentuate differences due to cell type representation [4, 5].

The recent advances in single-cell transcriptomics technology have enabled in-depth analysis of cell types and functional states within complex tissues. While various methods have been developed for single-cell RNAseq (scRNAseq), the invention of droplet-based sequencing (Drop-seq) was truly the game-changer in the field [6, 7]. Drop-Seq was designed for high-throughput scRNA-seq, allowing the analysis of hundreds of thousands of single cells per experiment while lowering the cost by orders of magnitude compared to previous methods. The technology was successfully commercialized into user-friendly kits and equipment, quickly gained popularity, and is now emerging as a common tool for cell biology. Two main features of Drop-seq, droplet partitioning and primer barcoding, are central to high-throughput analysis, as described below.

In Drop-seq, single cells are partitioned in nanoliter-sized aqueous droplets in oil/buffer emulsion, instead of in individual wells on a plate as some of the previous methods. The microfluidics design guides each droplet to enclose, ideally, one single-cell and one microbead carrying DNA barcode sequences as ID tags for individual cells and transcripts [6, 7] (*see* Fig. 1a, b). Cell lysis occurs within the droplets, as well as the subsequent mRNA binding to the barcoded primers on the microbeads, ensuring cell-specific and transcript-specific labeling of the first-strand cDNAs. Subsequently the cDNAs from all cells are pooled and amplified to construct the library for sequencing. The 10× Chromium platform is based on the same concept, but with many differences in workflow, primer design, and chemistry.

The key to cell-labeling and transcript quantification lies in the primer design. There are four parts of sequence in the original Drop-Seq primer: the PCR handles (for following amplification of cDNA), the barcode (to label the mRNA's cell-of-origin), the UMI (Unique Molecular Identifier for every transcript captured), and a 30-bp dT sequence (to capture mRNA via poly-A tails). The PCR handles are identical across all beads, allowing for pooled amplification regardless of cell of origin. Primers on the same bead share a barcode that is unique to that bead, so that all transcripts within the same droplet (from the same cell) would share this barcode. Each individual primer contains a unique UMI, designed to count the number of starting transcripts captured regardless of subsequent amplification steps (*see* Fig. 1c). Subsequent commercial versions are largely based on the same principle in primer design. The Drop-seq-based technology is transformational for our understanding of complex tissues of the central nervous system. In fact, the earliest demonstration of this breakthrough technique was the single-cell

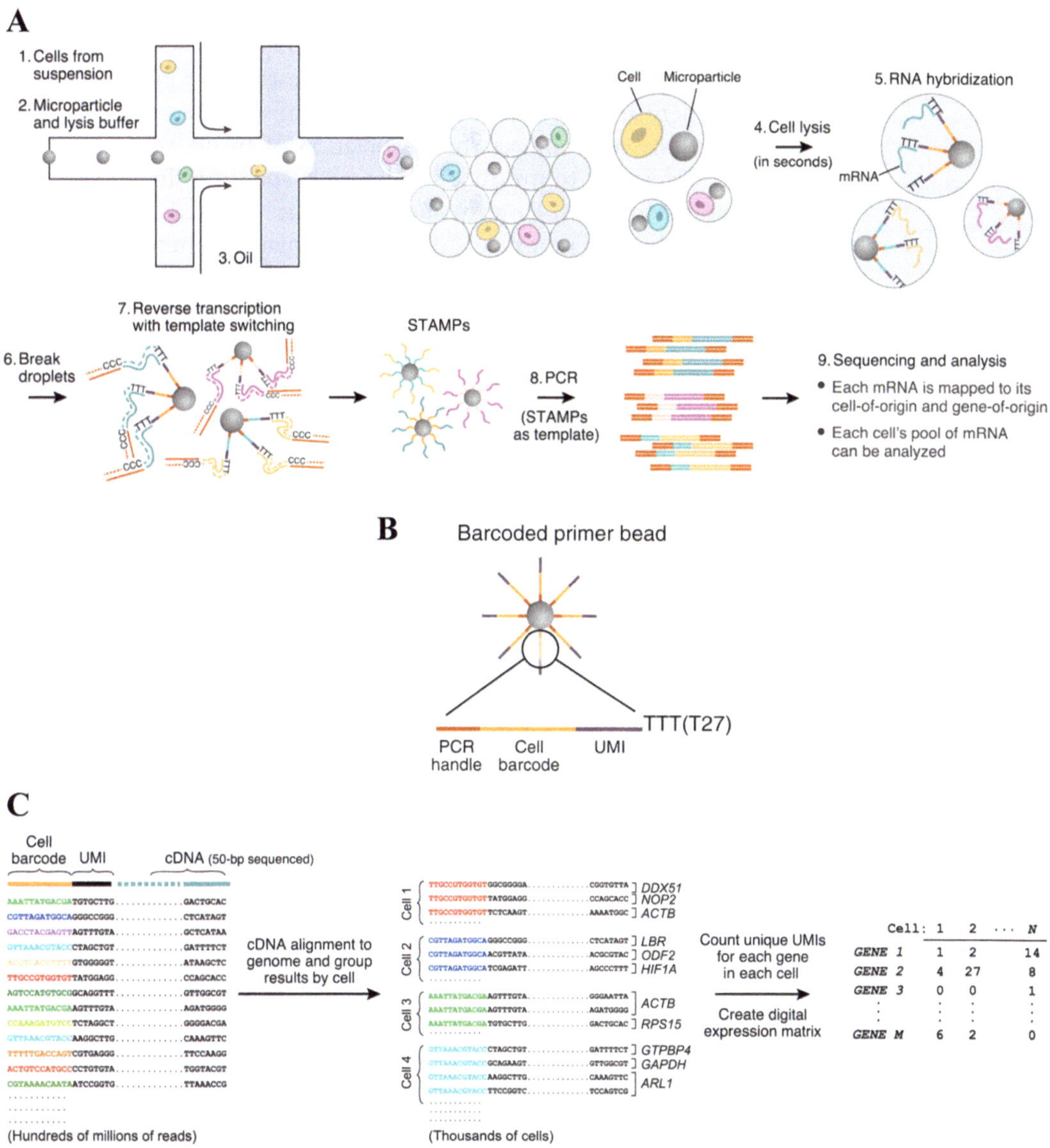

Fig. 1 Drop-Seq technology. (Reproduced from [6] with permission from Elsevier). Note that Drop-Seq and 10× Chromium platforms, while sharing the overall concepts, differs in various aspects both in workflow and in chemistry. (**a**) Drop-Seq workflow. (1) Dissociated cells and barcoded beads are flowed in the microfluidic device along with carrier oil. Three flows join and form droplets that co-encapsulate cell and barcoded bead. (2) In the droplet, the cell lyses instantly and (3) releases mRNAs to associate with primers on the bead. (4) Droplets are broken by destabilizing the oil–water interface. (5) mRNAs undergo reverse transcription in bulk. (6) cDNAs are amplified from *s*ingle-cell *t*ranscriptomes *a*ttached to *m*icro*p*articles and (7) sequenced and analyzed. (**b**) Schematic of a barcoded bead used in Drop-Seq. Each polymer-based bead carries hundreds of millions of DNA primers. A primer consists of four parts: PCR handle, barcode, UMI (Unique Molecular Identifier), and 30-bp dT sequence. (**c**) Droplet-based sequencing data analysis illustration. Each read from the sequenced library contains a cell barcode for cell-of-origin annotation, a UMI for transcript counting, and cDNA reads to be mapped to the reference genome. Using this information, the raw data is organized into a digital expression matrix, in which each number denotes the count of transcripts detected from one gene in a given cell

transcriptomics of the murine retina [6]. The trove of high-quality single-cell retina studies is rapidly expanding and provides an ever-increasing resource for the ocular research community [8–12]. There are, nevertheless, limitations of scRNA-seq methods.

ScRNA-seq requires the dissociation of tissue, often by enzymatic digestion, to produce single-cell suspension. Enzymatic dissociation involves lengthy incubation at elevated temperature, during which gene expression patterns may be altered [13], and biases toward cell populations with weaker cell–cell adhesion. Regardless of the method of dissociation, the process favors cell populations that are more likely to survive the process and selects against the more fragile or the less-accessible cell types. Last but not the least, scRNAseq requires fresh input samples, a major logistical difficulty for studying human samples [14–16].

The development of single-nucleus RNA sequencing (sNuc-seq) provided a solution to overcome the abovementioned limitations. One advantage of using sNuc-seq or its variations, such as Div-seq and SPLiT-seq [16, 17], is avoiding enzymatic cell dissociation altogether. Instead, sNuc-seq rapidly releases nuclei from samples with physical and chemical treatment, such as Dounce homogenizing in buffers with detergent. The variability is thus less affected, and importantly, frozen tissue can be used as input samples [14, 16]. The ability to utilize frozen tissues allows the possibility to tap into archived samples from human tissue banks and to minimize batch effects in designing experiments involving human samples. In the following sections, we describe in detail a demonstrated protocol using a commercially available droplet-based platform to analyze frozen ocular tissue by single-nucleus RNAseq (NucSeq) [18].

2 Materials

2.1 Cryosection

1. Research cryostat.
2. Tissue-Tek O.C.T. compound (Sakura).
3. Large forceps.
4. Fine forceps.
5. Small paint brush.
6. Specimen disk, 40 mm.
7. Low profile cryostat blade.
8. Razor blade.
9. SuperFrost plus microscope slides.
10. Dissection microscope.
11. 15-mL conical tubes.
12. 2-mL RNAse free microcentrifuge tubes.

2.2 RNA Quality Test

1. TRIzol™ reagent (Life Technologies).
2. Chloroform.
3. Isopropanol (RNase free).
4. 70% ethanol, prepare with RNase-free water.
5. 1.5 mL RNase-free microcentrifuge tubes.
6. RNA 6000 Nano kit (Agilent).
7. 2100 Bioanalyzer (Agilent).

2.3 Nuclei Extraction

1. Nuclei Isolation Buffer 1 (NIB1); 250-mM sucrose, 25-mM KCl, 5-mM MgCl2, 10-mM Tris buffer, pH 8.0. Prepare with DEPC-treated or RNase-free water and filter sterilize (0.22 μm). Store at 4 °C for up to 6 months.
2. 100-mM Dithiothreitol, molecular grade.
3. cOmplete™, mini, protease inhibitor cocktail, with EDTA (Roche).
4. 10% (v/v) Triton™ X-100, in nuclease-free water.
5. 20 U/μL SUPERase In™ RNase Inhibitor (Invitrogen).
6. 40 U/μL Ambion™ RNase Inhibitor, cloned (Invitrogen, 40 U/μL).
7. 1 mg/mL 4′,6-diamidino-2-phenylindole (DAPI).
8. UltraPure™ BSA (Invitrogen, 50 mg/mL).
9. Phosphate-Buffered Saline (10×) pH 7.4, RNase-free (Invitrogen).
10. Nuclease-free water 5-mL round-bottom polystyrene tubes, with 35-μm cell strainer snap cap.
11. (Optional) FlowMi cell strainer for 1000-μL pipette tips, 70 μm and 40 μm
12. 0.4% (w/v) Trypan Blue solution.
13. Glass homogenizer with loose pestle.
14. Hemocytometer or other cell counting device.

2.4 Library Construction Reagents

1. Chromium™ Single Cell 3′ GEM, Library & Gel Bead Kit v3 (10× Genomics).
2. Chromium™ Chip B Single Cell Kit (10× Genomics).
3. Chromium™ Multiplex Kit N Set A (10× Genomics).
4. SPRISelect Reagent (Beckman Coulter).
5. DNA Suspension Buffer; Tris–HCl 10 mM, EDTA 0.1 mM pH 8.0, Rnase-free.
6. 10% Tween 20.
7. Buffer EB (Qiagen).

8. 80% ethanol, freshly prepared.
9. Next GEM accessory kit (10× Genomics).
10. Chromium controller (10× Genomics).
11. Thermocycler.
12. High sensitivity DNA kit (Agilent).
13. Qubit fluorometer (Invitrogen).
14. Qubit dsDNA BR assay kit (Invitrogen).

3 Methods

3.1 Sample Processing and Quality Control

1. Flash freeze whole globes or dissected retinae from donor autopsy or animal dissection in liquid nitrogen (*see* **Notes 1** and **2**). Ship frozen tissue on dry ice and store at −80 °C.
2. For cryosection, precool the chamber temperature and cutting temperature to −23 °C. Prechill forceps, paint brush, and sample holder in the cryostat.
3. Label 15-mL Falcon conical tubes for collection of eye sections for nuclei extraction. Label 2-mL RNase free tubes for sections for RNA quality assessment. Precool tubes on dry ice.
4. Transfer the frozen globe to cryostat on dry ice; do not equilibrate the sample to cryostat temperature.
5. Promptly proceed to mounting the frozen globe onto specimen disk with O.C.T. compound. In a circular motion, squeeze a liberal layer of room temperature O.C.T. onto the prechilled specimen disk. Using large forceps holding the stub of the optic nerve, mount the frozen globe while the compound is still half transparent. Hold the globe in position until the compound solidifies completely.
6. Fasten the specimen disk to the cryostat arm. Adjust the angles to ensure the cutting plane is tangent to the globe at the base of the optic nerve stub. Trim off the stub with a clean razor blade.
7. Start trimming at 50–100-μm thickness. The initial sections would normally be the remaining optic nerve. Check the sections under a dissection microscope. Start collecting sections when RPE layer becomes visible (*see* Fig. 2).
8. Keep the collection tubes on dry ice and use fine forceps to transfer the frozen sections directly into the tubes. It is not necessary to save the shavings of frozen vitreous, which tend to break apart during transfer.
9. Collect 5–10 sections per tube, at total thickness of ~500 μm. Immediately bury the tubes in dry ice and store at −80 °C. Collect 2–3 peripheral sections in 2-mL RNase-free tubes for RNA quality assessment. Proceed to RNA extraction or store at −80 °C.

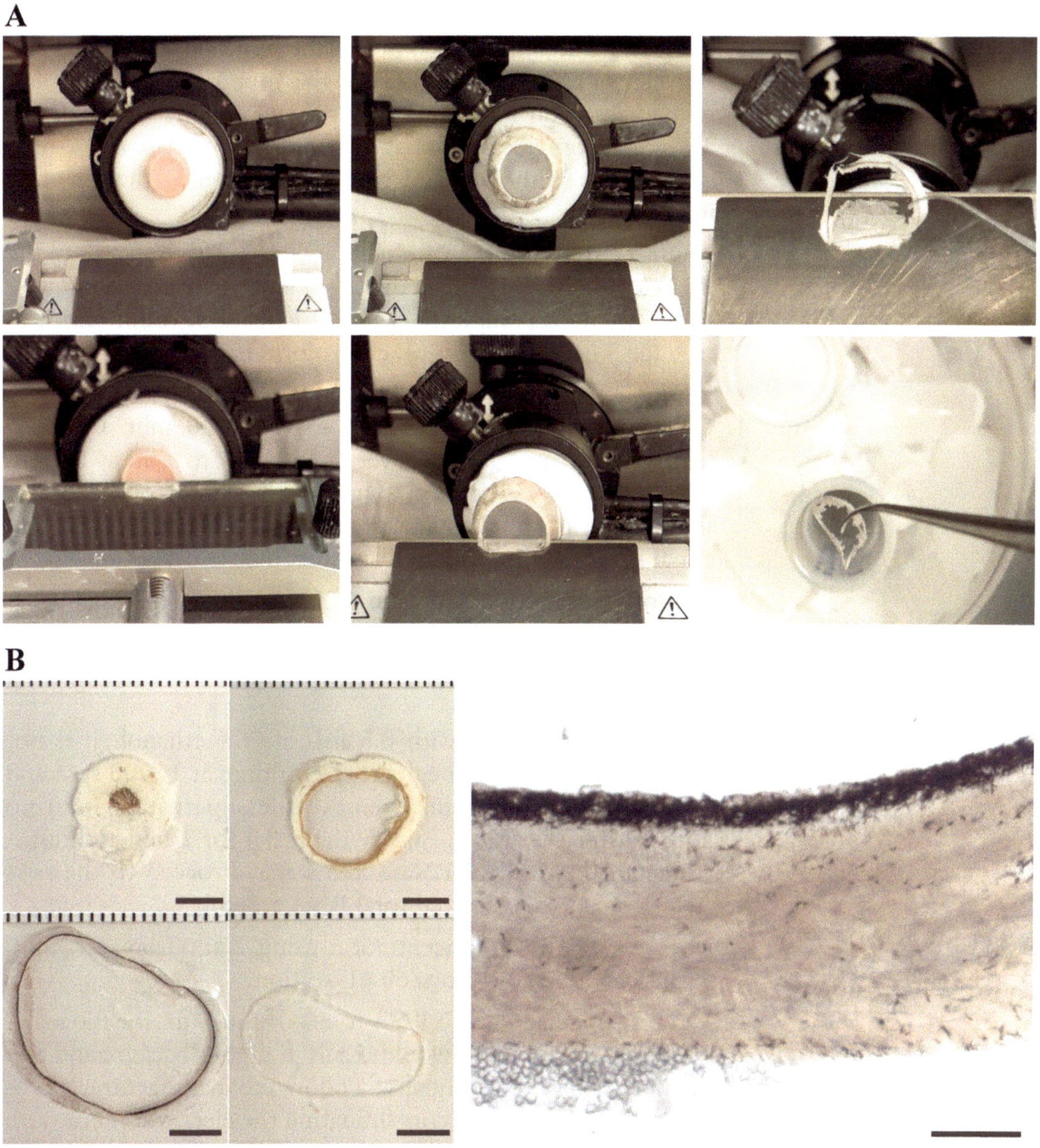

Fig. 2 Cryosection of whole eye globe for NucSeq. (**a**) Mounting and sectioning frozen whole globes. Left, rabbit eye sectioning (New Zealand White); middle, porcine eye sectioning; right, transferring frozen sections to precooled tubes on dry ice. Note the frozen vitreous often separates from the ring of ocular tissue, and it is not necessary to transfer vitreous. (**b**) Visible RPE layer in unstained cryosections. Upper left, human eye sections adjacent to the optic nerve. This is one of the initial sections with visible RPE and should be collected; upper middle, human eye section approximately a quarter of the diameter from the first visible RPE section; lower left, a section from a porcine eye; lower middle, a section from a NZW rabbit eye; right, unstained porcine eye section at 2.5× magnification. RPE layer is at the top. Scale bars, left and middle, 5 mm, right, 500 μm

3.2 RNA Quality Check

1. Precool a tabletop centrifuge to 4 °C.
2. Keep the 2 mL tube with peripheral sections on dry ice and transfer to chemical hood. Take the tube out of dry ice and immediately add 1-mL TRIzol™ reagent directly into the tube. TRIzol™ contains phenol and thus is highly toxic and corrosive; handle with care and properly dispose of the chemical waste.
3. Using a cut 1000p tip, carefully pipette up and down until the pigmented layer is visually dissolved and the remaining undissolved tissue is completely white. Incubate at room temperature for 5 min. Add 200-μL chloroform in the chemical hood. Mix well by shaking.
4. Centrifuge at 12,000 rpm and 4 °C for 20 min. Carefully transfer the top aqueous layer (~450 μL) to a new 1.5-mL RNase-free tube without touching the white protein layer separating the aqueous and organic solvent layer (pink). Add equal volume of isopropanol and mix by vortex.
5. Centrifuge at 12,000 rpm and 4 °C for 20 min. A small pellet should be visible at the bottom of the tube (*see* **Note 3**). Carefully remove the supernatant without disturbing the pellet.
6. Wash the pellet once with 0.5 mL of 75% ethanol. It is not necessary to dislodge the pellet. Centrifuge at 12000 rpm and 4 °C for 5 min. Carefully remove the supernatant until no liquid droplet is visible. Air dry the pellet for 2 min and resuspend in 20–30 μL of RNase-free water. Proceed to the next step or store the extracted total RNA at −80 °C.
7. Measure the RNA concentration using Nanodrop or Qubit. Typical yield is 20–40 ng/60 μL section.
8. Dilute a small aliquot of RNA to 50–100 ng/μL for Bioanalyzer input; overloading would result in higher background and seemingly lower RNA quality. Follow the manufacturer's protocol carefully to avoid contaminating the electrodes. Prewarm reagents to room temperature and prepare the ladder as instructed. Denature the diluted RNA aliquot at 70 °C for 2 min in a thermocycler, heat block, or water bath.
9. Prime and load the RNA 6000 nano chip and start the Bioanalyzer program. This step takes about 20–30 min to complete. A representative plot is shown in Fig. 3c. We recommend RNA integrity number ≥ 7 for NucSeq experiments.

3.3 Nuclei Extraction and Purification

1. To prevent RNA degradation during nuclei isolation, keep tissue sections on dry ice until addition of lysis buffer, maintain resuspensions and buffers on ice, and use recommended amounts of fresh RNase inhibitors. The nuclei extraction

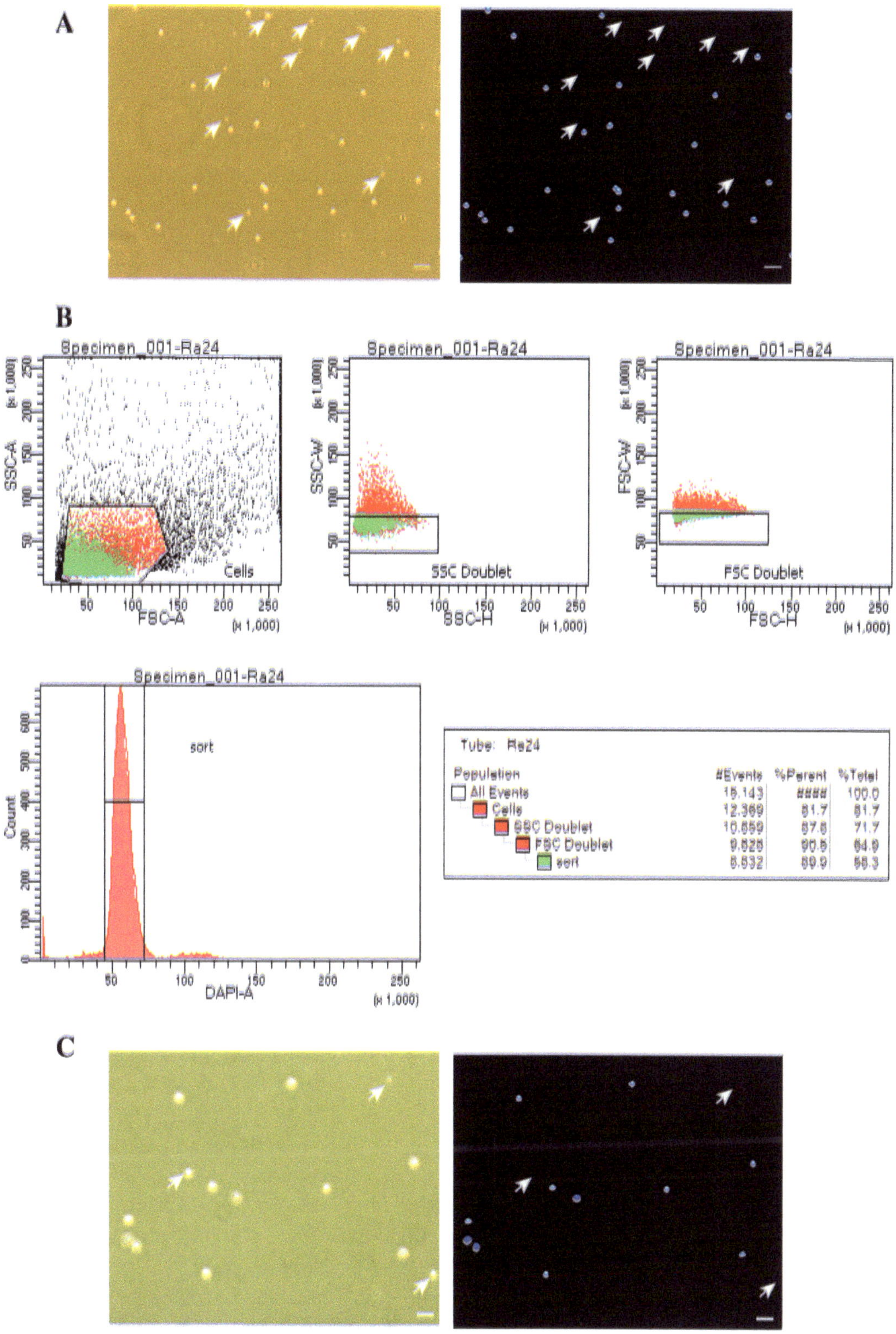

Fig. 3 Nuclei extraction from frozen rabbit eye sections. (**a**) Nuclei suspension after homogenization. Left, bright field view; right, DAPI staining. Arrows, cell debris without DNA (DAPI). Scale bars, 50 μm. (**b**) Representative FACS gating for 2 N DNA content. (**c**) Post-sort nuclei. Left, bright field view, right, DAPI (added post-sort). Arrows, cell debris without DNA. Scale bars, 25 μm

protocol is largely based on Krishnaswami et al. [19] with minor modifications. For human samples, perform all steps prior to FACS sorting in a BL2 biosafety cabinet.

2. Dissolve 1 tablet of cOmplete mini protease inhibitor in 10-mL Nuclei Isolation Buffer 1 (NIB1). Rock at room temperature for 5–10 min until the tablet is completely in solution. Vortex and place on ice. Add 10 μL of 1-mM DTT to chilled buffer and mix by vortex. This buffer is NIB2.
3. For each sample, prepare 3 mL of *supplemented* NIB2:

NIB2	2910 μL
10% v/v triton™ X-100	30 μL
SUPERase in™ RNase inhibitor	30 μL
Ambion™ RNase inhibitor	30 μL
1 mg/mL DAPI	0.6 μL

4. Mix by vortexing and keep on ice. This buffer should be prepared fresh right before nuclei extraction.
5. Chill a clean glass homogenizer and a *loose* pestle on ice. Prepare one set per sample.
6. Transfer one frozen tube with sections from dry ice to ice and immediately add 0.75 mL of *supplemented* NIB2. Use a cut 1000P tip to pipette the sample mixture up and down 5 times and transfer sample and buffer to chilled glass douncer. Add another 0.75 mL of *supplemented* NIB2 to rinse out the tube and transfer to douncer.
7. Using a chilled loose pestle, slowly dounce the sample 15 times. If pieces of tissue are trapped between the pestle and glass wall, slowly remove the pestle and use an RNase-free pipette tip to push the tissue into solution (*see* **Note 4**). Avoid creating vacuum inside the glass douncer. If the fibrous tissues are devoid of pigment before or during douncing, fish out the remaining tissue with a clean tip and continue with remaining douncing strokes.
8. Leave homogenate on ice for 5 min. Filter samples in prechilled 35-μm cell strainer cap tubes. It usually takes 3–4 caps per sample. Alternatively, filter samples 350–450 μL per filter using the FlowMi tip filters (4–5 per sample per size), start with 70 μm and followed by 40 μm.
9. Transfer filtered sample to a prechilled 2-mL tube. If processing more than 1 sample, keep this tube on ice and proceed to **steps 5–7** with other samples. We recommend keeping sample numbers low (not more than three per experiment).
10. Centrifuge at 500 g, 4 °C for 5 min, carefully remove the supernatant.

11. Resuspend pellet in 0.5 mL ice-cold *supplemented* NIB2 buffer. Centrifuge at 500 g, 4 °C for 5 min, carefully remove the supernatant, and resuspend again in 0.5-mL ice-cold supplemented NIB2 buffer.
12. (Optional) At this step or prior to **step 9**, transfer 5–10 μL of the sample to a glass slide, cover with a small coverslip, and check for nuclei morphology under a fluorescent microscope using the DAPI channel. An example of successful nuclei release is shown in Fig. 3a.
13. We recommend fluorescent-activated cell sorting (FACS) for removing cellular debris from the nuclei prep. In our experience ocular nuclei prep do not generally contain high levels of debris compared to other tissues, and other methods of purification (e.g., sucrose gradient) may be used as an alternative to FACS.
14. During centrifugation **steps 9** and **10**, prepare 1.5 mL of Nuclei Collection Buffer for each sample on ice: 150 μL of 10× RNase-free PBS, 300 μL of 100-mg/mL RNase-free BSA, 1.05-mL RNase-free water, and 7.5-μL RNase inhibitors. For each sample, prepare two 1.5-mL RNase-free tubes with 0.5-mL Nuclei Collection Buffer. Invert the tubes a few times to coat the entire tube with buffer.
15. Proceed promptly to FACS. Set collection and sample chamber both at 4 °C. If using human samples, make sure the FACS machine is compliant with biosafety regulations. We performed our experiments on BD FACS-ARIA III with a 70-μm nozzle. After normal startup procedures, load 0.5 mL of Nuclei Collection Buffer and run for 3 min.
16. Load the first nuclei sample. Set gate for size on forward and side scatter, followed by linear gate on DAPI. The histogram should show one sharp population representing 2 N DNA content. Representative plots are shown in Fig. 3b.
17. Collect 500,000 nuclei per tube. Do not overload the tubes as this will dilute the RNase inhibitor (*see* **Note 5**). Keep tubes with nuclei on ice and proceed immediately to library preparation (within 30 min after end of sort).

3.4 Single Nucleus Library Preparation, Sequencing, and Exploratory Analysis

1. Centrifuge sorted nuclei samples at 500 g, 4 °C for 7 min. At the end of centrifugation, promptly return the tubes on ice and carefully remove the supernatant, leave ~50 μL of the supernatant in the tube and resuspend the nuclei in the residual liquid. Pipette with a 20p tip for 10 times.
2. Transfer 5 μL of the resuspended nuclei to a new tube and add 5 μL of Trypan Blue solution. Mix well and load unto a hemocytometer. Count and record the density of nuclei under light

microscope. Adjust the nuclei density to 700–1200 nuclei/μL. Nuclei are not DAPI-stained at this point. A DAPI re-stained example of sorted ocular nuclei is shown in Fig. 3c.

3. Proceed with 10× Chromium Single Cell 3′ library construction kits (*see* Materials). Follow the detailed protocols from 10× Genomics. Depending on the target population, adjust the appropriate nuclei numbers per injection.
4. We follow the 10× protocol with one modification: at the cDNA amplification step, we consider the RNA content of nuclei to be ~25% of cells and adjust the PCR cycle numbers accordingly. For example, 10,000 nuclei of target recovery (~17,400 nuclei loaded) is treated as ~2500 cells, and we amplify the cDNA with 12 instead of 11 cycles.
5. Carefully record the sample identifiers during library preparation. The 10× platform is compatible with most common Illumina sequencers. It is important to follow the recommended instrument-specific loadingconcentrations for different sequencers specified by 10× Genomics.
6. Bioinformatic analysis of scRNA-seq and sNucSeq is a rapidly expanding and evolving field and is out of the scope of this chapter. While 10× Genomics offer convenient software packages (Cell Ranger and Loupe Cell Browser) for basic exploratory analysis (e.g., *see* Fig. 4), we encourage readers to consult guided clustering tutorials and publications for SEURAT from the Satija Lab (https://satijalab.org/seurat/v3.0/pbmc3k_tutorial.html) [20].

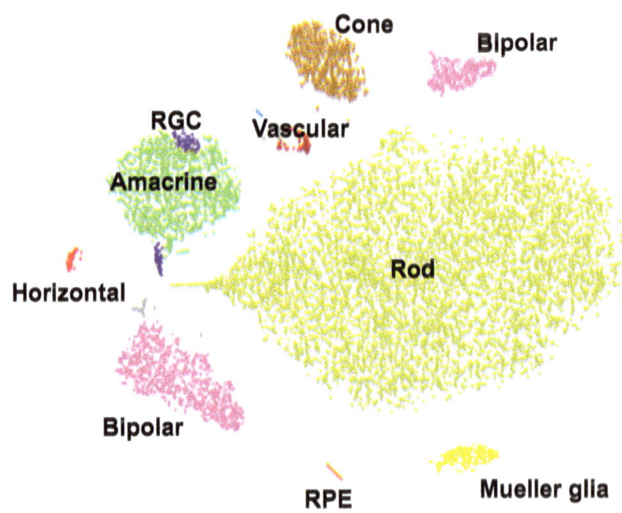

Fig. 4 Example of sNucSeq data. Ocular nuclei from adult domestic New Zealand white rabbits were analyzed by sNucSeq. Results from 16 K individual nuclei were analyzed in Cell Ranger and visualized on Loupe Cell Browser 2.0

4 Notes

1. The starting tissue quality is of utmost importance for NucSeq success. We recommend postmortem interval (PMI) < 5 h for donor samples before snap freezing. Lengthy PMI and slow freezing methods will result in poor nuclear morphology as well as low RNA integrity.
2. The frozen whole globe often cracks at the anterior segment. This normally does not affect the experimental procedures. Occasionally the crack runs parallel to the cutting plane and can impede consistent cryosections. In this case, it is advisable to "repair" the crack with O.C.T. compound before sectioning.
3. The RNA pellet from TRIzol extraction may appear to be brown or pink. This does not affect the subsequent analysis.
4. During douncing, RPE layer should gradually lose color as the cells are lysed and nuclei release. As a result, the nuclei resuspension may appear pinkish.
5. After sorting, the DAPI concentration in the collection tubes is highly diluted, and the nuclei will not appear fluorescent during the subsequent counting step.

References

1. Huang S (2009) Non-genetic heterogeneity of cells in development: more than just noise. Development 136(23):3853–3862
2. Li L, Clevers H (2010) Coexistence of quiescent and active adult stem cells in mammals. Science 327(5965):542–545
3. Shalek AK et al (2014) Single-cell RNA-seq reveals dynamic paracrine control of cellular variation. Nature 510(7505):363–369
4. Hwang B, Lee JH, Bang D (2018) Single-cell RNA sequencing technologies and bioinformatics pipelines. Exp Mol Med 50(8):96
5. Whitmore SS et al (2014) Transcriptomic analysis across nasal, temporal, and macular regions of human neural retina and RPE/choroid by RNA-Seq. Exp Eye Res 129:93–106
6. Macosko EZ et al (2015) Highly parallel genome-wide expression profiling of individual cells using nanoliter droplets. Cell 161(5): 1202–1214
7. Zheng GX et al (2017) Massively parallel digital transcriptional profiling of single cells. Nat Commun 8:14049
8. Buenaventura DF, Corseri A, Emerson MM (2019) Identification of genes with enriched expression in early developing mouse cone photoreceptors. Invest Ophthalmol Vis Sci 60(8):2787–2799
9. Lukowski SW et al (2019) A single-cell transcriptome atlas of the adult human retina. EMBO J 38(18):e100811
10. Peng YR et al (2019) Molecular classification and comparative taxonomics of foveal and peripheral cells in primate retina. Cell 176(5): 1222–1237. e22
11. Shekhar K et al (2016) Comprehensive classification of retinal bipolar neurons by single-cell transcriptomics. Cell 166(5):1308–1323. e30
12. Voigt AP et al (2019) Molecular characterization of foveal versus peripheral human retina by single-cell RNA sequencing. Exp Eye Res 184: 234–242
13. Huang HL et al (2010) Trypsin-induced proteome alteration during cell subculture in mammalian cells. J Biomed Sci 17:36
14. Grindberg RV et al (2013) RNA-sequencing from single nuclei. Proc Natl Acad Sci U S A 110(49):19802–19807
15. Habib N et al (2017) Massively parallel single-nucleus RNA-seq with DroNc-seq. Nat Methods 14(10):955–958
16. Habib N et al (2016) Div-Seq: single-nucleus RNA-Seq reveals dynamics of rare adult newborn neurons. Science 353(6302):925–928
17. Rosenberg AB et al (2018) Single-cell profiling of the developing mouse brain and spinal cord

with split-pool barcoding. Science 360(6385): 176–182

18. Orozco LD et al (2020) Integration of eQTL and a single-cell atlas in the human eye identifies causal genes for age-related macular degeneration. Cell Rep 30(4):1246–1259 e6

19. Krishnaswami SR et al (2016) Using single nuclei for RNA-seq to capture the transcriptome of postmortem neurons. Nat Protoc 11(3):499–524

20. Butler A et al (2018) Integrating single-cell transcriptomic data across different conditions, technologies, and species. Nat Biotechnol 36(5):411–420

Chapter 31

Vector Shedding and Immunogenicity Sampling in AAV-Based Gene Therapy for Retinitis Pigmentosa Patients

Ahra Cho

Abstract

Viral vectors are employed in gene therapy to deliver functional genes. It is often traceable in bodily secretions and excretions of the recipients. Methods of collecting, processing, and storing specimens need to be standardized to ensure effective regulation and monitoring of vector safety. Furthermore, these regulations are crucial in upholding the safety and efficacy of clinical trials and subsequent delivery of these treatments. This chapter discusses vector immunogenicity monitoring and methods of lacrimal, saliva, urine, blood, and serum sampling in patients with retinitis pigmentosa before and throughout the delivery of adeno-associated virus-based gene therapy.

Key words Vector shedding, Immunogenicity, Sampling, Gene therapy, Adeno-associated virus, Retinitis pigmentosa

1 Introduction

Gene therapy clinical trials are actively implemented both nationally and internationally. Approximately 2600 clinical trials involving gene therapy have been completed, approved, or are ongoing in 38 countries [1]. The subretinal injection of the adeno-associated virus (AAV2) vector harboring the cDNA of the *RPE65* gene was the first FDA-approved gene therapy for inherited disorders, namely, Leber congenital amaurosis [2].

AAV vectors are desirable modes of gene transfer and expression due to their persistence in the subretinal space and the lack of pathogenicity of the wild-type virus [3]. The development of transgenes and regulatory sequences has removed barriers associated with the small packaging capacity of vectors. The discovery of new serotypes further improved tissue specificity and their efficacy.

Stephen H. Tsang and Peter M. J. Quinn (eds.), *Retinitis Pigmentosa*,
Methods in Molecular Biology, vol. 2560, https://doi.org/10.1007/978-1-0716-2651-1_31,

Vector shedding is commonly collected through the sampling of peripheral blood, tear, saliva, and urine. Implementation of standardized methods for collecting and monitoring vector dissemination into the environment is necessary due to the inherent abilities of viral vectors to activate the immune response, establish latency, and carry out chromosomal integration followed by recombination. Continuous monitoring is crucial due to the development of vectors that ensure long-term transgene expression in host tissues.

In general, recipients of AAV vector-driven gene therapy are subject to extensive investigation because of the direct administration mode, high capsid diversity, and the various routes of delivery [4]. The conventional method of vector shedding for patients with retinitis pigmentosa is through the tear. The direct injection of the vector into the immune-privileged subretinal space is very unlikely to cause an immune response in the recipient. However, in the context of clinical trials, it is pertinent to assess immunogenicity to assess safety and efficacy. It is recommended that sampling is conducted before and after the vector administration at even intervals to account for latency [5].

Polymerase chain reaction (PCR) is commonly used to detect the vector DNA or RNA of the shed virus. To assess the potential risk of its pathogenic transmission, it is recommended that quantitative PCR (qPCR) is coupled with infectivity assays, which assess the ability or the pathogen to infect, to distinguish the intact from the degraded virus [6]. If there are no other indirect monitoring techniques available to make the distinction, it is recommended to err on the side of caution by assuming that the shed material is infectious. One can infer the infectivity of genetically modified organisms from the change in copy-numbers overtime on qPCR [5]. However, this option would not apply to non-replicating viral vectors such as AAV2.

The activation of adaptive immune responses associated with the vector is a significant factor impeding successful gene transfers. As such, monitoring the immune status before and after treatment by evaluating anti-AAV antibodies is necessary. The enzyme-linked immunosorbent assay (ELISA) rapidly quantifies most anti-AAV antibodies and AAV neutralizing transduction assay performs a functional analysis of the antibodies [7]. The enzyme-linked immunospot (ELISPOT) assay, which quantifies IFN-gamma producing cells, also demonstrates the degree of cellular immune response activation. Other methods include an ex vivo assay using specific immune-cell fractions from the peripheral blood sample [5].

2 Materials [5]

All materials used should be kept in a sterile condition and stored away from direct sunlight prior to use. They should be free of DNA, RNases, DNases, PCR inhibitors, and pyrogens that can cause the nucleic acid samples to disintegrate and compromise the integrity of the samples. Strict adherence should be observed to the expiration date of the equipment packaging.

2.1 Lacrimal Sampling Kit

- Sterile polyester fiber rod wick (2 mm × 15 mm polyester wick, Transorb Wick, Filtrona, Richmond, VA, ×2, one for each eye).
- Sterile forceps (×2, one for each eye).
- Safe-Lock CryoSafe tube (1.5 mL, ×3).
- Safe-Lock CryoSafe tube (1.5 mL, pre-filled with 1 mL phosphate-buffered saline (PBS) pH 7.4, without calcium, magnesium, or phenol red). Sample tubes should be chilled to 2–8 °C and kept on ice prior to sampling.
- Sterile, graduated pipettes (1 mL, ×2).
- Sterile, disposable scissors (×2).

2.2 Saliva Sampling Kit

- Sterile swab.
- Safe-Lock CryoSafe collection tubes (2 mL, ×3).
- CryoSafe adhesive labels.
- Sterile, graduated pipette (1 mL).

2.3 Urine Sampling Kit

- Sterile urine collection container (100 mL).
- Sterile urinary catheter (for female participants who are clinically indicated).
- Safe-Lock CryoSafe tubes (2 mL, ×3).
- CryoSafe adhesive labels.
- Sterile, graduated pipette (1 mL).

2.4 Blood Collection Kit

- Venipuncture blood collection set.
- Gold top blood collection tubes (5 mL, SST gel separator with silica clot activator and gel, ×2).
- Lavender top blood collection tube (4 mL, with dipotassium EDTA salt).

2.5 Blood Processing Kit

- Safe-Lock CryoSafe collection tubes (2 mL, ×3).
- CryoSafe adhesive labels.
- Sterile graduated pipette (1 mL).

2.6 Serum Processing Kit

- Safe-Lock CryoSafe tubes (2 mL, ×3).
- Sterile, graduated pipette (1 mL).

2.7 Other Necessary Items/Equipment

- Vortex.
- Centrifuge with a relative centrifugal force (RCF) of minimum 1100.
- 100% ethanol.
- CryoSafe, solvent-resistant permanent marker.
- Disinfected racks for Safe-Lock CryoSafe collection tubes and blood collection tubes.

3 Methods [5]

The following are the methods for the collection and processing of samples intended for clinical research nurses or research personnel with ophthalmic training and phlebotomy experience. Written consent of all participants must be obtained prior to sample collection. Appropriate personal protective equipment (PPE) should be worn throughout all sampling and processing procedures to avoid sample contamination, possible assay interference, and the transmission of viruses or other pathogens through bodily fluids. Samples should be de-identified with a code to protect the privacy of the participants and prevent bias in sample collection and processing. The code, sample type, visit type, date, and time of collection should be accurately recorded using a CryoSafe marker. The records should be kept in a secure, locked cabinet.

3.1 Lacrimal Sampling

1. Use the CryoSafe labels to label each collection tube pre-filled with phosphate buffered saline PBS, one for each eye.
2. Ensure the participant looks up throughout the procedure.
3. Start with the right eye. Gently pull the lower eyelid down and place the polyester fiber wick parallel to the cornea to avoid injury to the eye. Swab the inside with the wick.
4. Immediately place the wick in the CryoSafe tube pre-filled with PBS. Cut off the wick with the sterile scissors to fit in the tube if necessary.
5. Vortex the sample and hold on ice immediately.
6. Repeat **steps 3–5** for the left eye.
7. For the sample of the right eye, use sterile forceps to push the wick to the side of the tube to release as much fluid as possible. Discard the wick.

8. Use the sterile pipette to transfer the sample equally into three chilled Safe-Lock CryoSafe tubes. Label the tube using CryoSafe labels. Place the tubes on ice.
9. Repeat **steps 7–8** for the left eye.
10. Freeze the samples at −80 °C.

3.2 Saliva Sampling

1. Label each tube using the CryoSafe labels.
2. Ensure the participant did not consume any food or drink 1 h prior to sample collection. Do not use oral stimulants.
3. Have participant rinse mouth thoroughly with water and wait at least 10 min.
4. Ask the participant to tilt their head forward to allow saliva to passively fill the collection tube. Close the cap tightly.
5. Place the tube on ice immediately after collection.
6. Repeat **steps 4–5** two more times to collect a total of three 2-mL saliva samples.
7. Use the vortex to aliquot the supernatant and freeze at −80 °C.

3.3 Urine Sampling

1. Label each tube using the CryoSafe labels.
2. Ask the participant to wash hands thoroughly and then collect urine in the container mid-stream. Use a sterile urethral catheter for female participants who are clinically indicated.
3. Using the sterile pipettes, transfer 1 mL of urine into each of the three Safe-Lock CryoSafe tubes.
4. Freeze the samples at −80 °C.

3.4 Blood Sampling

1. Follow local procedures and guidelines to draw blood (venipuncture) using sterile venipuncture set.
2. Slowly fill the gold top, 5-mL tube. Place the cap of the tube. Gently invert five times. Repeat for the second collection.
3. Slowly fill the lavender top, 4-mL tube. Place the cap of the tube. Gently invert ten times.
4. Label each tube appropriately.
5. Do not freeze these samples.

3.5 Anticoagulated Blood Sample Processing

1. Use a sterile graduated pipette to transfer 1 mL of the whole blood sample into each of the three 2-mL Safe-Lock CryoSafe collection tubes. Close the caps tightly.
2. Label each tube using the CryoSafe labels.
3. Immediately, freeze the samples at −80 °C.

3.6 Serum Sampling from Whole Blood

1. Label three 2 mL Safe-Lock CryoSafe collection tubes using the CryoSafe labels.
2. Sample processing should occur within 2 h after collection.

3. Allow 15–30 min for the whole blood sample in the gold top tube to form a dense clot.
4. Use a refrigerated centrifuge at relative centrifugal force (RCF) of 1000–2000 × g for 10 min to isolate the clot.
5. Transfer approximately 1 mL of the supernatant into each of the three 2-mL Safe-Lock CryoSafe collection tubes. Close the caps tightly.
6. Immediately, freeze the samples at −80 °C.

4 Notes

1. Ensure participants are instructed ahead of time on how to prepare for the saliva sampling, i.e., no eating 1 h before sampling.
2. Clear verbalization of each step to the participant prior to performing them can encourage cooperation.
3. For children and infants who may have difficulty with passively filling the CryoSafe collection tubes, Children's Swab and Infant's Swab are recommended, respectively. These swabs are commercially available. After saliva is collected, the swabs should be cut with sterile scissors to fit in the collection tubes.
4. When slowly pipetting viscous fluids such as saliva, tilt the tube and aspirate slowly to avoid the formation of bubbles.
5. After collecting blood by venipuncture, slowly transfer the specimen into the collection tubes to reduce the risk of hemolysis.
6. Validation and quality control of all immunoassays are recommended for accurate results.

References

1. Ginn SL, Amaya AK, Alexander IE et al (2018 May) Gene therapy clinical trials worldwide to 2017: an update. J Gene Med 20(5): e3015
2. Hanna E, Remuzat C, Auquier P et al (2017) Gene therapies development: slow progress and promising prospect. J Mark Access Health Policy 5(1):1265293
3. Daya S, Berns KI (2008 Oct) Gene therapy using adeno-associated virus vectors. Clin Microbiol Rev 21(4):583–593
4. Le Guiner C, Moullier P, Arruda VR (2011) Biodistribution and shedding of AAV vectors. Methods Mol Biol 807:339–359
5. Barnard AR, Rudenko AN, MacLaren RE (2018) Vector shedding and immunogenicity sampling for retinal gene therapy. Methods Mol Biol 1715:359–371
6. Agency EM (2009) General principles to address virus and vector shedding. ICH considerations. European Medicines Agency, London, p 7
7. Martino AT, Herzog RW, Anegon I et al (2011) Measuring immune responses to recombinant AAV gene transfer. Methods Mol Biol 807: 259–272

Chapter 32

Current Management Options for Patients with Retinitis Pigmentosa

Abinaya Thenappan

Abstract

With an estimated prevalence of 1 in 4000 worldwide [1], retinitis pigmentosa (RP) comprises a spectrum of progressive inherited retinal disorders that can lead to blindness as early as age 30 [2]. Despite its relatively high prevalence and devastating consequences, RP does not have a definitive cure. Therapeutic attempts have been made with nutritional supplementation, but these strategies only have proven benefit in a limited number of patients with rare forms of RP. Thus, current standards of care involve regular follow-up, management of associated ocular pathology such as macular edema and cataracts, and genetic counseling and low vision rehabilitation. In recent years, gene therapy, visual prostheses, and stem cell therapy have emerged as FDA-approved treatments for RP, but these options are not yet widely used. Herein, this chapter will discuss the therapeutic strategies listed above that comprise the current standards of care and briefly discuss some emerging options.

Key words Cataracts, Cystoid macular edema, Gene therapy, iPSCs, Management, Nutrition, Prostheses, Retinitis pigmentosa, Treatment

1 Introduction

The most common hereditary retinal dystrophy, retinitis pigmentosa (RP), represents a genetically and phenotypically heterogeneous group of retinal disorders which instigate degeneration of first rod, then cone, photoreceptors [3]. The typical clinical features of RP are nyctalopia and peripheral vision loss, and the classic triad of exam findings include optic disk pallor, bone-spicule retinal pigmentation, and arteriolar attenuation. Despite its devastating consequences, RP does not have any established treatment protocols to halt disease progression or restore vision.

Therapeutic attempts have been made with vitamin and nutritional supplementation, but these strategies only have proven benefit in rare forms of RP. Thus, current standards of care include supportive and conservative strategies, with a reliance on regular

Stephen H. Tsang and Peter M. J. Quinn (eds.), *Retinitis Pigmentosa*,
Methods in Molecular Biology, vol. 2560, https://doi.org/10.1007/978-1-0716-2651-1_32,

follow-up to identify and manage the collateral complications of RP, such as macular edema or cataracts. Additionally, genetic counseling and low vision rehabilitation are essential to help patients make informed decisions and cope with the limitations of severe vision loss.

Emerging therapies such as gene therapy, visual prostheses, and stem cell therapy have shown significant progress over the past few years, but these therapeutic modalities are not yet widely used. Ongoing efforts to optimize the safety, efficacy, and sustainability of these investigational technologies are promising. This chapter will describe the current standards of care summarized above and briefly dive into promising therapeutic modalities for the future.

2 Nutritional Supplementation

Nutritional supplementation, including lutein, vitamin A, docosahexaenoic acid (DHA), calcium channel blockers, and ascorbic acid, has been explored to have a possible supportive role in RP. Unfortunately, although some studies report modest benefit, others report no detectable difference in clinically relevant measures [4–6].

Specifically, the most widely recommended nutritional supplement for patients with RP is vitamin A. Critical to the structural and functional integrity of photoreceptors, vitamin A deficiency or abnormal vitamin A metabolism has unsurprisingly been considered to play a role in the underlying pathophysiology RP [7]. However, a therapeutic role for vitamin A supplementation remains controversial. One randomized controlled trial assigned 601 patients with RP to one of four groups receiving 15,000 IU/day of vitamin A, 15,000 IU/day of vitamin A plus 400 IU/day of vitamin E, trace amounts of both vitamins, or 400 IU/day of vitamin E [8]. Although the study revealed a marginally lower rate of decline of ERG amplitudes with vitamin A supplementation, no effect was documented in regard to clinically relevant measures of visual function such as visual field loss or visual acuity change. Interestingly, vitamin E supplementation actually accelerated the decline of ERG amplitudes [8]. These findings, coupled with the toxicity and teratogenicity of high dose vitamin A supplementation, have discouraged clinicians from using vitamin A or E supplementation as a mainstay of treatment.

More recently, omega 3 fatty acids have been investigated for potential therapeutic benefit. Omega 3 fatty acids have been shown to accumulate in the brain and eye in late fetal and early neonatal life [9], and in particular, high levels of docosahexaenoic acid (DHA) are found in the retina and continue to serve as support for retinal photoreceptor outer segment membranes throughout life. In fact, studies have shown that patients with RP have low levels of DHA

[10]. However, a systematic review of six randomized controlled trials concluded that DHA supplementation is not associated with significant benefit in RP [11]. Thus, it is generally recommended that patients with RP consume a diet rich in omega 3 fatty acids, but supplemental DHA is not prescribed.

In three rare, secondary forms of RP, nutritional supplementation can actually serve as a definitive cure:

1. Abetalipoproteinemia is an autosomal recessive disorder caused by defective intestinal absorption of fat-soluble vitamins. As early as infancy, signs and symptoms including failure to thrive, malnutrition, and steatorrhea manifest. As an individual with this condition ages, spinocerebellar ataxia, peripheral neuropathy, and muscle weakness resembling a diffuse neuromuscular disease develops. Abetalipoproteinemia is also associated with various ophthalmologic manifestations, including RP. Supplementation with fat-soluble vitamins (specifically A, E, and K) has been shown to restore reverse ERG abnormalities and improve retinal function and dark adaptation [12].
2. Phytanic acid oxidase deficiency, also known as Refsum disease, is an autosomal recessive disorder which causes anosmia as well as RP. The disorder is caused by defective metabolism of phytanic acid, which can accumulate in the retinal pigment epithelium and lead to photoreceptor cell degeneration. Dietary modification, including avoiding food rich in phytol and phytanic acid (i.e., beef, lamb, seafood, dairy products), can slow disease progression and result in stabilization of retinal function [13]. Plasmapheresis may also be necessary.
3. Alpha tocopherol transfer protein (α-TTP) deficiency is a genetic syndrome associated with defective intracellular transport of α-tocopherol, the most biologically active form of vitamin E. Abnormalities of the α-TTP gene have been identified as a cause of RP [14]. In patients with this mutation, disease progression can be slowed with vitamin E supplementation [15].

3 Managing Associated Ocular Pathology

Comprehensive management of RP includes regular follow-up with ophthalmic examinations to detect vision-threatening collateral consequences of RP, most frequently cystoid macular edema and cataract development. Timely and appropriate ancillary treatments for these secondary complications is imperative to preserving patients' remaining vision.

3.1 Cystoid Macular Edema

In later stages of RP, patients can develop cystoid macular edema (CME) that compromises central vision. Because these patients likely already have severe peripheral field loss, timely and appropriate management of CME is imperative to preserve central acuity. However, because the underlying mechanism of CME due to RP is poorly characterized and likely multifactorial, numerous treatment protocols have been proposed and the optimal therapy remains debated. In most cases, carbonic anhydrase inhibitors, oral or topical, are regarded as reliable first-line treatment options. These drugs promote fluid reabsorption across the retinal pigment epithelium by stimulating active transport across the blood–retina barrier and decreasing leakage [16]. Patients who are not responsive to carbonic anhydrase inhibitors may benefit from steroids (intravitreal or oral), intravitreal anti-VEGF agents, grid laser photocoagulation, or pars plana vitrectomy [17].

It is important to note that acetazolamide has no effect on vision or ERG changes in patients without CME [18] and is associated with a wide spectrum of side effects, including peripheral numbness/tingling, malaise, gastrointestinal upset, kidney stones, and altered taste sensation. Methazolamide is another oral carbonic anhydrase inhibitor which has a more favorable side effect profile; however, it has been shown to be less effective overall [19]. An additional limitation of oral carbonic anhydrase inhibitors is that they cannot be used for more than several weeks because extended use is associated with rebound edema [20, 21].

Topical carbonic anhydrase inhibitors like dorzolamide are typically not trialed as a first-line treatment due to their reported reduced efficacy in treating macular edema and improving visual acuity when compared to oral carbonic anhydrase inhibitors [22]. However, they are an effective alternative for patients who are unable to tolerate the systemic side effects of acetazolamide. For the same reason, they are preferred as a first-line option in pediatric and elderly populations. It has also been suggested that, unlike acetazolamide, dorzolamide can sustain improvement in CME for up to 15 months [23].

In terms of imaging modalities to detect CME and monitor for treatment efficacy, fluorescein angiography was the mainstay option prior to the advent of optical coherence tomography (OCT). OCT has since been shown to be more sensitive in detecting macular edema in these patients [24]. OCT is further preferred as it is quick and noninvasive.

3.2 Posterior Subcapsular Cataracts

A common anterior segment complication of RP is the development of a cataract, particularly a posterior subcapsular lens opacity. In fact, it has been shown that 35–51% of adults with RP develop posterior subcapsular cataracts [25, 26]. Because of uncertain visual outcomes and increased surgical risk, the decision to proceed with cataract extraction in these patients can be challenging.

According to a recent study, cataract extraction with implantation of a new intraocular lens improves visual acuity in a majority of RP patients with a preoperative visual acuity of 20/200 or better [27]. Patients with a preoperative acuity of 20/400 or worse typically experience modest objective improvement (though they do report subjective improvement), likely due to macular involvement of their underlying RP [27]. 10–2 visual fields and OCT imaging are important preoperative tests that can be used to assess the macula and predict postoperative visual potential. Preoperative evaluation of lens stability is also important as zonular instability is common among RP patients undergoing cataract extraction [27]. Patients should be counseled that their visual field or disease progression will not change.

3.3 Refractive Errors

Refractive errors such as myopia and astigmatism are common in RP [28]. Routine ophthalmic examinations and accurate measurement of refractive errors are imperative, especially for patients with end-stage RP. A careful measurement of the refractive error can also suggest a specific inheritance pattern of RP. For example, there is evidence that patients with myopia of at least 2 diopters are more likely to have X-linked RP [29].

4 Counseling

Regular follow-up with RP patients is essential to provide support and offer counseling as necessary. For example, clinicians can help guide patients who have been prescribed retinotoxic medications such as erectile dysfunction drugs, isotretinoin, phenothiazines, hydroxychloroquine, tamoxifen, and vigabatrin, as these medications should be used with caution [3]. Additionally, genetic counseling and low vision rehabilitation serve as important cornerstones of regular follow-up visits.

The goal of genetic counseling is to use pedigree analysis and the patient's genotype to educate the patient about the likely inheritance pattern and the chance that the trait will be passed onto future generations or expressed in other family members. This information can inform a patient's decision-making about future plans, including family planning and clinical intervention.

Low vision rehabilitation can help target specific functional limitations that a patient may experience in everyday life. A few examples of devices that can help patients compensate for a constricted visual field include visual field awareness devices, high-intensity lamps, filters, and magnifiers. Also, tinted glasses can be used in bright environments to improve contrast sensitivity. Patients should be oriented toward rehabilitation institutions as their disease progresses, as low vision services and mobility training can help RP patients live more independently and learn new professional skills [30].

5 Emerging Treatment Modalities

5.1 Gene Therapy

Gene therapy involves intracellular delivery of genomic material to replace or silence a known mutation with the goal of eliciting a therapeutic benefit. One of the most successful delivery systems studied for RP are viral vectors, specifically adenovirus, lentivirus, and adeno-associated virus [31]. Using a virus as a carrier, genes are delivered to outer retinal cells via a subretinal injection, which requires iatrogenic retinal detachment. Although pieces of the viral genome are intentionally damaged to ensure safety, viral vectors carry intrinsic immunogenicity that incites an inflammatory response.

Non-viral delivery systems include liposomes, polypeptides, polymers, and compacted nanoparticles [32]. These methods tend to be more cost-effective, accessible, and have the advantage of reduced immunogenicity. However, they face other challenges including inefficient cell membrane transport and intracellular degradation. Non-viral delivery systems are not yet a feasible option, but continuing advances in engineering technologies have made non-viral delivery systems a promising approach for the future.

In terms of RP, the retina is an attractive target for gene therapy due to its immune privilege and compartmentalization [33], which reduces systemic absorption. Thus, although gene therapy is not yet widely used for RP, it is an emerging option that can be attempted in early stages of the disease in a limited number of patients. The proportion of treatable RP patients with gene therapy is estimated to be 5–20% [34]. If feasible, gene therapy in early stages is ideal as it can preserve as many intact photoreceptors as possible. However, its uncertain efficacy and accompanying surgical risks have discouraged its use in early stages, and it is typically attempted only in advanced disease.

Targeted genome editing is a subset of gene therapy that aims to correct the specific disease-causing mutation. The clustered regularly interspaced short palindromic repeat (CRISPR)/Cas9, an RNA-guided DNA cleavage system, is a well-known genome editing tool that has promising potential for the future. Although most cases of RP are monogenic, targeted genome editing for RP has faced a number of obstacles due to the pronounced genetic diversity and considerable overlap in causative genes and mutations with other retinal dystrophies. Not only are there limited target genes and indicated patients, but targeted genome editing requires invasive administration methods and has been shown to have modest efficacy at best.

In summary, gene therapy has the potential to achieve a definitive cure for RP patients, but it currently faces limitations such as modest efficacy and limited target genes. Ongoing research and development suggest that it can be a promising therapeutic option in the future.

5.2 Retinal Prosthesis

RP is a disease characterized by a dramatic and progressive decline in the number of photoreceptors. In patients without any remaining photoreceptors left, retinal prosthesis can be explored as a treatment option. In a nutshell, these prostheses are electrical devices that can stimulate the remaining retinal cells by applying an electrical charge by an electrode. These devices can be implanted in the epiretinal, subretinal, or suprachoroidal spaces.

Two devices, Argus II and Alpha-IMS, are currently commercially available and have documented long-term clinical trial results. The Alpha-IMS implant is a subretinal implant that showed significant improvement in visual performance in 45% of the 29 enrolled patients for 6 years [34]. The ARGUS II implant is an epiretinal implant which has been used in several hundred RP patients worldwide with bare or no light perception vision since its approval. It is a surgically implantable array of epiretinal microelectrodes that obtains visual data from an eyeglass-mounted camera. This information is converted into action potentials, which are then transmitted to the brain through the optic nerve. Studies have shown modest visual improvement including orientation, mobility, target localization, and even reading of letters [35], but there is still wide variability in functional outcomes among patients. Surveillance studies have demonstrated safety, tolerability, and sustainability of outcome in up to 5 years of follow-up [36].

Despite encouraging clinical trial results, the patients who have trialed these devices only regained rudimentary vision, and only patients with end-stage disease are currently indicated [36]. Significant developments in the electronic technology are needed for retinal prostheses to achieve more clinically meaningful widespread use.

5.3 Stem Cell Transplantation

Cell transplantation is the process of introducing progenitor cells (retinal photoreceptor precursors or stem cells) into a patient to replace diseased cells in the retina and regenerate a population of healthy retinal cells. Stem cells can come from embryonic stem cells, induced pluripotent stem cells (iPSCs), or an endogenous origin. Autologous iPSCs and iPSC-derived retinal precursor cells carry the benefit of evading immunologic or ethical issues; however, a big drawback is that the disease may recur after transplantation. As of now, only a small number of clinical trials are currently exploring their role in RP, so autologous iPSCs are not yet a feasible therapy. However, further technical advancement and experience from other applications may allow iPSCs to serve as a future therapeutic option.

6 Conclusion

RP represents a group of progressive retinal dystrophies that can result in devastating visual consequences and eventual blindness. However, there are no established standard treatment modalities to date that can prevent or reverse visual loss for these patients. Nutritional supplementation in rare forms of RP, treating associated ocular pathology, and appropriate counseling comprise current standards of care, Gene therapy, visual prosthesis, and stem cell transplantation are reserved for investigational purposes in advanced disease. With increasing knowledge about specific mutations and the driving biochemical mechanisms, RP is a compelling target for novel technologies, and clinicians are optimistic that a definitive cure is on the horizon.

References

1. Hartong DT, Berson EL, Dryja TP (2006) Retinitis pigmentosa. Lancet 368(9549): 1795–1809. https://doi.org/10.1016/S0140-6736(06)69740-7
2. Berson EL (1993) Retinitis pigmentosa: the Friedenwald lecture. Invest Opthal Vis Sci 34(5):1655–1676
3. Bowling B, Kanski JJ (2016) Kanskis clinical ophthalmology: a systematic approach. Elsevier, Amsterdam
4. Hoffman DR et al (2014) Four-year placebo-controlled trial of docosahexaenoic acid in X-linked retinitis pigmentosa (DHAX trial): a randomized clinical trial. JAMA Ophthalmol 132(7):866–873. https://doi.org/10.1001/jamaophthalmol.2014.1634
5. Hoffman DR et al (2004) A randomized, placebo-controlled clinical trial of docosahexaenoic acid supplementation for X-linked retinitis pigmentosa. Am J Ophthalmol 137(4): 704–718. https://doi.org/10.1016/j.ajo.2003.10.045
6. Berson EL et al (2004) Clinical trial of docosahexaenoic acid in patients with retinitis pigmentosa receiving vitamin A treatment. Arch Ophthalmol 122(9):1297–1305. https://doi.org/10.1001/archopht.122.9.1297
7. Wald G, Zeavin BH (1956) Rod and cone vision in retinitis pigmentosa. Am J Ophthalmol 42(4 Part 2):253–269. https://doi.org/10.1016/0002-9394(56)90377-4
8. Marmor MF (1993) A randomized trial of vitamin A and vitamin E supplementation for retinitis pigmentosa. Arch Ophthalmol 111(11): 1460–1461. author reply 1463-5
9. Innis SM (2003) Perinatal biochemistry and physiology of long-chain polyunsaturated fatty acids. J Pediatr 143(4 Suppl):S1–S8. https://doi.org/10.1067/s0022-3476(03)00396-2
10. Hoffman DR et al (2015) Docosahexaenoic acid slows visual field progression in X-linked retinitis pigmentosa: ancillary outcomes of the DHAX trial. Invest Ophthalmol Vis Sci 56(11): 6646–6653. https://doi.org/10.1167/iovs.15-17786
11. Hodge WG et al (2006) The evidence for efficacy of omega-3 fatty acids in preventing or slowing the progression of retinitis pigmentosa: a systematic review. Can J Ophthalmol 41(4):481–490. https://doi.org/10.1016/S0008-4182(06)80012-8
12. Gouras P, Carr RE, Gunkel RD (1971) Retinitis pigmentosa in abetalipoproteinemia: effects of vitamin A. Investig Ophthalmol 10(10): 784–793
13. Wierzbicki AS et al (2002) Refsum's disease: a peroxisomal disorder affecting phytanic acid alpha-oxidation. J Neurochem 80(5): 727–735. https://doi.org/10.1046/j.0022-3042.2002.00766.x
14. Yokota T et al (1996) Retinitis pigmentosa and ataxia caused by a mutation in the gene for the alpha-tocopherol-transfer protein. N Engl J Med 335(23):1770–1771. https://doi.org/10.1056/NEJM199612053352315
15. Schuelke M et al (1999) Treatment of ataxia in isolated vitamin E deficiency caused by alpha-tocopherol transfer protein deficiency. J Pediatr

134(2):240–244. https://doi.org/10.1016/s0022-3476(99)70424-5
16. Moldow B et al (1998) The effect of acetazolamide on passive and active transport of fluorescein across the blood-retina barrier in retinitis pigmentosa complicated by macular oedema. Graefes Arch Clin Exp Ophthalmol 236(12):881–889. https://doi.org/10.1007/s004170050175
17. Bakthavatchalam M et al (2018) Treatment of cystoid macular edema secondary to retinitis pigmentosa: a systematic review. Surv Ophthalmol 63(3):329–339. https://doi.org/10.1016/j.survophthal.2017.09.009
18. Greenstein VC et al (1993) The effects of acetazolamide on visual function in retinitis pigmentosa. Invest Ophthalmol Vis Sci 34(1):269–273
19. Fishman GA et al (1994) Effect of methazolamide on chronic macular edema in patients with retinitis pigmentosa. Ophthalmology 101(4):687–693. https://doi.org/10.1016/s0161-6420(94)31277-2
20. Apushkin MA et al (2007) Rebound of cystoid macular edema with continued use of acetazolamide in patients with retinitis pigmentosa. Retina 27(8):1112–1118. https://doi.org/10.1097/IAE.0b013e31805f6b79
21. Fishman GA, Glenn AM, Gilbert LD (1993) Rebound of macular edema with continued use of methazolamide in patients with retinitis pigmentosa. Arch Ophthalmol 111(12):1640–1646. https://doi.org/10.1001/archopht.1993.01090120062023
22. Grover S et al (1997) Efficacy of dorzolamide hydrochloride in the management of chronic cystoid macular edema in patients with retinitis pigmentosa. Retina 17(3):222–231. https://doi.org/10.1097/00006982-199705000-00009
23. Fishman GA, Apushkin MA (2007) Continued use of dorzolamide for the treatment of cystoid macular oedema in patients with retinitis pigmentosa. Br J Ophthalmol 91(6):743–745. https://doi.org/10.1136/bjo.2006.107466
24. Apushkin MA, Fishman GA, Janowicz MJ (2004) Monitoring cystoid macular edema by optical coherence tomography in patients with retinitis pigmentosa. Ophthalmology 111(10):1899–1904. https://doi.org/10.1016/j.ophtha.2004.04.019
25. Heckenlively J (1982) The frequency of posterior subcapsular cataract in the hereditary retinal degenerations. Am J Ophthalmol 93(6):733–738. https://doi.org/10.1016/0002-9394(82)90469-x
26. Fishman GA, Anderson RJ, Lourenco P (1985) Prevalence of posterior subcapsular lens opacities in patients with retinitis pigmentosa. Br J Ophthalmol 69(4):263–266. https://doi.org/10.1136/bjo.69.4.263
27. Dikopf MS et al (2013) Cataract extraction outcomes and the prevalence of zonular insufficiency in retinitis pigmentosa. Am J Ophthalmol 156(1):82–88. e2. https://doi.org/10.1016/j.ajo.2013.02.002
28. Sieving PA, Fishman GA (1978) Refractive errors of retinitis pigmentosa patients. Br J Ophthalmol 62(3):163–167. https://doi.org/10.1136/bjo.62.3.163
29. Fishman GA, Farber MD, Derlacki DJ (1988) X-linked retinitis pigmentosa. Profile of clinical findings. Arch Ophthalmol 106(3):369–375. https://doi.org/10.1001/archopht.1988.01060130395029
30. Shah P et al (2018) Low vision services: a practical guide for the clinician. Ther Adv Ophthalmol 10:2515841418776264. https://doi.org/10.1177/2515841418776264
31. Bulcha JT et al (2021) Viral vector platforms within the gene therapy landscape. Signal Transduct Target Ther 6(1):53. https://doi.org/10.1038/s41392-021-00487-6
32. Ramamoorth M, Narvekar A (2015) Non viral vectors in gene therapy- an overview. J Clin Diagn Res 9(1):GE01–GE06. https://doi.org/10.7860/JCDR/2015/10443.5394
33. Benhar I, London A, Schwartz M (2012) The privileged immunity of immune privileged organs: the case of the eye. Front Immunol 3:296. https://doi.org/10.3389/fimmu.2012.00296
34. Stingl K et al (2015) Subretinal visual implant alpha IMS--clinical trial interim report. Vision Res 111(Pt B):149–160. https://doi.org/10.1016/j.visres.2015.03.001
35. Dias MF et al (2018) Molecular genetics and emerging therapies for retinitis pigmentosa: basic research and clinical perspectives. Prog Retin Eye Res 63:107–131. https://doi.org/10.1016/j.preteyeres.2017.10.004
36. da Cruz L et al (2016) Five-year safety and performance results from the Argus II retinal prosthesis system clinical trial. Ophthalmology 123(10):2248–2254. https://doi.org/10.1016/j.ophtha.2016.06.049

Chapter 33

Challenges of Treatment Methodologies and the Future of Gene Therapy and Stem Cell Therapy to Treat Retinitis Pigmentosa

Angela Y. Chang

Abstract

Retinitis pigmentosa (RP) is a heterogeneous group of hereditary retinal degenerations for which there is currently no cure. Studies investigating the use of gene therapy, gene editing, and stem cells as potential treatment strategies have shown promising results in animal models and some early clinical trials. Even still, major barriers still exist, including the ability to develop therapies that can target the wide range of mutational etiologies and phenotypic presentations that encompass RP. Additionally, effective screening and early diagnosis are crucial for maximum therapeutic potential, especially because many therapeutic agents require a baseline level photoreceptor function.

Key words CRISPR/Cas9, Gene-editing technology, Gene therapy, Inherited retinal disease, Pluripotent stem cells, Retinal dystrophy, Retinitis pigmentosa, Stem cell therapy

1 Introduction

Retinitis pigmentosa (RP) encompasses a group of inherited retinal dystrophies that lead to progressive loss of rod and cone photoreceptors and retinal degeneration in later stages. The disease frequently begins with loss of rod photoreceptors followed by cone photoreceptors. Clinically, RP typically manifests with nyctalopia in adolescence, visual field scotomas in young adulthood, and decreased visual acuity and visual field constriction in later stages [1, 2]. Central vision is usually lost by the sixth decade [1]. On exam, the retina commonly displays bone-spicule degeneration in the mid-periphery, optic disk pallor, and retinal arteriole attenuation [1, 2]. RP specifically involves the outer nuclear layer of the retina, where the rod and cone photoreceptor cell bodies are found [1]. In later stages of the disease, other retinal layers may also undergo degeneration [1]. RP is associated with angle-closure

Stephen H. Tsang and Peter M. J. Quinn (eds.), *Retinitis Pigmentosa*,
Methods in Molecular Biology, vol. 2560, https://doi.org/10.1007/978-1-0716-2651-1_33,

glaucoma, high myopia, cystoid macular edema, and posterior subcapsular cataract [2].

RP has a worldwide prevalence of 1 in 4000, with over 1 million people affected [1]. Over 45 different genes have been implicated in RP, and they demonstrate various inheritance patterns including autosomal dominant (30–40%), autosomal recessive (50–60%), and X-linked (5–15%) [1]. Additionally, 40% of RP cases are attributable to mutations in genes not yet identified [1]. Less frequently, RP can display non-Mendelian inheritance patterns [1].

Currently, there is no cure for RP, and there are no treatments that can stop retinal degeneration. However, supplementation with vitamin A, vitamin E, and omega 3 fatty may preserve visual function and slow disease progression [1]. The integrity of cone photoreceptors, that are crucial for the sharp vision and daily living, depends on rod photoreceptor health. Various hypotheses regarding the close relationship between rod and cone health have been proposed. Cones depend on trophic factors produced by rods, rod degeneration leads to cone nutrient deficiency, and rod degeneration leads to oxidative stress that impacts cones [3, 4]. Thus, many treatment strategies seek to prevent rod degeneration and thus preserve cone function. Many recent studies and clinical trials involving use of gene therapy, gene editing, and stem cell therapy have been promising for treatment of RP.

2 Materials

1. Gene Therapy.
   - (a) Intravitreal vs subretinal injection.
   - (b) Adeno-associated virus (AAV) vs lentivirus (LV) vectors vs DNA nanoparticles.
2. Gene Editing.
   - (a) CRISPR/Cas9.
   - (b) Cas9 DNA endonuclease.
   - (c) Guide RNA (gRNA).
   - (d) DNA repair at non-homologous end joining (NHEJ) or high-fidelity homology-directed repair (HDR).
   - (e) Protospacer adjacent motif (PAM) sequence.
3. Stem Cell Therapy.
   - (a) Autologous induced pluripotent stem cells.
   - (b) Human embryonic stem cells (hESCs).
   - (c) Induced pluripotent stem cells (iPSCs).
4. Therapy for Advanced Photoreceptor Degeneration.
   - (a) Retinal prostheses (i.e., Argus II Retinal Prosthesis System).

3 Methods

3.1 Gene Therapy

Gene therapy involves suppressing or inactivating a mutated gene and then delivering a novel or replacement gene that can rectify the existing mutation. Often, genetic material corresponding to the wild-type protein is delivered to restore the absent protein function. Monogenic mutations in target genes leading to complete or near complete absence of function are particularly amenable to treatment by gene therapy, since they do not require gene knockdown. Additionally, since there is little-to-no native protein function, there is less risk of protein overexpression with administration of gene therapy. Protein overexpression can lead to unwanted side effects including retinal toxicity. In contrast, gain-of-function mutations that frequently exhibit a dominant inheritance pattern are less amenable to treatment by gene therapy since a two-step process of gene knockdown of the abnormal gene product then subsequent gene administration is required.

Most commonly, gene therapy for ophthalmic diseases involves gene delivery through retinal injections. There are two types of retinal injections: intravitreal and subretinal. Intravitreal injections are made directly in the vitreous cavity, resulting in delivery close to the ganglion cells. Intravitreal injections are particularly useful when the gene needs to be delivered to the inner layers of the retina [5]. Complications from intravitreal injections include endophthalmitis, retinal detachment, uveitis, and iritis [6]. Subretinal injections result in a transient retinal detachment that allows for delivery between the photoreceptors and the retinal pigment epithelium. Thus, subretinal injections are preferred when the gene needs to be delivered to the outer layers of the retina [5]. Even though subretinal injections are more invasive than intravitreal injections, the treatment can directly reach the photoreceptors, leading to protein translation and expression [7]. Additionally, subretinal injections exhibit greater penetration of the target cells [7]. Since most inherited retinal degenerations, including RP, result in mutations in this region, subretinal injections are the most used modality for gene therapy [5].

Although use of injections for gene delivery is promising, its efficacy is inherently highly variable; gene therapy may only reach a subset of photoreceptors, leading to variable treatment outcomes [6, 8]. Additionally, the distribution of photoreceptors in the retina varies along with the island of vision, with the highest density of cone photoreceptors in the central macular area [6]. This region is responsible for the sharpest vision and color vision, which may have significant impacts on one's quality of life and ability to accomplish activities of daily living. However, this region is the last to be affected in RP, with rod photoreceptors in the periphery affected early on in the disease process. These factors are important to consider, as gene therapy is most effective when the photoreceptors still have residual function.

Retinal gene therapy has been administered using adeno-associated virus (AAV) and lentivirus as vectors for gene delivery, with use of AAV being the most common [7]. The use of AAV vectors to deliver retinal gene products has been the delivery modality of choice, since they are able to provide efficient transduction with minimal safety concerns [9]. They are advantageous in that they are non-pathogenic, display low viral integration frequency and immunogenicity, and can transduce nondividing cells [7, 9]. AAV serotypes 2, 5, 7, 8, and 9 are capable of transducing photoreceptors with AAV8 being particularly efficient [7, 9]. One major limitation to using AAV vectors is that they are restricted by the amount of DNA they can carry to about 4.8 kb of single-stranded DNA [9], limiting the subset of mutations they can treat. Additionally, they display a slow onset of expression; the conversion of the single-stranded DNA genome to double-stranded DNA can take weeks to occur [7]. Compared to AAV, lentivirus (LV) vectors have increased cloning capacity of up to 10 kb [7]. They also transduce both dividing and non-dividing cells. However, unlike AAV, LV vectors tend to integrate into the host genome. Although the eye is an immune privileged site, systemic spread of the AAV or LV vectors can lead to an inflammatory response and immunosuppression of gene therapy. Studies have shown that even at low titers, antibodies are able to neutralize vector transduction [6]. AAV vectors have also been found to have higher amounts of systemic shedding with intravitreal injections than subretinal injections [6].

Since use of AAV vectors is limited by the size of the DNA vector that can be efficiently delivered, inclusion of the full native DNA sequence may be impractical for effective gene delivery. While gene therapy can be administered with cDNA expression vectors, cDNA vectors can lead to protein overexpression and subsequent toxicity. Inclusion of noncoding genomic DNA sequences in the vector may help reduce overexpression and improve therapeutic outcomes [10]. One study showed that including native intronic sequences in gene therapy led to improvements in rod function and preservation of cone function in a subset of RP involving mutations in the rhodopsin gene [10]. The use of compacted DNA nanoparticles to administer gene therapy has also been explored as a method to overcome AAV vector size limitations [10].

3.1.1 Gene Therapy for Loss-of-Function RP

Many types of X-linked RP are particularly well suited for gene therapy, because they result in gene knockouts or complete loss of function and the affected gene size is often small enough to be delivered using an AAV vector. A subset of RP involves a loss-of-function mutation in the retinitis pigmentosa 2 (RP2) gene, and they encompass 10–15% of RP cases exhibiting an X-linked pattern for inheritance [11]. The small size of the RP2 coding sequence (1050 bp) makes it ideal for AAV vector delivery. With use of AAV-based gene therapy, one group was able to rescue cone degeneration in mouse models [11].

Another subset of RP that encompasses 70–80% of mutations demonstrating an X-linked pattern of inheritance involves mutations of the retinitis pigmentosa GTPase regulator (RPGR) gene [9]. Overall, they account for 10–20% of all RP cases [9]. 80% of RPGR mutations occur in exon ORF15, and these mutations typically lead to protein truncation [9]. Because these mutations typically lead to loss of function and ORF15 has a size of 3.5 kb, this subset of RP is amenable to gene therapy with AAV vectors. A major challenge with this method, however, is construction of a stable vector that leads to adequate gene expression without mutations that could lead to off-target effects and toxicity. The ORF15 region is particularly unstable because it is purine rich, increasing the likelihood of spontaneous mutations during vector cloning [9]. One method to increase the stability of the vector includes codon optimization, which does not change the amino acid sequence [9]. Following optimization of the ORF15, several clinical trials for RPGR gene therapy have been initiated and are currently in process (ClinicalTrials.gov identifiers: NCT03116113, NCT03252847, NCT03316560). The therapies in the three trials differ in the AAV viral capsid and coding sequence of the delivered gene.

The efficacy of gene therapy is also dependent on transduction efficiency and timing of the treatment [8]. Protein overexpression can lead to toxicity while under expression may lead to insufficient production of the functional gene and incomplete rescue [10]. The stage at which the gene therapy is administered could also influence treatment outcomes. Gene therapy given early before retinal degeneration has occurred can prevent disease onset, and therapy given in early stages of retinal degeneration can preserve remaining visual function or halt disease progression. One challenge with using gene therapy to treat RP is that since RP begins by affecting rod photoreceptors in the periphery, patients may present only after they become symptomatic, when significant photoreceptor loss has already occurred. Gene therapy is not effective at end stages of the disease when few or no photoreceptors remain [8]; there needs to be a sufficient number of photoreceptors remaining to utilize the replaced protein. Even still, there may be a broad window in which gene therapy may be effective. The autosomal recessive mutation of the gene PDE6B is responsible for 36,000 new cases of RP worldwide each year [8]. This mutation leads to deficiency of rod cGMP-phosphodiesterase, leading to cGMP accumulation and subsequent cell death [1, 8]. One study demonstrated that gene therapy in mouse models with this mutation preserved visual function for at least 1 year at in both early and later stages of RP [8].

3.1.2 Gene Therapy for Gain-of-Function RP

While gene therapy is promising for loss-of-function mutations, its use in subtypes of RP demonstrating autosomal dominant modes of inheritance present more of a challenge. Autosomal dominant mutations typically correspond to gain-of-function mutations that necessitate a two-step process of gene knockout or knockdown and subsequent replacement of the affected gene. Twenty-four genes have been implicated in autosomal dominant RP, and most are mutations in the rhodopsin gene [12]. The P23H mutation in *rhodopsin* is the most common form of autosomal dominant RP in the USA [13].

Various knockdown strategies have been demonstrated in murine models and may be promising as future therapeutic methods. One method to conduct gene knockdown is by silencing the mutant RNA transcript with ribozyme-directed cleavage and subsequent gene therapy [13]. Ribozymes can cleave allele-specific RNA transcripts without affecting the wild-type transcript. In murine models carrying the P23H mutation, ribozyme-directed cleavage of mutant transcripts delivered through recombinant AAV vectors has been shown to slow the rate of photoreceptor degeneration, even with significant photoreceptor loss [13].

Suppression of mutant proteins can also be done on the transcriptional level with zinc fingers. Transcriptional repression silences both mutant and wild-type genes, without specificity for the particular mutation in the rhodopsin (RHO) gene [14]. This approach may be favorable since it is applicable to the heterogeneous group of autosomal dominant mutations that can lead to RP while also suppressing residual wild-type protein activity [14].

Both methods of gene suppression can slow disease progression, but they still require gene supplementation with the wild-type gene [15]. A major challenge is that it is difficult to control level of protein expression to achieve sufficient gene rescue without retinal toxicity [14]. In the ribozyme-directed approach, wild-type copies of the gene are not affected, further complicating the appropriate amount of gene replacement needed.

3.2 Gene Editing

The challenges associated with gene therapy for autosomal dominant forms of RP, which require the two-step process of gene knockdown and subsequent gene delivery, has led to studies investigating use of gene editing for in vivo functional correction. CRISPR/Cas9 gene editing technology appears particularly promising for tailored RP treatment, since it can efficiently target desired transgene sequences. The Cas9 DNA endonuclease can be directed by a guide RNA sequence to a target DNA site, where it induces a double-stranded break. Subsequent repair of the DNA can occur through non-homologous end joining (NHEJ) or high-fidelity homology-directed repair (HDR) if a DNA template is present, allowing for correction of mutations at the target site. Genome editing with HDR has not yet been optimized at a therapeutically beneficial rate, primarily because HDR is unfavorable in postmitotic cells [16]. Thus, therapeutic strategies have focused on utilizing the error-prone NHEJ repair pathway; NHEJ is prone to indels that lead to frameshift mutations and subsequent gene knockouts.

One form of RP involves a dominant S334ter mutation in rhodopsin (*Rho*) that leads to premature termination of protein translation. This mutation is only expressed in rod photoreceptors [15]. One group demonstrated that CRISPR/Cas9 gene editing can be used for selective ablation of the mutant gene, preventing retinal degeneration, and improved visual function [15]. The CRISPR/Cas9 targeted a PAM sequence unique to the transgene, selectively ablating the transgene while allowing for residual WT *Rho* function. Thus, there was wild-type *Rho* activity without accumulation of the mutant gene that leads to toxic effects.

Aside from using CRISPR/Cas9 technology for gene knockouts using NHEJ, use of the high-fidelity HDR directed repair has also been explored as a treatment strategy. One group demonstrated that HDR directed repair in RP10 mouse models carrying autosomal recessive mutation in PDE6B led to improved visual function in the treated eye relative to the untreated eye [4]. Additionally, this group used electroporation for delivering the CRISPR/Cas9 plasmids, overcoming cargo size limitations of AAV vectors and potential immunogenicity [4]. Even though this type of therapy has not been replicated in larger animals or human clinical trials, these studies are promising for development of future therapies that utilize gene editing.

3.2.1 Challenges to Using Gene Editing for RP Treatment

One challenge to using CRISPR/Cas9 for therapeutic treatment is delivering all the components necessary for the gene editing with AAV vectors through a subretinal injection; AAV vectors are limited by the amount of DNA they carry to about 4.8 kb, and CRISPR/Cas9 components are typically larger than 5 kb [4, 9, 17]. A potential solution is packaging the components into separate AAV vectors, but this strategy reduces the efficiency of the gene editing because the coinfection of cells would then be required to deliver all components [4, 17]. The use of Cas9 genes from other species, which may be small enough to be packaged into AAV vectors, may also be used to overcome these existing limitations [17]. Additionally, while this therapy appears promising, it is unknown whether the genomic changes conferred by CRISPR/Cas9 gene editing will have lasting effects with long-term photoreceptor survival [15].

Another challenge associated with gene editing is the mutational heterogeneity associated with RP; the PAM sequences must be optimized for each individual mutation so therapies cannot be broadly used for all subtypes of RP. One group, however, used CRISPR/Cas9 to silence the autosomal dominant P23H mutation associated with RP in mouse models [17]. The CRISPR/Cas9 system was used to target exon 1 of the mutant gene to knock down expression of the mutant protein in mouse model [17]. Since this system targeted *Rho* as a whole, their method resulted in mutation-independent targeting of the rhodopsin gene that can be applied to the heterogeneous group of mutations affecting *Rho*.

Additionally, to account for mutational heterogeneity, CRISPR/Cas9 technology has also been used to target proteins upstream of the implicated mutant protein, such as the neural retina leucine zipper (*Nrl*) gene, for gene-independent therapy. *Nrl* is a key protein in photoreceptor development that leads to generation of rods and plays a role in rod homeostasis [16]. The use of CRIPSR/Cas9 to disrupt *Nrl* expression interferes with normal rod development and results in reprogramming of rods, leading them to gain cone-like features [16]. Additionally, the disruption of *Nrl* improves rod function and preserves cone function [16]. Since RP begins with rod degeneration, which is then followed by cone loss, this strategy may be widely applicable to the heterogenous group of mutations that cause RP.

The use of CRISPR/Cas9 technology in vivo also comes with safety concerns, particularly with potential immune responses to the bacterial-derived Cas9 and its potential for off-target effects. Additionally, since this technology is so new, little is known about long-term side effects of its use in humans and whether persistent expression of CRISPR/Cas9 components may lead to unwanted consequences [16].

3.3 Stem Cell Therapy

The use of stem cell therapy to replace degenerated photoreceptors is another domain that offers immense potential for RP treatment. Most studies thus far have been done in mouse models but demonstrate therapeutic potential. One study demonstrated how use of adult bone marrow-derived lineage-negative hematopoietic stem cells can incorporate into degenerating retinal vasculature and provide vasculotrophic and neurotrophic factors, preventing cone degeneration in rd1 and rd10 mouse models [18, 19]. It is thought that these factors upregulate a series of anti-apoptotic genes that slow photoreceptor degeneration [18]. The effects were observed for up to 6 months and most efficacious when the treatment was applied before complete retinal degeneration [18]. One factor to note is that the stem cells are not actually differentiating into photoreceptors, and they do not rescue photoreceptors already lost [19]. Another study has shown evidence of autologous induced pluripotent stem cells differentiating into tissue morphologically and functionally similar to retinal pigment epithelium tissue in mouse models, leading to improved vision [20]. Another group showed that identification of the optimal ontogenetic stage for stem cell transplantation facilitates the integration and differentiation of stem cells into rod photoreceptors to improve visual function in mouse models [21].

Although most studies to date have been in animal models, there have been emerging clinical trials investigating the therapeutic potential in humans. One study evaluating quality of life of RP patients who received intravitreal injections of bone marrow-derived stem cells reports significant improvement in visual function 3 months after treatment but no statistical difference from baseline at 12 months [22].

One major challenge to stem cell therapy is its safety profile, particularly with risk of tumorigenesis. Another challenge is facilitating proper differentiation of the stem cells into newly formed photoreceptors and integrating them into the neural circuit to restore visual function. Subretinal transplantation of human embryonic stem cells (hESC) has demonstrated medium- to long-term safety profiles in studies involving use of hSEC-derived RPE in Stargardt's macular dystrophy and age-related macular degeneration [23]. These results are promising for their potential application to other macular dystrophies including RP. However, the use of hESC comes with a host of challenges including ethical dilemmas to using human embryos, risk of immune rejection, and risk of tumorigenesis.

An alternative to hESC is through use of stem cells from an autologous source from the patient. The use of induced pluripotent stem cells (iPSCs) from the patient would address the ethical and immune-mediated concerns to using hESC, but the patient's own cells harbor the deleterious disease-causing mutation. The use of gene editing technology such as CRISPR/Cas9 is one method that could be used to rectify these mutations before these cells are used therapeutically. One study has demonstrated the use of CRISPR/Cas9 to repair a RPGR point mutation implicated in RP in a patient's iPSCs [24]. These results are promising for future treatment options involving autologous stem cell therapy.

3.4 Therapy for Advanced Photoreceptor Degeneration

For patients with advanced photoreceptor degeneration, gene therapy, gene editing technology, and stem cell therapy may not be enough to produce therapeutic benefit since there are too few photoreceptors remaining. The use of retinal prostheses in these patients has been explored as a potential method to preserve or retain residual visual function. These devices can target various points in the visual pathway, with many targeting the subretinal layer [25–27].

Devices such as the Argus II Retinal Prosthesis System have been shown to restore some vision in patients completely blind and with profound visual loss from RP, allowing for improved performance on visual function tests [28, 29]. It has been FDA approved for patients with severe to profound RP [30]. Patients wear glasses containing a camera that captures light. It then projects light patterns onto the retina as a series of electrode stimulation patterns [28]. Additionally, the Argus II System has been shown to have long-term safety profiles in study patients [28, 29]. Prosthetic devices are emerging as promising therapeutic options for patients with significant retinal degeneration and can be beneficial given proper patient counseling, training, and management of expectations [30].

4 Conclusion

While there is currently no cure for RP, therapeutic strategies involving gene therapy, gene editing, and stem cells have shown promising results in animal models. Some of these treatment strategies are also being investigated in human clinical trials. Many of these treatments work best in early stages of RP, when there has not been significant photoreceptor degeneration. However, since patients with RP may not become symptomatic until later stages of the disease, when significant retinal degeneration has already occurred, screening and early diagnosis is essential for maximizing therapeutic potential. For patients with near or complete blindness from RP, retinal prostheses may be a potential therapeutic option to restore some visual function.

References

1. Hartong DT, Berson EL, Dryja TP (2006) Retinitis pigmentosa. Lancet (London, England) 368(9549):1795–1809. https://doi.org/10.1016/s0140-6736(06)69740-7
2. Zhang Q (2016) Retinitis pigmentosa: progress and perspective. Asia Pac J Ophthalmol (Phila) 5(4):265–271. https://doi.org/10.1097/apo.0000000000000227
3. Narayan DS, Wood JP, Chidlow G et al (2016) A review of the mechanisms of cone degeneration in retinitis pigmentosa. Acta Ophthalmol 94(8):748–754. https://doi.org/10.1111/aos.13141
4. Vagni P, Perlini LE, Chenais NAL et al (2019) Gene editing preserves visual functions in a mouse model of retinal degeneration. Front Neurosci 13:945. https://doi.org/10.3389/fnins.2019.00945
5. Dalkara D, Goureau O, Marazova K et al (2016) Let there be light: gene and cell therapy for blindness. Hum Gene Ther 27(2):134–147. https://doi.org/10.1089/hum.2015.147
6. Ochakovski GA, Bartz-Schmidt KU, Fischer MD (2017) Retinal gene therapy: surgical vector delivery in the translation to clinical trials. Front Neurosci 11:174–174. https://doi.org/10.3389/fnins.2017.00174
7. Moore NA, Morral N, Ciulla TA et al (2018) Gene therapy for inherited retinal and optic nerve degenerations. Expert Opin Biol Ther 18(1):37–49. https://doi.org/10.1080/14712598.2018.1389886
8. Koch SF, Tsai YT, Duong JK et al (2015) Halting progressive neurodegeneration in advanced retinitis pigmentosa. J Clin Invest

125(9):3704–3713. https://doi.org/10.1172/jci82462

9. Martinez-Fernandez De La Camara C, Nanda A, Salvetti AP et al (2018) Gene therapy for the treatment of X-linked retinitis pigmentosa. Expert Opin Orphan Drugs 6(3): 167–177. https://doi.org/10.1080/21678707.2018.1444476
10. Han Z, Banworth MJ, Makkia R et al (2015) Genomic DNA nanoparticles rescue rhodopsin-associated retinitis pigmentosa phenotype. FASEB J 29(6):2535–2544. https://doi.org/10.1096/fj.15-270363
11. Mookherjee S, Hiriyanna S, Kaneshiro K et al (2015) Long-term rescue of cone photoreceptor degeneration in retinitis pigmentosa 2 (RP2)-knockout mice by gene replacement therapy. Hum Mol Genet 24(22):6446–6458. https://doi.org/10.1093/hmg/ddv354
12. Rossmiller B, Mao H, Lewin AS (2012) Gene therapy in animal models of autosomal dominant retinitis pigmentosa. Mol Vis 18: 2479–2496
13. LaVail MM, Yasumura D, Matthes MT et al (2000) Ribozyme rescue of photoreceptor cells in P23H transgenic rats: long-term survival and late-stage therapy. Proc Natl Acad Sci U S A 97(21):11488–11493. https://doi.org/10.1073/pnas.210319397
14. Mussolino C, Sanges D, Marrocco E et al (2011) Zinc-finger-based transcriptional repression of rhodopsin in a model of dominant retinitis pigmentosa. EMBO Mol Med 3(3):118–128. https://doi.org/10.1002/emmm.201000119
15. Bakondi B, Lv W, Lu B et al (2016) In vivo CRISPR/Cas9 gene editing corrects retinal dystrophy in the S334ter-3 rat model of autosomal dominant retinitis pigmentosa. Mol Ther 24(3):556–563. https://doi.org/10.1038/mt.2015.220
16. Yu W, Mookherjee S, Chaitankar V et al (2017) Nrl knockdown by AAV-delivered CRISPR/Cas9 prevents retinal degeneration in mice. Nat Commun 8:14716. https://doi.org/10.1038/ncomms14716
17. Latella MC, Di Salvo MT, Cocchiarella F et al (2016) In vivo editing of the human mutant rhodopsin gene by electroporation of plasmid-based CRISPR/Cas9 in the mouse retina. Mol Ther Nucleic Acids 5(11):e389. https://doi.org/10.1038/mtna.2016.92
18. Otani A, Dorrell MI, Kinder K et al (2004) Rescue of retinal degeneration by intravitreally injected adult bone marrow-derived lineage-negative hematopoietic stem cells. J Clin Invest 114(6):765–774. https://doi.org/10.1172/JCI21686
19. Smith LEH (2004) Bone marrow-derived stem cells preserve cone vision in retinitis pigmentosa. J Clin Invest 114(6):755–757. https://doi.org/10.1172/JCI22930
20. Li Y, Tsai Y-T, Hsu C-W et al (2012) Long-term safety and efficacy of human-induced pluripotent stem cell (iPS) grafts in a preclinical model of retinitis pigmentosa. Mol Med 18(1): 1312–1319. https://doi.org/10.2119/molmed.2012.00242
21. MacLaren RE, Pearson RA, MacNeil A et al (2006) Retinal repair by transplantation of photoreceptor precursors. Nature 444(7116): 203–207. https://doi.org/10.1038/nature05161
22. Siqueira RC, Messias A, Messias K et al (2015) Quality of life in patients with retinitis pigmentosa submitted to intravitreal use of bone marrow-derived stem cells (Reticell-clinical trial). Stem Cell Res Ther 6(1):29–29. https://doi.org/10.1186/s13287-015-0020-6
23. Schwartz SD, Regillo CD, Lam BL et al (2015) Human embryonic stem cell-derived retinal pigment epithelium in patients with age-related macular degeneration and Stargardt's macular dystrophy: follow-up of two open-label phase 1/2 studies. Lancet (London, England) 385(9967):509–516. https://doi.org/10.1016/s0140-6736(14)61376-3
24. Bassuk AG, Zheng A, Li Y et al (2016) Precision medicine: genetic repair of retinitis pigmentosa in patient-derived stem cells. Sci Rep 6(1):19969. https://doi.org/10.1038/srep19969
25. Zrenner E, Bartz-Schmidt KU, Benav H et al (2011) Subretinal electronic chips allow blind patients to read letters and combine them to words. Proc Biol Sci 278(1711):1489–1497. https://doi.org/10.1098/rspb.2010.1747
26. Stingl K, Bartz-Schmidt KU, Besch D et al (2013) Artificial vision with wirelessly powered subretinal electronic implant alpha-IMS. Proc Biol Sci 280(1757):20130077–20130077. https://doi.org/10.1098/rspb.2013.0077
27. Chow AY, Bittner AK, Pardue MT (2010) The artificial silicon retina in retinitis pigmentosa patients (an American Ophthalmological Association thesis). Trans Am Ophthalmol Soc 108: 120–154
28. Ho AC, Humayun MS, Dorn JD et al (2015) Long-term results from an epiretinal prosthesis to restore sight to the blind. Ophthalmology

122(8):1547–1554. https://doi.org/10.1016/j.ophtha.2015.04.032

29. Humayun MS, Dorn JD, da Cruz L et al (2012) Interim results from the international trial of Second Sight's visual prosthesis. Ophthalmology 119(4):779–788. https://doi.org/10.1016/j.ophtha.2011.09.028

30. Finn AP, Grewal DS, Vajzovic L (2018) Argus II retinal prosthesis system: a review of patient selection criteria, surgical considerations, and post-operative outcomes. Clin Ophthalmol 12:1089–1097. https://doi.org/10.2147/OPTH.S137525

Chapter 34

Ocular Injection Techniques for Retinitis Pigmentosa: Intravitreal, Subretinal, and Suprachoroidal

Ioana Scherbakova, Sara D. Ragi, and Tarun Sharma

Abstract

Ocular gene therapy represents an emerging and promising therapeutic approach for the treatment of several of the inherited retinal diseases. Currently, the focus has been to investigate monogenic inherited retinal disorders. Genetic and cellular therapies can be delivered to the eye by various injection techniques, including those that are intravitreal, subretinal, and suprachoroidal. Each of these three delivery methods are discussed with regard to their historical background, indications, surgical steps, and follow-up.

Key words Gene therapy, Inherited retinal diseases, Intravitreal injection, Ocular injection, Retinitis pigmentosa, Suprachoroidal injection, Subretinal injection

1 Introduction

During the last decade or more, there has been a surge in establishing genetic causes for inherited retinal diseases (IRDs). Identification of the causative gene for IRDs has led to gene therapies with the hope of mitigating disease progression and preserving vision for affected individuals. In December 2017, the US Food and Drug Administration approved the first gene therapy for the treatment of *RPE65* gene mutation-associated retinal dystrophy [1].

Currently, there are several ongoing gene therapy trials (phase I/II or phase III) for IRDs. The most common approach for gene therapy is the delivery of the normal gene with a viral vector inside the eye. To deliver the gene to the retina, the viral vector is injected either into the vitreous cavity (intravitreal injection) or subretinal space (after vitreous surgery or via the suprachoroidal space). The goal of this chapter is to describe the steps involved in each of the delivery techniques.

Stephen H. Tsang and Peter M. J. Quinn (eds.), *Retinitis Pigmentosa*,
Methods in Molecular Biology, vol. 2560, https://doi.org/10.1007/978-1-0716-2651-1_34,

2 Methods

2.1 Intravitreal Injection

2.1.1 Background

Over the last decade, intravitreal injections have become one of the most common intraocular procedures. The first description of an intravitreal injection was in 1911 by Ohm, who successfully treated two patients with retinal detachments by intravitreal injections of sterile air [2]. Three decades later, antibiotics began to be injected intravitreally to treat endophthalmitis [3]. The first medication to be FDA-approved for intravitreal injection was fomivirsen sodium in 1998; an antiviral for the treatment of CMV retinitis [4]. Since the early 2000s, off-label intravitreal injections of anti-VEGF agents have been used in the management of retinal diseases including neovascularization due to age-related macular degeneration and macular edema due to diabetes or retinal vein occlusion [5].

Gene therapy is a recent medical development, with the first therapeutic trial of gene therapy approved in 1990 for a form of severe combined immunodeficiency disease (ADA-SCID) [6]. Since 2017, when the first virus vector-based gene therapy was FDA-approved for treatment of *RPE65* mutation-associated retinal dystrophy, numerous gene therapies have been under investigation for treatment of inherited retinal diseases. Viral vectors can be targeted directly to the eye and are most commonly delivered either by subretinal or intravitreal injection in order to be close to the pathologic retinal cells. Compared to subretinal injection, which is an operative procedure, intravitreal injection has the advantage of being simpler to perform. Intravitreal injection can be done safely in an office setting and carries low risks, principally of endophthalmitis. Despite the greater ease of administration, however, intravitreal delivery of gene therapy has had limited success in animal models of outer retinal disease, likely because of decreased access to the target cells due to dilution of viral vector in the vitreous and the cellular barrier between the vitreous and the outer retina [7].

Intravitreal injections are performed by first anesthetizing and sterilizing the ocular surface. Then, a small injection needle is inserted through the sclera and pars plana into the vitreous cavity. After the medication or viral vector is delivered and the needle is removed, patients are monitored to ensure that they have formed vision and a follow-up plan is established. We will consider the applications of intravitreal injections in gene therapy, the injection technique, possible complications, and other special considerations related to this targeted delivery method.

2.1.2 Applications in Gene Therapy

Retinal gene therapy trials, active and completed, employing intravitreal injections are as follows. Information was obtained from the Clinical Trials online registry at https://clinicaltrials.gov on 14 February 2020.

1. Retinitis Pigmentosa
   (a) Dose-escalation Study to Evaluate the Safety and Tolerability of GS030 in Subjects with Retinitis Pigmentosa (PIONEER): Clinicaltrials.gov identifier NCT03326336
   (b) RST-001 Phase I/II Trial for advanced Retinitis Pigmentosa: Clinicaltrials.gov identifier NCT02556736
   (c) Study to Evaluate Safety and Tolerability of QR-421a in Subjects with RP due to Mutation in Exon 13 of the USH2A Gene (Stellar): Clinicaltrials.gov identifier NCT03780257
   (d) A Study to Evaluate the Safety and Tolerability of QR-1123 in Subjects With Autosomal Dominant Retinitis Pigmentosa Due to the P23H Mutation in the RHO Gene (AURORA): Clinicaltrials.gov identifier NCT04123626
2. X-Linked Juvenile Retinoschisis
   (a) Study of RS1 Ocular Gene Transfer for X-linked Retinoschisis: Clinicaltrials.gov identifier NCT02317887
   (b) Safety and Efficacy of rAAV-hRS1 in Patients with X-linked Retinoschisis (XLRS): Clinicaltrials.gov identifier NCT02416622
3. Leber Hereditary Optic Neuropathy
   (a) Efficacy Study of GS010 for the treatment of vision loss up to 6 months from onset in LHON due to the ND4 Mutation (RESCUE) Clinicaltrials.gov identifier NCT02652767
   (b) Efficacy Study of GS010 for Treatment of Vision Loss from 7 months to 1 year from onset in LHON due to the ND4 Mutation (REVERSE): Clinicaltrials.gov identifier NCT02652780
   (c) EAP GS010 Single Patient: Clinicaltrials.gov identifier NCT03672968
   (d) Efficacy & Safety Study of Bilateral IVT Injection of GS010 in LHON Subjects Due to the ND4 Mutation for up to 1 Year (REFLECT): ClinicalTrials.gov identifier NCT03293524
4. Leber Congenital Amaurosis
   (a) Multi-dose study for Efficacy, Safety, Tolerability, Exposure of QR-110 in LCA1 Clinicaltrials.gov identifier NCT03913143
5. Age-Related Macular Degeneration
   (a) Safety and Tolerability Study of AAV2-sFLT01 in Patients with neovascular Age-Related Macular Degeneration (AMD) ClinicalTrials.gov identifier NCT01024998

(b) AAVCAGsCD59 for the Treatment of Wet AMD: ClinicalTrials.gov identifier NCT03585556

(c) Treatment of Advanced Dry Age Related Macular Degeneration with AAVCAGsCD59: ClinicalTrials.gov identifier NCT03144999

(d) ADVM-022 Gene Therapy for Wet AMD (OPTIC): ClinicalTrials.gov identifier NCT03748784

(e) RGX-314 Gene Therapy for Neovascular AMD Trial: ClinicalTrials.gov identifier NCT03066258

(f) A Study of Genetic and Environmental Factors and Their Effect on Response to Treatment With Lucentis (Ranibizumab) for Wet AMD: ClinicalTrials.gov Identifier: NCT00469352

6. Refractory Retinoblastoma

(a) Evaluate Safety and the Oncolitic Adenovirus VCN-01 Activity in Patients with Refractory Retinoblastoma (RTB): ClinicalTrials.gov identifier NCT03284268

2.1.3 Techniques of Intravitreal Injection

1. *Office-based or operating room*: The choice is based on the clinician's preference and/or the practice pattern in the country. In a retrospective study, the risk of endophthalmitis appeared to be similar in office-based examination room compared to operating room settings (0.035% and 0.065%, respectively) [8].
2. *Pupillary dilation*: Before beginning the procedure, the patient may have their pupils dilated in order to allow for examination of the fundus after injection, although expert opinions differ as to whether post-injection fundus examination is necessary [5]. Dilation can be performed with a combination of one drop of 1–2.5% phenylephrine and one drop of 0.5–1% tropicamide.
3. *Informed consent*: The team should explain the procedure, its benefits, and risks and obtain written informed consent.
4. *Procedural time out*: Before the injection, verify the identity of the patient, eye (quick fundus examination), and the type of the injection.
5. *Local anesthesia*: One drop of 0.5% tetracaine or 0.5% proparacaine may be used. A sterile cotton tip soaked in liquid anesthetic may be applied to the intended site of injection for 5 s. If anesthetic gel is used, be aware that it interferes with povidone-iodine contact with the conjunctival surface and therefore limits its sterilizing effect.
6. *Povidone-iodine*: Sterilize the ocular surface using a few drops of 5% povidone-iodine or a 10-mL flush of the same solution

[9]. Allow the antiseptic solution to remain on the ocular surface for at least 30 s and up to 5 min. Povidone-iodine may also be applied to eyelids and eyelashes prior to introducing a sterile speculum. There is no need to use pre-injection topical antibiotics.

7. *Surgical masks and gloves*: During the procedure, physicians and those assisting may wear surgical masks or may simply minimize speaking, coughing, and sneezing in order to avoid contaminating the ocular surface with oral flora. Patients should minimize speaking, as well. Those performing the injection clean their hands commonly and wear clean gloves.
8. *Use of a sterile speculum*: Retract the eyelids away from ocular surface either manually or, preferably, using a sterile speculum. This prevents contact of the lid margin or eyelashes with the shaft of the needle and therefore minimizes the risk of endophthalmitis.
9. *Needle selection*: The preferred needle is 30-gauge or smaller and 18 mm in length or shorter.
10. *Injection procedure* (*see* Fig. 1): The injection site is in the inferotemporal quadrant, 4 mm from the limbus in phakic patients and 3.5 mm from the limbus in aphakic or pseudophakic patients. Instruct the patient to look in the nasal-superior direction. Insert the needle perpendicular through the sclera and pars plana, directed toward the center of the globe. Inject the drug (around 0.05 mL) into the mid-vitreous cavity at a moderately slow speed; a rapid injection can cause the needle to come off the syringe. As the needle is removed, a sterile cotton applicator is immediately placed over the injection site to prevent any reflux. The needle should be disposed in a sharp disposal container.
11. *Post-injection irrigation*: Use povidone-iodine 5% to cover the conjunctival surface. Thoroughly irrigate the conjunctival sac with copious balanced salt solution, and gently remove the speculum.

2.1.4 Post-Injection Monitoring and Follow-Up

1. Examine the fundus to assess for any procedure-related complications and pulsation of the optic disk.
2. An eye patch is not necessary after the injection but may be used based on the physician and patient's preferences.
3. The influx of volume from an intravitreal injection may cause a rise in intraocular pressure and temporary nonperfusion. This can lead to a transient decrease in vision lasting less than 1 or 2 min which does not require treatment. However, if the intraocular pressure remains high or if vision loss persists, consider anterior chamber paracentesis. Patients with ocular

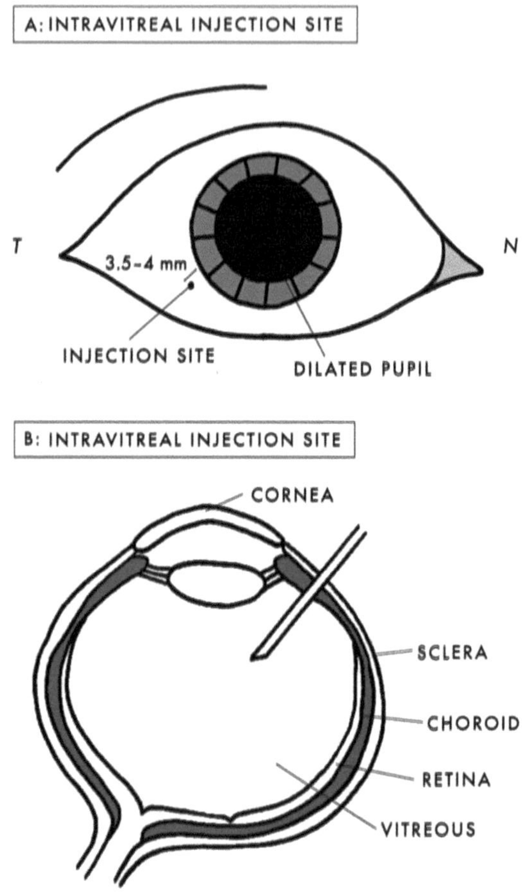

Fig. 1 Schematic presentation of intravitreal injection. (**a**) Frontal facing schematic with injection site and dilated pupil indicated. (**b**) Lateral view of the intravitreal injection schematic with insertion of the needle shown perpendicular through the sclera and pars plana, directed toward the center of the globe

hypertension or glaucoma may require close monitoring of the intraocular pressure.

4. The use of post-injection topical antibiotics is not universally agreed-upon but is practiced by many clinicians.
5. Follow-up plans vary for each patient, but all patients must be educated about the symptoms of infection or retinal detachment and asked to present for immediate care if they experience loss of vision, light sensitivity, severe eye pain, or severe eye redness.
6. If performing bilateral injections, repeat each step for the second eye, though many physicians may prefer to do a second procedure on a different day.

2.1.5 Complications

1. *Subconjunctival hemorrhage*: Subconjunctival hemorrhage is the most common complication of intravitreal injection. Although the condition is benign and painless, the appearance of blood under the conjunctiva can be cosmetically upsetting. Subconjunctival hemorrhage can occur immediately post-procedure due to the trauma of the injection or later as a result of inflammation following the injection. Systemic hypertension is a risk factor for subconjunctival hemorrhage after intravitreal injection [10].
2. *Floaters*: Many patients experience floaters following intravitreal injections, possibly due to air bubbles or syringe lubricant oil droplets. Patients should be counseled that this is normal, but symptoms of numerous flashing lights or scotomas should be evaluated further as these could indicate a retinal tear or detachment. Benign floaters normally resolve within days or weeks.
3. *Endophthalmitis*: Endophthalmitis presents as severe ocular inflammation due to infection after surgery, injection, or ocular trauma. Signs include anterior chamber cell and flare, posterior segment vitritis, and hypopyon. If untreated, endophthalmitis can cause severe visual loss or blindness. Bacterial infection of the vitreous cavity following intravitreal injection is rare, with an incidence around 0.05% [11, 12]. The most common causative organisms are *Staphylococcus* and *Streptococcus* species, both of which can be found in the upper respiratory tract [11]. As such, refraining from speaking during the procedure and/or wearing face masks are the best methods for preventing respiratory droplet transmission and are helpful in preventing procedure-related infections.
4. *Pseudo-endophthalmitis*: Pseudo-endophthalmitis refers to the appearance of endophthalmitis-like symptoms after an intravitreal injection in the absence of infection. This condition has been associated with intravitreal injections of triamcinolone acetonide, a corticosteroid used to treat refractory macular edema and inflammatory eye diseases [13, 14]. It is thought that steroid particles in the anterior chamber and vitreous cavity can cause floaters may simulate inflammatory cells. Pseudoendophthalmitis is characterized by anterior vitreous haze, hypopyon, and impaired vision without periorbital inflammation or pain. The condition resolves without treatment and vision returns to normal within weeks.
5. *Retinal detachment*: Retinal detachment is uncommon after intravitreal injections, with a prevalence between 0.0% and 0.9% per injection [15]. This complication is thought to be largely related to underlying retinal conditions such as CMV retinitis, abnormal retinal anatomy, or previous ocular surgeries [16].

6. *Intraocular hemorrhage*: Retinal hemorrhage, vitreous hemorrhage, or hyphema may occur infrequently following intravitreal injections. This complication may often be related to the underlying ocular pathology rather than the injection procedure [16]. Patients with polypoidal choroidal vasculopathy or on anticoagulants area at higher risk of submacular hemorrhage following intravitreal anti-VEGF injections [17].
7. *Cataract*: The development and progression of cataract is associated with intravitreal triamcinolone injection [18]. By 1 year after injection, posterior subcapsular cataract formation becomes visually significant in almost half of eyes [19].
8. *Uveitis*: Intraocular inflammation in the form of uveitis or iritis is uncommon and has been reported after administration of cidofovir or fomivirsen for CMV retinitis and ovine hyaluronidase for vitreous hemorrhage [16].
9. *Ocular hypertension*: Transient ocular hypertension is common and can occur after intravitreal injections of any agent. Sustained hypertension, however, can cause retinal artery occlusion or damage to retinal ganglion cells [16]. This condition is more commonly associated with corticosteroid injections [16]. In addition, multiple treatments with VEGF inhibitor injections can lead to consistently elevated intraocular pressure, often with delayed onset after 10 or more injections [20].
10. *Hypotony*: An intraocular pressure of less than 6 mm Hg is a rare complication of intravitreal injection and has mainly been found in eyes treated with cidofovir and fomivirsen antiviral injections [16].

2.1.6 Special Considerations

1. *Chlorhexidine Versus Povidone-Iodine*: Povidone-iodine is the most common topical antiseptic preparation for intravitreal injection. However, it can cause ocular surface irritation and, rarely, patients can be allergic to the agent. An alternative antiseptic is aqueous chlorhexidine, which is safe and effective when used in concentrations less than or equal to 1% [21]. About 6.6% of patients receiving 5% povidone-iodine coupled with anesthetic report moderate to severe eye irritation [22], and povidone-iodine can also cause hyperemia and punctate epitheliopathy [23]. Notably, aqueous chlorhexidine (0.1%) has been found to result in less post-injection discomfort than povidone-iodine antisepsis [24] and is similarly effective as an antiseptic [23].
2. *Pre-filled syringes*: Since 2018, both ranibizumab and aflibercept have both been approved by the FDA for administration from single-use, pre-filled syringes. The use of pre-filled syringes eliminates the need for the physician to prepare and draw up the medication and has been found to result in a decreased

risk of culture-positive endophthalmitis, possibly because the fewer steps necessary to prepare the injection results in decreased exposure of the syringe and ocular surface to aerosolized oral bacteria [25].

3. *Silicone droplets*: Intravitreal injections can lead to the presence of silicone oil droplets in the vitreous cavity. The droplets do not have adverse effects, are asymptomatic, are not associated with any particular agent, and are thought to be caused by silicone oil lubricant on the syringes or needles used for intravitreal injections [26]. The use of luer cone rather than staked-on syringes [27] and the use of pre-filled syringes for intravitreal injections have led to reduced incidence of and silicone oil droplets [28].

2.2 Subretinal Injection

2.2.1 Background

The subretinal space, a potential space, is located between RPE cells and photoreceptors (part of neurosensory retina) [29]. Subretinal injection was first used in mouse models of hereditary retinal degeneration [29]. In dystrophic RCG rat models, transplanted human fetal RPE cells were injected subretinally to rescue photoreceptor cells. Later, in subjects with age-related macular degeneration, RPE cell suspensions were transplanted after the removal of choroidal neovascular membrane resulting in preservation of neurosensory retinal function.

Subretinal injection to deliver gene therapy is considered more effective than intravitreal injections for the treatment of inherited retinal disease caused by mutations in photoreceptors or RPE genes [29]. Subretinal injection allows the delivery of viral vectors into a targeted space so that a direct contact is established with the plasma membrane of the photoreceptor and RPE cells [29]. Additionally, a lower dose is required to accurately target cells in the subretinal space. Theoretically, virus vector delivery may lead to toxicity and immune responses; however, the subretinal space is a closed anatomic region with greater immune privilege allowing for greater safety in delivering viral vectors directly to RPE and/or photoreceptor cells [29].

Currently, subretinal drug delivery technique is being explored for the administration of gene therapy and cell therapy in several clinical trials.

2.2.2 Applications in Gene Therapy

Retinal gene therapy trials, active and completed, employing subretinal injections are as follows. Information was obtained from the Clinical Trials online registry at https://clinicaltrials.gov on 14 February 2020:

1. Achromatopsia: Clinicaltrials.gov identifiers: NCT02610582, NCT02935517, NCT02599922, NCT02935517

2. Age-related Macular Degeneration: Clinicaltrials.gov identifiers: NCT03846193, NCT01494805, NCT01344993, NCT01301443, NCT02463344, NCT03178149, NCT00788177, NCT02557451, NCT02002377, NCT01896284, NCT03468296, NCT00304954, NCT03585556, NCT02357342, NCT03699618, NCT02732899, NCT00538538, NCT02321241, NCT02762188, NCT01644513, NCT02713204, NCT00021736, NCT03034772, NCT00333476
3. Choroideremia: Clinicaltrials.gov identifiers: NCT02671539, NCT02407678, NCT03496012, NCT01461213, NCT03507686, NCT03584165, NCT02553135, NCT01461213, NCT03507686, NCT03584165, NCT02553135, NCT02077361, NCT01325181, NCT01971190
4. Leber Congenital Amaurosis: Clinicaltrials.gov identifiers: NCT00821340, NCT00481546, NCT03872479, NCT03920007, NCT00643747, NCT03920007, NCT00643747, NCT00749957, NCT00999609, NCT00516477
5. Retinal Arterial Macro-aneurysm: Clinicaltrials.gov identifiers: NCT02120066
6. Retinitis Pigmentosa: Clinicaltrials.gov identifiers: NCT01505062, NCT03374657, NCT02464436, NCT03374657, NCT02464436, NCT01482195, NCT02903576
7. Stargardt Macular Dystrophy: Clinicaltrials.gov identifiers: NCT02941991, NCT01345006, NCT01367444, NCT01469832, NCT01367444, NCT01469832
8. Diabetic Macular Edema: Clinicaltrials.gov identifiers: NCT03975088, NCT00682539, NCT01292798, NCT00989989

2.2.3 Technique (See Fig. 2) [30]

1. Subretinal delivery of viral vector involves three-port pars plana vitrectomy, internal limiting membrane staining, and using intraoperative OCT during subretinal injection.
2. Using a dual-bore 41 G/23 G Teflon tipped cannula, a parafoveal bleb (avoiding any major blood vessels) is created first with balanced salt solution (BSS), and thereafter through the same self-sealing retinotomy site, a slow infusion of viral vector (dose, 0.1 mL) is done into the subretinal space under foot-pedal control.
3. To avoid any air bubbles entering the subretinal space, the cannula tip is flushed with BSS, outside the eye.

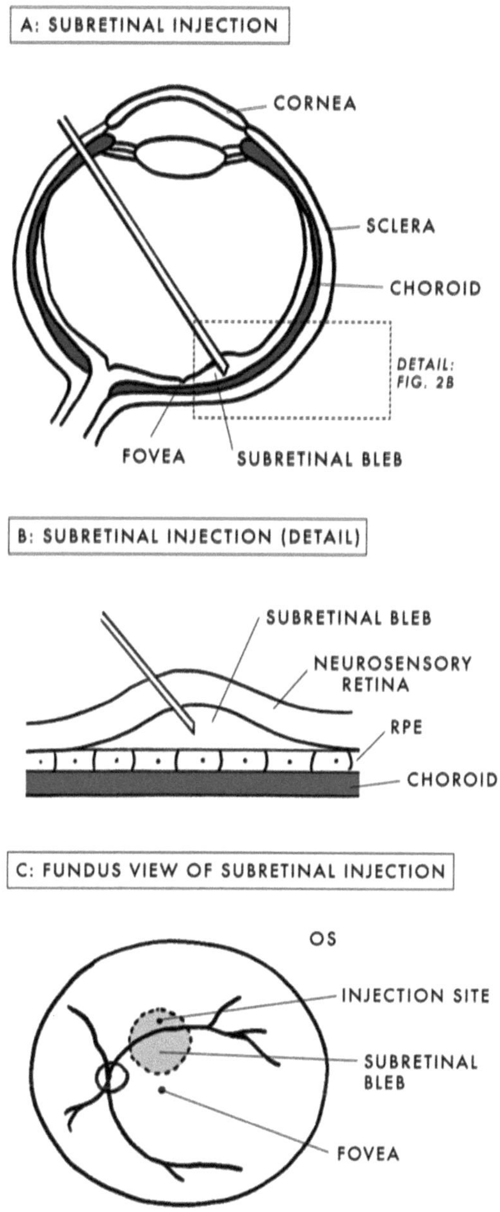

Fig. 2 Schematic presentation of subretinal injection. (**a**) Lateral facing schematic with injection site and subretinal bleb indicated. (**b**) Detailed cross-sectional view of the subretinal injection schematic to clearly identify the subretinal bleb. (**c**) Fundus view of the subretinal injection schematic

4. In the end, the vitreous cavity was washed or irrigated to remove refluxed free-floating adeno-associated virus (AAV) particles, if any.
5. The eye is usually left filled with fluid, and sclerotomies were sutured.

2.2.4 Post-Injection Monitoring and Follow-Up [30]

1. Oral peri-operative steroids are administered starting 2 days before surgery and continued with a tapering dosage in the postoperative period for 3 weeks.
2. At each follow-up visit, examine for cataract, increased intraocular pressure, retinal tear or retinal detachment, macular hole, epiretinal membrane, intraocular inflammation, etc.

2.3 Suprachoroidal Injection

2.3.1 Background

The suprachoroidal space is the most recent location to come under study for the administration of therapeutics to the posterior segment of the eye. The suprachoroidal space is a potential space about 30-μm thick between the sclera and the choroid and goes circumferentially around the eye, extending from the ora serrata anteriorly to the optic nerve posteriorly [31]. It contains various components including collagen, elastic fibers, fibrocytes, melanocytes, ganglion cells, and nerve plexi [32]. Injection into this potential space allows for rapid delivery of drugs and gene therapies to the posterior segment without vitrectomy, the creation of a hole in the retina, or entrance into the inner eye and the associated risks of endophthalmitis, retinal tears or detachment, and traumatic cataract [33]. Suprachoroidal injection allows drugs to reach the choroid and retina selectively and medications do not spread to the anterior chamber, lens, cornea, or conjunctiva, where they can cause unwanted side effects [32]. As a result, the suprachoroidal space is being investigated for the delivery of gene therapies and the administration of other pharmacotherapies to the posterior segment.

Suprachoroidal injections are being widely studied to deliver steroids, small molecules, and biomaterials. In February 2019, the FDA accepted a new drug application for Xipere (Clearside Biomedical), a triamcinolone acetonide ophthalmic suspension, for suprachoroidal injection using a proprietary injector [34]. Currently, several clinical trials are under way to investigate the suprachoroidal injection of triamcinolone acetonide with and without aflibercept for the treatment of macular edema and non-infectious uveitis. Studies have also evaluated the suprachoroidal injection of bevacizumab for patients with choroidal neovascularization [35]. Suprachoroidal injection techniques are also being studied in the treatment of ocular melanoma [34]. Synthetic viral nanoparticles conjugated to infrared-activated small molecules can bind selectively to neoplastic cells and target these cells for destruction with an ophthalmic laser. Injection of these nanoparticles into the suprachoroidal space may allow for less invasive, non-surgical delivery of therapeutic agents to target tissues in the retina and choroid, such as a choroidal melanoma. The suprachoroidal space may also be used to allow sustained drug delivery to the posterior pole. Biomaterials, such as polymers with controlled-release characteristics, may be injected suprachoroidally and used to create long-lasting drug delivery systems [36]. A light-activated gel has been investigated in animal models for the sustained suprachoroidal delivery of bevacizumab, which is used to treat choroidal neovascularization [37].

Research on suprachoroidal delivery of retinal gene therapies is in early stages. Preclinical trials in animal models demonstrated that suprachoroidal delivery of adenoviral vectors can be used successfully for ocular gene transfer [38, 39]. Suprachoroidal approaches are also being studied as a means to deliver medications and cell-based therapy to the subretinal space, such as in the delivery of human umbilical cord tissue-derived cells to the subretinal space for the treatment of geographic atrophy due to age-related macular degeneration [40]. Techniques are in development to deliver gene therapies to the subretinal space via suprachoroidal approaches [41]. While direct subretinal approaches require vitrectomy and can result in retinal detachment, the suprachoroidal approach may be a safer means of subretinal access as it does not require vitrectomy or retinotomy [40].

2.3.2 Applications in Gene Therapy

Although there are no current clinical trials involving suprachoroidal injection of retinal gene therapies, the following active and completed trials involve suprachoroidal injections or suprachoroidal access to the subretinal space. Information was obtained from the Clinical Trials online registry at https://clinicaltrials.gov on 14 February 2020:

1. Diabetic Macular Edema
   (a) Suprachoroidal Injection of Triamcinolone Acetonide for Management of Diabetic Macular Edema (SCI): Clinicaltrials.gov identifier NCT04069780
   (b) Suprachoroidal Injection of CLS-TA Alone or With Aflibercept in Subjects With Diabetic Macular Edema (HULK): ClinicalTrials.gov identifier NCT02949024
   (c) Suprachoroidal CLS-TA With Intravitreal Aflibercept Versus Aflibercept Alone in Subject With Diabetic Macular Edema (TYBEE): ClinicalTrials.gov identifier NCT03126786
2. Macular Edema Following RVO
   (a) Suprachoroidal Injection of Triamcinolone Acetonide With IVT Aflibercept in Subjects With Macular Edema Following RVO (TANZANITE): ClinicalTrials.gov identifier NCT02303184
   (b) Suprachoroidal Injection of Triamcinolone Acetonide With IVT Anti-VEGF in Subjects With Macular Edema Following RVO (TOPAZ): ClinicalTrials.gov identifier NCT03203447

(c) Suprachoroidal Injection of Triamcinolone Acetonide With IVT Anti-VEGF in Subjects With Macular Edema Following RVO (TOPAZ): ClinicalTrials.gov identifier NCT03203447

(d) Suprachoroidal Injection of Triamcinolone Acetonide With IVT Aflibercept in Subjects With Macular Edema Following RVO (SAPPHIRE): ClinicalTrials.gov identifier NCT02980874

3. Non-Infectious Uveitis

   (a) Safety Study of Suprachoroidal Triamcinolone Acetonide Via Microneedle to Treat Uveitis: ClinicalTrials.gov identifier NCT01789320

   (b) Suprachoroidal Injection of CLS-TA in Subjects Non-infectious Uveitis (AZALEA): ClinicalTrials.gov identifier NCT03097315

4. Macular Edema Following Non-Infectious Uveitis

   (a) Suprachoroidal Injection of Triamcinolone Acetonide in Subjects With Macular Edema Following Non-Infectious Uveitis (DOGWOOD) ClinicalTrials.gov identifier NCT02255032

   (b) Suprachoroidal Injection of CLS-TA in Subjects With Macular Edema Associated With Non-infectious Uveitis (PEACHTREE): ClinicalTrials.gov identifier NCT02595398

5. Age-Related Macular Degeneration

   (a) A Study to Evaluate the Safety and Clinical Response of Subretinal Administration of CNTO 2476 in Participants With Geographic Atrophy (PRELUDE): ClinicalTrials.gov identifier NCT02659098

6. Macular Edema or Degeneration from Various Pathologies

   (a) Suprachoroidal Injection of Triamcinolone Acetonide Using Custom Made Needle to Treat Macular Diseases and Non Infectious Posterior Uveitis ClinicalTrials.gov identifier NCT03606733

2.3.3 Technique

Various techniques have been used to perform suprachoroidal injections in animal subjects and human cadaver eyes. One method involves creating a scleral incision, inserting a catheter into the suprachoroidal space, injecting the material or drug of interest, and suturing the scleral incision to close [33]. More commonly, however, trials for suprachoroidal drug delivery involve the use of microinjectors, with the drug injected just beneath the scleral surface into the suprachoroidal space [42, 43]. Microinjectors can also

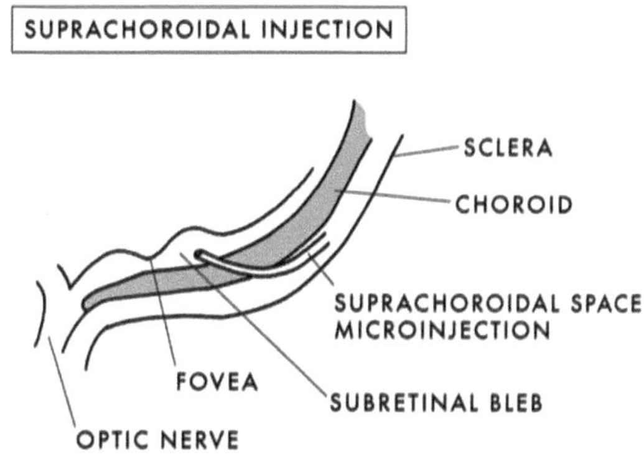

Fig. 3 Schematic presentation of subretinal injection. Microinjectors can also be used to access the subretinal space by a suprachoroidal approach

be used to access the subretinal space by a suprachoroidal approach, as shown in Fig. 3.

Multiple approaches and injectors are in development, each with an associated injection technique. The FDA has cleared Xipere (Clearside Biomedical), a triamcinolone acetonide formulation, for suprachoroidal injection using a proprietary injector. The injection is performed in the pars plana, 4–5 mm from the limbus, in approximately the same location as for an intravitreal injection. The injector is held perpendicularly to the sclera and constant, firm pressure is maintained on the plunger [44]. The sclera is dimpled down with the hub of the needle and the drug is injected slowly and consistently.

The following technique was used for suprachoroidal injection of triamcinolone acetonide in patients with noninfectious uveitis (www.ClinicalTrials.gov, NCT01789320) [45]:

1. The eye is dilated.
2. Topical anesthetic is applied.
3. A speculum is placed, and the eye is sterilized.
4. A single injection of 4 mg of a proprietary triamcinolone acetonide preparation (Triesence®, Alcon) is administered approximately 4 mm posterior to the limbus, into the suprachoroidal space of the study eye via a proprietary microinjector (Clearside Biomedical). The microinjector is a 1-mL syringe attached via a Luer lock to a commercially purchased cannula that was cut down to an approximately 1 mm in length and a 30-gauge needle.
5. After injection, the subjects remained in the clinic for approximately 3 h for observation. The study eye was assessed immediately after injection, 1 h afterward, and 3 h afterward by indirect ophthalmoscopy.

2.4 Conclusion

The field of ocular gene therapy is exciting and rapidly growing, with numerous ongoing clinical trials exploring the role of gene therapy in various retinal diseases. Several injection techniques have been developed, including subretinal and intravitreal injections. Suprachoroidal delivery of genetic and cellular therapies is being actively investigated. Genes introduced into the retina by injection can treat inherited retinal diseases by replacing deficient genes and allowing for the restoration of normal retinal function. In acquired retinal diseases such as age-related macular degeneration, locally delivered gene therapies may allow for enhanced modulation of existing cellular proteins and may lead to better disease control.

In the future, we hope to see advancement in this arena focusing on refining viral vectors, cell lines, developing newer surgical instruments, improving intraoperative imaging, and optimizing surgical delivery techniques. New methods of surgical delivery are being explored, including sub-internal-limiting-membrane (sub-ILM) delivery of gene therapy, wherein an AAV vector is placed in a surgically hydrodissected space between the ILM and neural retina [46]. Alongside these new technical developments, we will have data regarding the natural history of disease progression to define the clinical end points against which the efficacy of interventional trials can be measured.

References

1. Fischer A (2017) FDA approves novel gene therapy to treat patients with a rare form of inherited vision loss. US Food and Drug Administration, https://www.fda.gov/news-events/press-announcements/fda-approves-novel-gene-therapy-treat-patients-rare-form-inherited-vision-loss. Accessed 27 Jan 2020
2. Ohm J (1911) Über die Behandlung der Netzhautablösung durch operative Entleerung der subretinalen Flüssigkeit und Einspritzung von Luft in den Glaskörper [On the treatment of retinal detachment by surgical evacuation of subretinal fluid and injection of air into the vitreous]. Albrecht Von Graefes Arch Für Ophthalmol 79(3):442–450
3. Schneider J, Frankel SS (1947) Treatment of late postoperative intraocular infections with intraocular injection of penicillin. Arch Ophthalmol 37:304–307
4. DeLap R (1998) Vitravene Approval Letter. U.S. Food and Drug Administration. https://www.accessdata.fda.gov/drugsatfda_docs/nda/98/20961_Vitravene_Approv.pdf. Accessed 27 Jan 2020
5. Avery RL, Bakri SJ, Blumenkranz MS et al (2014) Intravitreal injection technique and monitoring. Retina 34(Suppl 12):S1–S18. https://doi.org/10.1097/IAE.0000000000000399
6. Blaese RM, Culver KW, Miller AD et al (1995) T lymphocyte-directed gene therapy for ADA- SCID: initial trial results after 4 years. Science 270(5235):475–480
7. Gupta PR, Huckfeldt RM (2017) Gene therapy for inherited retinal degenerations: initial successes and future challenges. J Neural Eng 14(5):051002. https://doi.org/10.1088/1741-2552/aa7a27
8. Tabandeh H, Boscia F, Sborgia A et al (2014) Endophthalmitis associated with intravitreal injections: office-based setting and operating room setting. Retina 34(1):18–23. https://doi.org/10.1097/IAE.0000000000000008
9. Doshi RR, Bakri SJ, Fung AE (2011) Intravitreal injection technique. Semin Ophthalmol 26(3):104–113. https://doi.org/10.3109/08820538.2010.541318
10. Yun C, Oh J, Hwang S-Y et al (2015) Subconjunctival hemorrhage after intravitreal injection of anti-vascular endothelial growth factor. Graefes Arch Clin Exp Ophthalmol 253:1465–1470

11. McCannel CA (2011) Meta-analysis of endophthalmitis after intravitreal injection of anti-vascular endothelial growth factor agents: causative organisms and possible prevention strategies. Retina 31(4):654–661. https://doi.org/10.1097/IAE.0b013e31820a67e4
12. Bhavsar AR, Ip MS, Glassman AR et al (2007) The risk of endophthalmitis following intravitreal triamcinolone injection in the DRCRnet and SCORE clinical trials. Am J Ophthalmol 144(3):454–456
13. Nelson ML, Tennant MT, Sivalingam A et al (2003) Infectious and presumed noninfectious endophthalmitis after intravitreal triamcinolone acetonide injection. Retina 23(5): 686–691
14. Sutter FK, Gillies MC (2003) Pseudo-endophthalmitis after intravitreal injection of triamcinolone. Br J Ophthalmol 87(8): 972–974
15. Karabag RY, Parlak M, Cetin G et al (2015) Retinal tears and rhegmatogenous retinal detachment after intravitreal injections: its prevalence and case reports. Digit J Ophthalmol 21(1):8–10. https://doi.org/10.5693/djo.01.2014.07.001
16. Jager RD, Aiello LP, Patel SC et al (2004) Risks of intravitreous injection: a comprehensive review. Retina 24(5):676–698
17. Shin YI, Sung JY, Sagong M et al (2018) Risk factors for breakthrough vitreous hemorrhage after intravitreal anti-VEGF injection in age-related macular degeneration with submacular hemorrhage. Sci Rep 8(1):10560. https://doi.org/10.1038/s41598-018-28938-1
18. Cekiç O, Chang S, Tseng JJ et al (2005) Cataract progression after intravitreal triamcinolone injection. Am J Ophthalmol 139(6):993–998
19. Thompson JT (2006) Cataract formation and other complications of intravitreal triamcinolone for macular edema. Am J Ophthalmol 141(4):629–637
20. Pershing S, Bakri SJ, Moshfeghi DM (2013) Ocular hypertension and intraocular pressure asymmetry after intravitreal injection of anti-vascular endothelial growth factor agents. Ophthalmic Surg Lasers Imaging Retina 44(5):460–464. https://doi.org/10.3928/23258160-20130909-07
21. Hamill MB, Osato MS, Wilhelmus KR (1984) Experimental evaluation of chlorhexidine gluconate for ocular antisepsis. Antimicrob Agents Chemother 26(6):793–796
22. Trinavarat A, Atchaneeyasakul LO, Nopmaneejumruslers C et al (2006) Reduction of endophthalmitis rate after cataract surgery with preoperative 5% povidone-iodine. Dermatology 212(Suppl 1):35–40
23. Merani R, McPherson ZE, Luckie AP et al (2016) Aqueous chlorhexidine for intravitreal injection antisepsis: a case series and review of the literature. Ophthalmology 123(12): 2588–2594. https://doi.org/10.1016/j.ophtha.2016.08.022
24. Oakley CL, Vote BJ (2016) Aqueous chlorhexidine (0.1%) is an effective alternative to povidone-iodine for intravitreal injection prophylaxis. Acta Ophthalmol 94(8):e808–e809. https://doi.org/10.1111/aos.12981
25. Storey PP, Tauqeer Z, Yonekawa Y et al (2019) The impact of prefilled syringes on endophthalmitis following intravitreal injection of ranibizumab. Am J Ophthalmol 199:200–208. https://doi.org/10.1016/j.ajo.2018.11.023
26. Bakri SJ, Ekdawi NS (2008) Intravitreal silicone oil droplets after intravitreal drug injections. Retina 28(7):9961–9001
27. Scott IU, Oden NL, VanVeldhuisen PC et al (2009) SCORE Study Report 7: incidence of intravitreal silicone oil droplets associated with staked-on vs luer cone syringe design. Am J Ophthalmol 148(5):725–732, e7
28. Sassalos TM, Paulus YM (2019) Xy31Prefilled syringes for intravitreal drug delivery. Clin Ophthalmol 13:701–706. https://doi.org/10.2147/OPTH.S169044
29. Xue K, MacLaren RE (2018) Ocular gene therapy for choroideremia: clinical trials and future perspectives. Expert Rev Ophthalmol 13(3): 129–138
30. Schon C, Biel M, Michalakis S (2014) Retinal gene delivery by adeno-associated virus (AAV) vectors: strategies and applications. Eur J Pharm Biopharm 95(Part B):343–352
31. Del Amo EM, Rimpelä AK, Heikkinen E et al (2017) Pharmacokinetic aspects of retinal drug delivery. Prog Retin Eye Res 57:134–185
32. Rai Udo J, Young SA, Thrimawithana TR et al (2015) The suprachoroidal pathway: a new drug delivery route to the back of the eye. Drug Discov Today 20(4):491–495. https://doi.org/10.1016/j.drudis.2014.10.010
33. Habot-Wilner Z, Noronha G, Wykoff CC (2019) Suprachoroidally injected pharmacological agents for the treatment of chorio-retinal diseases: a targeted approach. Acta Ophthalmol 97(5):460–472. https://doi.org/10.1111/aos.14042
34. Clearside Biomedical (2019) Clearside Biomedical announces license agreement with aura biosciences for suprachoroidal space microinjector designed to optimize ocular oncology drug delivery. https://ir.

clearsidebio.com/news-releases/news-release-details/clearside-biomedical-announces-license-agreement-aura. Accessed 23 Sept 2019

35. Morales-Canton V, Fromow-Guerra J, Longoria SS et al (2013) Suprachoroidal microinjection of bevacizumab is well tolerated in human patients. Invest Ophthalmol Vis Sci 54:3299
36. Einmahl S, Savoldelli M, D'Hermies F et al (2002) Evaluation of a novel biomaterial in the suprachoroidal space of the rabbit eye. Invest Ophthalmol Vis Sci 43(5):1533–1539
37. Tyagi P, Barros M, Stansbury JW et al (2013) Light-activated, in situ forming gel for sustained suprachoroidal delivery of bevacizumab. Mol Pharm 10(8):2858–2867. https://doi.org/10.1021/mp300716t
38. Ding K, Shen J, Hafiz Z et al (2019) AAV8-vectored suprachoroidal gene transfer produces widespread ocular transgene expression. J Clin Invest 130:4901–4911. https://doi.org/10.1172/JCI129085
39. Peden MC, Min J, Meyers C et al (2011) Ab-externo AAV-mediated gene delivery to the suprachoroidal space using a 250 micron flexible microcatheter. PLoS One 6(2): e17140. https://doi.org/10.1371/journal.pone.0017140
40. de Smet MD, Lynch JL, Dejneka NS et al (2018) A subretinal cell delivery method via suprachoroidal access in minipigs: safety and surgical outcomes. Invest Ophthalmol Vis Sci 59:311–320
41. Gyroscope Therapeutics (2019) Gyroscope Therapeutics merges with Orbit Biomedical creating a leading retinal gene therapy company. https://gyroscopetx.com/wp-content/uploads/2019/04/Gyroscope-and-Orbit-Merger-Final-11.4.19.pdf. Accessed 23 Sept 2019
42. Olsen TW, Feng X, Wabner K et al (2011) Pharmacokinetics of pars plana intravitreal injections versus microcannula suprachoroidal injections of bevacizumab in a porcine model. Invest Ophthalmol Vis Sci 52(7):4749–4756. https://doi.org/10.1167/iovs.10-6291
43. Patel SR, Lin ASP, Edelhauser HF et al (2011) Suprachoroidal drug delivery to the back of the eye using hollow microneedles. Pharm Res 28: 166–176
44. Barakat M (2019) The hands-on technique for suprachoroidal injection. Retina Specialist. https://www.retina-specialist.com/article/the-handson-technique-for-suprachoroidal-injection. Accessed 27 Jan 2020
45. Goldstein DA, Do D, Noronha G et al (2016) Suprachoroidal corticosteroid administration: a novel route for local treatment of noninfectious uveitis. Transl Vis Sci Technol 5:14
46. Gamlin PD, Alexander JJ, Boye SL et al (2019) SubILM injection of AAV for gene delivery to the retina. Methods Mol Biol 1950:249–262. https://doi.org/10.1007/978-1-4939-9139-6_14

Chapter 35

Surgical Approach with Pars Plana Vitrectomy for Subretinal Gene Therapy

Mark P. Breazzano, Sean A. Batson, Stephen H. Tsang, and Royce W. S. Chen

Abstract

Gene therapy is emerging as a treatment for inherited diseases including retinitis pigmentosa. Through surgery, specifically with pars plana vitrectomy, the subretinal space can be accessed to directly administer this treatment. The goal herein is to provide an overview of this approach.

Key words Gene therapy, Inherited retinal diseases, Pars plana vitrectomy, Subretinal technique, Retinitis pigmentosa

1 Introduction

Pars plana vitrectomy (PPV) is a commonly performed procedure for managing a variety of diseases by accessing the vitreous cavity and posterior segment. This chapter addresses the subretinal injection as well as the necessary preceding PPV for gene therapy, particularly as this treatment emerges for inherited retinal diseases including specific types of retinitis pigmentosa.

2 Materials

1. Conventional apparatus for pars plana vitrectomy.
2. Standard surgical draping and operative room attire.
3. Extension tubes.
4. Syringes.
5. Subretinal injection cannula.

Stephen H. Tsang and Peter M. J. Quinn (eds.), *Retinitis Pigmentosa*,
Methods in Molecular Biology, vol. 2560, https://doi.org/10.1007/978-1-0716-2651-1_35,

3 Methods

3.1 Preoperative Surgical Protocols

An operating room using standard sterile precautions is expected for subretinal gene therapy. A complete history and physical examination, in coordination with an anesthesiologist, is generally acquired. Written informed consent detailing the risks, benefits, and alternatives of the procedure should be appropriately obtained from the patient and/or guardian (using interpreter services if appropriate), preferably in clinic beforehand. Preoperative administration of immunosuppressive therapy, such as oral prednisone dosed 1 mg/kg/day, may be advised in some cases for several days before surgery. Active infection is ideally excluded clinically. At the time of surgery, the correct patient, laterality, and procedure should be confirmed, typically with a formal "time out"—either with a verbalized or written checklist during review of the consent. Availability and correct equipment, including the drug for gene therapy, should all be verified before proceeding with surgery. The eye is dilated with topical ophthalmic drops, which may include phenylephrine 2.5%, tropicamide 1%, and cyclopentolate 1% solutions. Preoperative topical broad-spectrum antimicrobial medication, such as moxifloxacin or ofloxacin, is typically administered. Topical 5% povidone-iodine solution is applied to the ocular surface, while the surrounding tissue including eyelids and lashes are thoroughly cleaned with sterile gauzes and cotton swabs, respectively, each three times with 10% povidone-iodine solution. No individual gauze or cotton swab is typically used to clean the same area more than once.

3.2 Anesthesia

Direct and consistent communication with the anesthesiologist is critical. Monitored anesthetic care using select sedatives and a local ophthalmic "block" is usually all that is required for this surgery, while general anesthesia can be considered for special circumstances. These authors prefer an anesthetic consisting of 2% lidocaine and 0.75% bupivacaine with or without hyaluronidase (4.5: 4.5:1 ratio) that is injected locally into sub-Tenon's space. However, a retrobulbar or peribulbar anesthetic injection that is performed prior to sterile draping may also be reasonable. Blunt Westcott scissors and conjunctival forceps are used to make a small incision in the inferonasal fornix, followed by access with an 18-gauge curved cannula that is used to follow the contour of the globe posteriorly, with subsequent injection of the anesthetic. Careful but limited dissection below the plane of Tenon's tissue and superficial to the sclera is ideal for maximal anesthetic effect and without "ballooning" of the overlying conjunctiva. A subtle amount of cautery may be necessary for hemostasis, particularly with eyes having fragile blood vessels or for patients currently proceeding with antiplatelet or anticoagulant medications.

3.3 First Incision

The surgical microscope, corresponding foot pedals, seat and bed height, and any other factors influencing surgeon posture or technical aspects of the surgery should be adjusted to accommodate maximal ergonomics as well as patient safety. Confirmation of instrumentation including a 25-gauge vitrectomy setup is made. Then, the first trocar with its cannula in adults is placed 4.0 mm (for phakic eyes, or 3.5 mm for aphakic or pseudophakic eyes) posterior to the limbus (distance is adjusted for children) into the vitreous cavity in the inferotemporal quadrant. We prefer displacement of the conjunctiva using conjunctival forceps or a cotton swab, with an insertion parallel to the limbus for several millimeters, followed by perpendicular insertion into the vitreous cavity for the remaining aspect of the maneuver. The infusion line connected and primed with the vitrectomy machine is then run and temporarily clamped (to minimize influx of air bubbles later), followed by placement into the inferotemporal cannula. After confirmation of insertion in the vitreous cavity, generally with a light pipe from the nasal direction for illumination outside the eye, the infusion line is opened. The next two trocars are used to similarly place cannula at 2:30 and 9:30 clock positions at the same distance from the limbus. Vigilance for ongoing physiologic ocular pressure and functionality of the vitrectomy apparatus at all times is important. Clear and open communication with the operating room staff is also advisable throughout the entire procedure.

3.4 Vitrectomy

The vitrector and light pipe are inserted into the superior cannula and directed toward the mid-vitreous cavity, just into view from direct visualization with the operating microscope. Vitrectomy settings are generally configured with moderate vacuum and high cut rates. The anterior portion of the vitrectomy is initiated by beginning with the vitreous adjacent to the cannula opening, as the vitrector is rotated 360 degrees within this zone of peripheral vitreous. The anterior vitreous is gradually cleared circumferentially behind, but with careful attention not to interfere with, the lens in phakic eyes. The infusion and contralateral ports are also cleared of vitreous diligently, as to minimize fluctuations in pressure intraoperatively as well as the possibility of retinal tears and detachments due to traction from adherent vitreous at these sclerotomy sites.

Next, posterior visualization, either with a contact lens or non-contact method, is established. Many patients have their posterior hyaloid attached to the optic nerve and posterior retina, though some may have separation of the vitreous. Confirmation of its status could be performed with diluted triamcinolone injected into the vitreous cavity, though this step has not been extensively investigated in the setting of subretinal gene therapy. Maneuvers for separating an attached posterior hyaloid include close approximation of the vitrector to the vitreomacular attachment interface near the papillomacular bundle or alternatively, the edge of the optic disk. Ensuring cut settings are off and with high vacuum, the vitrector is slowly lifted toward the periphery. Depending on the adherence of the interface, the number of attempts necessary to achieve elevation of the posterior hyaloid can be variable. It is important that the hyaloid is lifted circumferentially around the optic nerve and macula, but it does not need to be brought fully into the periphery. Close examination of the entire retina, including the periphery with scleral depression, is typically warranted to evaluate for any retinal tears or breaks or other conditions that may require treatment such as laser retinopexy. The intended site for injection at the macula should be inspected closely, possibly with assistance of a surgical tool (e.g., a flexible loop or membrane scraper) to ensure absence of vitreoschisis and that posterior cortical vitreous has been removed. If a membrane or other adherent tissue is present, it should be removed. Peeling of the internal limiting membrane is generally not advised. The use of dyes, like triamcinolone, in this setting may require additional investigation before routine use with subretinal gene therapy injection.

3.5 Subretinal Injection

Following the PPV, the subretinal gene therapy injection can begin. Extra subretinal injection cannula, extension tubes, and syringes should be available. A variety of injection cannulae are compatible for 25-gauge vitrectomy systems including 38-gauge and 41-gauge tips. It is important that the selected injection cannula is no larger than the vitrectomy cannula. The extension tube should meet length and diameter requirements as specified appropriately for the respective medication. The typical biocompatible syringe is 1 mL, disposable, and should contain the gene therapy medication as supplied by the pharmacy within the allotted timeframe. The medication-filled syringe should be inspected to confirm absence of particulates, cloudiness, or discoloration. Sterility and integrity of all instruments should also be verified. The syringe of medication is attached to the extension tube, which itself is connected to the subretinal injection cannula. The medication syringe is then slowly pushed so that the entire three-piece apparatus is devoid of air (fully replaced with medication) and the pre-designated amount of medication intended to be injected is left in the syringe. The surplus medication used to clear the line of air is safely injected into a sterile container and then discarded with care not to deform or contaminate the injection cannula.

The intraocular pressure should be reduced (e.g., to approximately 10 mm Hg) to allow for an increase in volume from the injected medication. The assistant should take hold of the medication syringe while the surgeon obtains the subretinal injection cannula and prepares for insertion into the vitreous cavity (*see* Fig. 1). The line should be clear of any kinks, tight connections between pieces verified, and priming of medication confirmed.

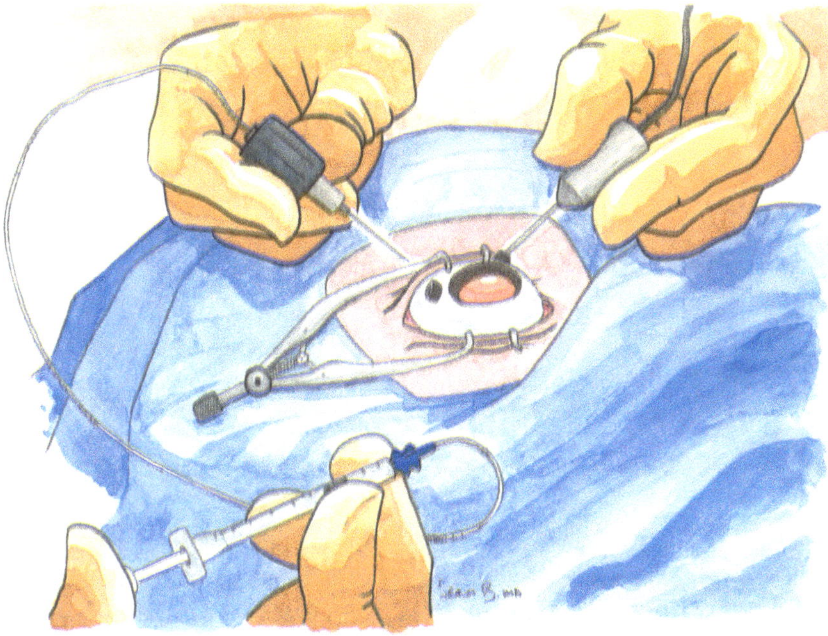

Fig. 1 Arrangement of draped patient, surgeon, and assistant. The patient and his/her eye are draped under sterile conditions. A speculum is in place to hold open the operative eye, and cannula have already been placed for the vitrectomy. Note the surgeon is located superior to the patient's head and is holding the light-pipe (typically in the non-dominant hand) and the subretinal injection cannula (typically in the dominant hand), ready for placement through the superior cannula into the mid-vitreous cavity. The assistant is holding the syringe of gene therapy medication, prepared for pushing on its plunger when appropriate

The injection site is then identified, generally adjacent to the superior arcade, and at least several millimeters away from the center of the fovea. The patient's anatomy and ease of access are considered to determine the exact site for injection. Areas of retinal atrophy or pigmentary change, for example, should be preferentially avoided, if possible. Arteriolar retinal vessels should also be avoided to prevent substantial hemorrhage. Once the subretinal injection cannula is safely advanced into the vitreous cavity, the tip is placed into neurosensory retina (with slight draping over the tip) without full perforation or extension to retinal pigment epithelium (*see* Fig. 2). Once placement of the cannula tip at this specific anatomic location is achieved by the surgeon, the assistant begins slowly and steadily injecting the medication while the surgeon watches for a bleb to begin to form. Any resistance or absence of bleb formation may warrant inspection for blockage or misplacement. Once the injection is completed, the assistant should continue to push the plunger for several seconds to ensure full medication administration. Bleb appearance can vary between patients. A different appropriate site is sometimes used to inject any remainder of medication that is not accomplished at the first site.

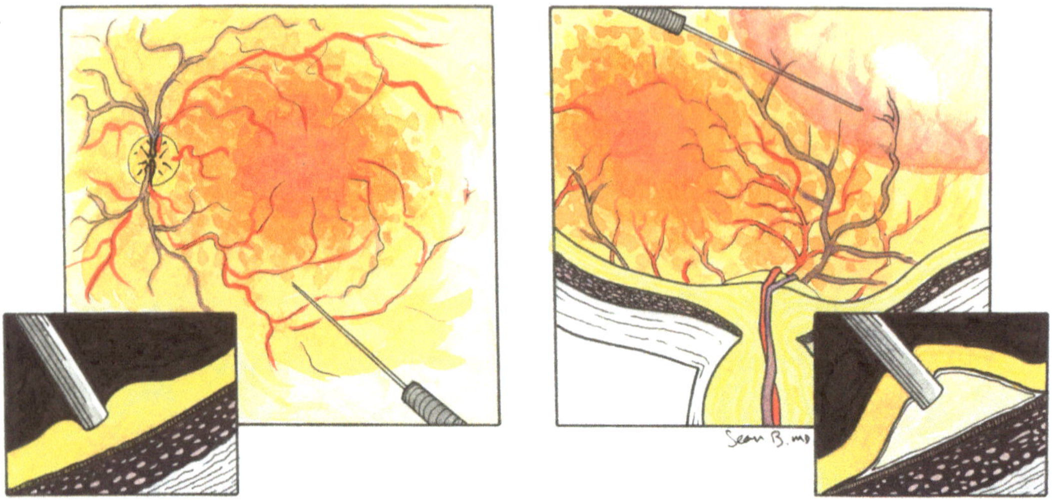

Fig. 2 Schematic during the moments of subretinal gene therapy injection. Left panel: The subretinal injection cannula is advanced through the vitreous toward the intended appropriate site of administration, typically near the superior arcade avoiding arteriolar vessels and away from the fovea. The cannula tip is placed specifically in the middle of neurosensory retina, avoiding perforation (cross section, bottom left). Right panel: The assistant slowly applies pressure to the medication syringe plunger as the surgeon holds steady and observes bleb formation. The cannula tip is now within the bleb itself, but never touching the retinal pigment epithelium or other tissues deep to the neurosensory retina (cross section, bottom right)

3.6 Conclusion of Surgery

Once the injection is completed, an air–fluid exchange is performed using a backflush or soft-tip cannula directed away from the bleb to avoid medication removal and after increasing the intraocular pressure (e.g., to 30 mm Hg). The periphery is closely examined again for any abnormalities and treated (with a modality such as endolaser) if appropriate.

All instrumentation including each cannula is removed from the eye, and the sclerotomies are closely examined. Any sign of leakage may warrant either a single interrupted 7-0 or 8-0 absorbable suture to be placed through an individual sclerotomy. Topical ointment with or without subconjunctival administration of antibiotic and steroid medication are considered. The eye is patched with a hard-plastic shield overlying it and taped into place. Supine positioning, as much as the patient can tolerate, with rest is directed for 24 h. Topical broad-spectrum antibiotic, steroid, and cycloplegic drops are typically administered by the patient or caregiver beginning on the first postoperative day. Postoperative oral steroid can also routinely be considered for several days immediately following surgery.

4 Notes

Subretinal gene therapy [1], like any other techniques, has complications, some of which are shared with other interventions. Cataract formation may be accelerated after vitrectomy and particularly from misdirected trocar insertion. In our experience, it is important that trocar is aimed vertically and posteriorly during insertion to avoid contact with the phakic lens. A subretinal hemorrhage can partially be avoided by creating the retinal bleb away from larger blood vessels. If this bleeding does occur, immediate and temporary elevation in intraocular pressure with the infusion can help minimize its extent. If a macular hole develops or becomes evident during the surgery, peeling of the internal limiting membrane (ILM) may be warranted with gas exchange and subsequent face down positioning. Identification of retinal detachment warrants its appropriate, respective management; careful maneuvers including sufficient anterior vitrectomy and fully circumferential clearance of vitreous from the sclerotomies may help prevent this complication. Inflammation is expected, but a disproportionate amount on examination should prompt consideration of infection, which can be devastating if not recognized and treated promptly. However, adequate antimicrobial and titrated steroid coverage as outlined above typically mitigates most inflammation.

Conflicts of Interest

Stephen H. Tsang receives financial support from Abeona Therapeutics, Inc and Emendo. He is also the founder of Rejuvitas and is on the scientific and clinical advisory board for Nanoscope Therapeutics.

Reference

1. Peng Y, Tang L, Zhou Y (2017) Subretinal injection: a review on the novel route of therapeutic delivery for vitreoretinal diseases. Ophthalmic Res 58 (4):217–226

INDEX

Stephen H. Tsang and Peter M. J. Quinn (eds.), *Retinitis Pigmentosa*,
Methods in Molecular Biology, vol. 2560, https://doi.org/10.1007/978-1-0716-2651-1,

M

N

O

P

Q

R

S

T

U

V

W

Z

MIX
Papier aus verantwortungsvollen Quellen
Paper from responsible sources
FSC® C105338

If you have any concerns about our products,
you can contact us on
ProductSafety@springernature.com

In case Publisher is established outside the EU,
the EU authorized representative is:
Springer Nature Customer Service Center GmbH
Europaplatz 3, 69115 Heidelberg, Germany

Printed by Libri Plureos GmbH
in Hamburg, Germany